THE
POWER
OF
CHANGE

A Mennonite Girl's Footprints in Asia

Marcy (Weber) Ninomiya

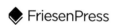 FriesenPress

One Printers Way
Altona, MB R0G 0B0
Canada

www.friesenpress.com

ISBN
978-1-03-912814-9 (Hardcover)
978-1-03-912813-2 (Paperback)
978-1-03-912815-6 (eBook)

1. *Biography & Autobiography, People with Disabilities*

Distributed to the trade by The Ingram Book Company

CONTENTS

ABBREVIATIONS & ACRONYMS

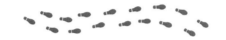

AAN	ASEAN Autism Network
AAR	Association for Aid and Relief, Japan
APCD	Asia-Pacific Development Centre on Disability
ARVN	Army of the Republic of Vietnam
ASEAN	Association of Southeast Asian Nations
BMF	Biwako Millennium Framework for Action
CA	Canadian Academy
CBR	Community-Based Rehabilitation
CRPD	Convention on the Rights of Persons with Disabilities
CWS	Church World Service
DPI	Disabled Peoples' International
DPI AP	Disabled Peoples' International for Asia and the Pacific
ESCAP	Economic Social Commission for Asia and the Pacific
HI	Handicap International
IL	Independent Living
JICA	Japan International Cooperation Agency
JCSWL	Japan Christian Social Work League

KGU	Kwansei Gakuin University
KSSSC	Kobe Seirei Social Service Community
Kyodan	United Church of Christ in Japan
LWR	Lutheran World Relief
MCC	Mennonite Central Committee
MCCO	Mennonite Central Committee Ontario
MOU	Memorandum of Understanding between Governments
MYF	Mennonite Youth Fellowship
NLF	National Liberation Front
NGO	Non-Government Organization
NPO	Non-Profit Organization
NVA	North Vietnamese Army
RMC	Rockway Mennonite Collegiate
SJMC	St. Jacobs Mennonite Church
UN	United Nations
UNESCAP	United Nations Economic and Social Commission for the Asia-Pacific
UNESCO	United Nations Educational, Scientific and Cultural Organization
UNHCR	United Nations High Commissioner for Refugees
VC	Viet Cong
VNCS	Vietnam Christian Service
WHO	World Health Organization
WLU	Wilfrid Laurier University

INTRODUCTION

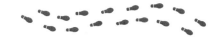

My life journey has been like a river constantly flowing. I needed courage to step into the river and trust in God. I grew up on a farm with a Mennonite family near the Grand River in the village of Conestogo, Ontario, Canada. Now I find myself retired in St. Jacobs, in the neighbouring town beside the same river where I first stepped out in faith.

Through the river water woven in my travels, I have encountered different cultures, languages, and religions. I believed in the power of change on the other side of the ocean. There was excitement, anxiety, uncertainty, and sometimes fear but I stepped forward in the stream trusting in God's protection. As a consequence, my life has been enriched.

Most of my adult life has been spent in Asia where I worked as a nurse in Vietnam during the war, married a Japanese, lived in Japan, and had a family of three children who are now living in Canada. My footprints continued in Thailand and Myanmar.

I hope that this autobiography will be an inspiration and you will enjoy living my experiences brought to life through letters written to my family and from memory. Many of the letters are not in full format since I only included certain information. My footprints circled the globe ending where I began, a witness to the power of change.

CHAPTER 1

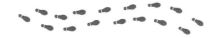

My Life in the Village of Conestogo

I grew up in a unique setting. If I went out the front door, I was in the village of Conestogo; if I went out the back door, I was on the farm.

When I was a child in the 1950s, the village of Conestogo had a population of 367 and boasted the Trail's End Hotel where the first settlers in the 1820s stayed, a general store that included the post office, Lutheran and United churches, and a two-room elementary school. I attended the same school that my father graduated from.

Our farm was small by Canadian standards but it gave me the best of two worlds. Dad did mixed farming as well as running the Conestogo dairy. The farm animals included one horse, some pigs, a few chickens, and twenty cows that provided milk for the village. Dad's horse drawn wagon could be seen delivering milk throughout the village every morning. It was a rare privilege to accompany him on his delivery route and deposit the bottles in the milk boxes of the homes. When the government made pasteurized milk mandatory in the early 1960s, Dad knew his days with the dairy were phasing out, so he decided to try raising turkeys.

When Dad, Nelson Weber, said goodbye to the dairy in 1964, he was already successfully raising turkeys. My two younger brothers, Clare and Robert, and I soon found ourselves helping feed the poults and doing other farm chores. In time, Weber's turkeys became the preferred turkey on the local market, in fact, Zehrs supermarkets began only buying our turkeys.

Besides farming, my parents were committed to the Mennonite church. Mennonites are known for their commitment to community, for living lives of simplicity and generosity, and for their work in peace, justice, and reconciliation. Although my parents were raised in a conservative environment, driving horse and buggy, both sets of parents were excommunicated from their church because one had bought a car and the other had gotten a telephone. This resulted in them joining a more liberal church in the Mennonite faith.

My parent's life continued to reflect simple living. My mother made all her clothes, my father's shirts, and the children's clothing from basic patterns. I recall having my coat remade from my mother's coat. Comforters and quilts were made from the leftover pieces of cloth; I would find pieces of my dress material in a finished quilt. Mom always said, "Waste not, want not." Even though nothing seemed to be wasted, my parents were always generous to those in need.

Most Mennonite's vegetable gardens and fruit orchards produced enough for their families until the next planting season. I grew up on food from our farm. My mother canned both vegetables and fruit: vegetables like onions, squash, pumpkins, potatoes, and cabbage were stored in the cool basement to extend their lives.

We also belonged to what my mother called "the beef ring", which consisted of forty conservative Mennonite farm families, each taking a turn donating a cow for forty weeks. Every week, each family received a different cut of the beef so that at the end of the forty weeks, a family would have eaten a whole cow. The amount of beef received every week filled a large metal basin. Mom canned some, but it fed our family of eight (two brothers, Clare and Robert, and three sisters, Brenda, Donna, and Susan), a hired man to help with the farming, and my paternal grandparents.

We had one hand pump for water in an alcove off the kitchen, our only source of water in the house except for a tap in the basement. Water had to be carried in large basins to wash dishes. Bathing meant a sponge bath in the alcove off the kitchen. We used a "pit privy" outside until winter set in, which meant using a pail with a toilet seat in the basement beside the coal bin. How well I recall going down the steps to the basement in the middle of the night only to be greeted by a surprised skunk at the foot of the stairs! Dad had forgotten to close the basement window, and two skunks had "fallen" into our basement. What a luxury to have a bathroom with a bath and flush toilet installed about four years later!

This idyllic life, surrounded by a caring Christian family on the farm and by friends in the community was to be envied. Then, at the age of eight, my world changed. Hemorrhages in my legs, frequent nose bleeds, and abdominal pain necessitated hospitalization and surgery. I woke up after an appendectomy, feeling nauseous: my nurse thought I was just being difficult, so she fed me a bowl of clear soup, which I immediately threw up, only to be scolded for the mess I had made! I decided then that I was going to become a nurse one day but not be like this one! Unfortunately, my family could not visit me at this time because three of them were sick with the mumps.

Because my health continued to decline, my family doctor consulted three pediatricians who discussed my health at the foot of my bed. The next day my pastor visited me, and he told me that my doctor had contacted him and said that he could not do anything more for me; my only hope was prayer. When he left after praying with me, I started bargaining with God. I was not going to die; I would do whatever God's plan was for me if He spared my life. In my mind, I was going to become a nurse and go to Asia. The Vacation Bible School stories of Asia had always fascinated me, especially India and China. Yes, I was going to get better and go to Asia as a nurse!

Recovery was slow, with complete bedrest for four months, followed by using a wheelchair for two months. Friends and relatives visited frequently: an elderly neighbour played checkers with me every day—until winning became a challenge for him. Two years later, I had a full recovery thanks to the power of prayer. Many years later I learned that a neighbouring church minister had once cancelled his sermon and held a prayer meeting for my healing. What a humbling experience!

At the age of thirteen, on the last day of summer Vacation Bible School, the teacher asked each one of us what we hoped to do with our lives. My immediate response was, "I want to be a nurse and go to Asia."

My parents felt that education was a priority for their children, but I found myself at a crossroad the night before high school began. My mother's back pain made it very difficult for her to function: my help was desperately needed at home. The night before school started, it was finally agreed that I could go to high school if I worked before and after school. I was ecstatic to be able to attend Elmira District Secondary School for Grade 9. I got up early in the morning to help feed the turkeys, and then after school I helped my mother and looked after my younger sisters.

Because finances were tight, Mom and I read an ad in the newspaper with interest regarding selling greeting cards. I replied, and soon after began selling greeting cards. I filled a suitcase with samples and walked through the villages of Conestogo and St. Jacobs taking orders. The profits of doing this for three years supplemented my monthly stipend in nurses' training until I graduated.

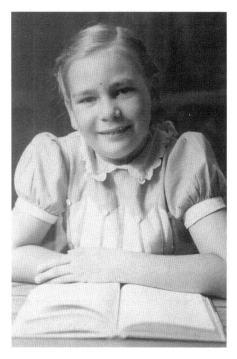

Childhood photo

The next three of my high school years were at Rockway Mennonite Collegiate (RMC) in Kitchener. Dad wanted his children to have a Christian education no matter what sacrifice it meant on his part. RMC got considerable publicity when I got third prize in the National Cherry Pie Contest in my senior year. It was tempting to pursue studies in Home Economics, but I felt my commitment was to follow through with my covenant to God. So, in 1961, I was accepted into the Kitchener-Waterloo Hospital School of Nursing three-year program. Our class of sixty-five students made history for being the largest class, having the first male student, and a set of twins. The three years of residence life was challenging with its rigid rules, which included no wearing pants in or out of residence. Our day began with chapel at seven a.m. and an inspection on exiting: no hair on the collar, a hair net in place, and polished brown shoes!

In hindsight, we did need boundaries. We studied and worked hard, but we also played hard. As student nurses we functioned as regular staff, at times covering all three shifts. My first experience with bedside care, which included a bed bath, is still vivid in my memory. It was quite intimidating. When preparing the toothbrush and toothpaste, I noticed a tube beside the toothbrush on the bedside table and was ready to squeeze some "toothpaste" onto the toothbrush, when the patient noticed that the tube was hemorrhoid cream! How embarrassing!

One night, after coming off an evening shift, a few of us decided to take my large orange stuffed camel—received as a door prize at a recent Christmas party—to Emergency, cover it with a white sheet, and page our favourite intern on call, on whom we all had a crush. Of course, we were nowhere to be found when he arrived. Fortunately, we never got caught! Rules were made to be broken.

Our training involved experience in each specialty area. Much of my time in the nursery was on the night shift with two fun classmates. One time, when we were all changing diapers, one was busy talking while changing the diaper on a male baby, triggering urination that shot up in the air. Unfortunately for my friend, her mouth was open in conversation, looking in my direction, when the stream of urine went straight into her mouth! Caught off guard, she said, "Where did that come from?" We laughed so hard! We learned fast from experience.

My training years ended with my placement in the O.R. (operating room). I vividly remember being on call one evening when a bachelor was scheduled for an emergency bronchoscopy: he had made chicken stew and then swallowed "something," making it difficult to breathe. Looking down the scope, one could read "Grade A" on the metal tag. He had cooked the whole chicken with the tag on, and then swallowed the tag! No wonder he had difficulty breathing. I really enjoyed working in the O.R., and I was delighted to be assigned there after graduation in August 1964.

Applying for Voluntary Service

By January 1965, I felt strongly that God was prodding me to follow through with my covenant with Him. I made an appointment with Harvey Taves, Executive Director of the Mennonite Central Committee Ontario (MCCO) in Kitchener, for a term of voluntary service. Mennonite Central Committee (MCC) was a worldwide ministry with headquarters in Akron, Pennsylvania with the motto to share God's love, and compassion for all, in the name of Christ, by responding to basic human needs through relief and development and working for peace and justice. They partnered with local churches and organizations in fifty countries around the world, which provided opportunities for volunteers as needed. I decided to volunteer as a nurse wherever there was an opening, with the term depending on the global location.

After a lengthy interview, Mr. Taves said that there were two positions available. One was in the O.R. in Haiti for a two-year term, and the other was a three-year term in a hospital/clinic setting in Vietnam. On reviewing the job description for Vietnam, he felt that it required a nurse with more experience. He thanked me for my willingness to serve and said that he would forward my application to the MCC headquarters in Pennsylvania: they would be in contact with me. Meanwhile, I submitted my application with two references and anxiously waited for a response.

On March 3, 1965, I received a letter from Urbane Peachey, Secretary of Personnel Services of the MCC office in Akron, Pennsylvania which stated:

> We are pleased, Miss Weber to accept you for assignment and believe that you will be prepared to serve significantly in one of our nursing assignments. Plan to begin by June 15, the first orientation of the summer.

The next correspondence from Akron, dated April 14, 1965, read:

> We still want to be sensitive to the geographical area to which you feel led or interested. We are suggesting a different location for which we feel you would be well qualified.

We are proposing a three-year term to the Nhatrang Hospital and Clinic in Vietnam. I will try to give you helpful background and interpretation of our thinking concerning this. We have been in Vietnam for ten years in material aid work. We have been there for a shorter period of time in the medical program at Nhatrang. We have just sent a doctor to Vietnam out of our April orientation. The major concern which you and others would have, is the matter of safety and security. MCC's work has progressed without interruption during the time of the political turbulence in Vietnam.

Robert Miller has sent us a telegram from Vietnam requesting us to follow through with the assignment proposal. The present nurse Marva Hasselblad is terminating this month. This raises a question of whether you would be able to go before June 15, if it were possible to secure your visa in time.

I am eager that you will be able to consider this under God's providence and trust that you will be able to respond affirmatively to this need. We have really tried to review and evaluate your file very carefully and believe that you would be very well-qualified to step into the role that is needed there and also that you have the kind of personal qualities that are needed for assignment in this area. Your four years of French will be very valuable because the western language generally spoken there is French. You would learn considerable Vietnamese during your assignment there as well.

After reading the letter, I needed to pray seriously. Haiti was a two-year commitment, but Vietnam was three. Although Vietnam represented Asia, where I had always felt I would go, the front page of our daily newspaper generally carried news of the Vietnamese war. Would MCC really send volunteers there given the seriousness of this conflict? My mother and I decided that the news said one thing, but MCC would be aware of the situation at the project site, so I responded to the Akron office that I was willing to serve in Vietnam.

MCC's response was almost immediate. On April 21, 1965, Urbane Peachey wrote:

> We are very grateful that you have felt led to respond affirmatively to the Vietnam assignment. Mennonite Travel Service is writing to you immediately with passport-visa instructions. I think we should have you come to Akron for special orientation by the morning of May 27. Because we will not have a regular orientation session going at the time, we will arrange a special series of appointments here and give you time for reading.

Then, correspondence dated April 28, 1965, arrived from Doris Longacre, the wife of Paul Longacre, MCC's director in Vietnam, welcoming me and giving advice as to what to take for my three-year term:

> If your friends and relatives are like ours, many of them are concerned about your coming to a warlike place like this. True, there are some tensions here, but generally we have a fairly normal day to day routine. There is much meaningful service you can give in the name of Christ, and He controls our lives and is our protection here just as anywhere else.
>
> We hope that you will bring with you an enthusiasm for learning the Vietnamese language. I am just finishing seven months of study, six hours a week and feel that every minute I have spent with it has been more than worthwhile. It's a difficult language at best, but the ability to communicate is basic to anything one tries to do, and therefore any time one spends learning the language helps to increase one's effectiveness. Taking time for part-time formal study with a teacher during your first several months will give you a basis for picking up more and more phrases as you work with the Vietnamese patients in the months following.
>
> We just welcomed Dr. Linford Gehman at the beginning of this week. It's two more months before Dr. Carl Yoder and

his family leave, so Dr. Gehman will have a good chance to
become established in the program here. Now we're looking
forward to your coming. We hope you have a good trip.

My time working in the O.R. at Kitchener-Waterloo Hospital was suddenly running out. I handed in my resignation with tears. I needed two weeks to prepare a three years' supply of personal effects, medical books, etc. before arriving in Akron on May 26.

I devoured the information forwarded by MCC about Vietnam because my knowledge was limited to what I read in the newspapers.

Vietnam is a small country in Southeast Asia with a 4,000-
year history with South China origin. After being ruled for
1000 years by the Chinese, it became a republic in 1955 after
emerging from a century of French colonial rule. Several
decades of internal conflict retarded self-development.
The population of 21 million includes many tribal people
(Montagnards) numbering close to 1 million who occupy
the central highland regions and are ethnically distinct from
the Vietnamese of the coastal and lowland areas.

Buddhism, ancestor worship, spirit worship, etc. are
the major religions. Catholicism is the most powerful
Christian religion with approximately 1.5 million members;
Protestantism claims about 30,000 members.

The people are considered courteous and peace loving,
and they are anxious for educational opportunities.
Vietnam is a rice-exporting country and not yet overpopu-
lated. The climate in summer varies between 80-100 degrees
and 60-80 degrees in the winter months. Highland areas
are cooler.

The language of the country is Vietnamese, with tribal
languages spoken by those groups. English is rapidly replac-
ing French as a main second language. All workers are
encouraged to learn as much Vietnamese as possible, start-
ing with several months of part-time study at the beginning

of the term. The language is difficult, but a little proficiency is a great aid to effective work and communication.

I was eager to read the description of the medical project at Nhatrang and what my responsibilities would entail.

The Nhatrang medical clinic and hospital are run by a board composed of Vietnamese pastors of the Evangelical Church: MCC provides the professional staff of three: national workers number five to seven with on-the-job training, two interpreters, one cleaning lady, and one chaplain complete the staff. The daily outpatient clinic serves 130-200, mostly poor fisherman and farmers: a small minority of tribal people come from villages that have been resettled out of mountain areas to locations near Nhatrang. There are beds for twenty inpatients now using a nearby building as well and running a census of thirty to thirty-five. The building consists of one open ward, clinic room, doctor's office, O.R., and a partially equipped lab. New facilities are under construction for an improved clinic, increased storage, and seven to ten more beds. Also, semi-permanent housing for more tuberculosis (TB) patients is being planned. At present, about fifteen TB patients live on the grounds in order to receive daily medicines. Others under regular supervision and treatment come from town at regular intervals. Currently we have about sixty TB patients under treatment.

The Nhatrang medical project serves as a general clinic and hospital: major surgery is done at the provincial hospital four kilometres away or at the American army hospital ten kilometres away: both provide chest X-rays, lab work, and orthopedic consultation and surgery: eye surgery is done here. Institute Pasteur, Nhatrang, seven kilometres away, is a Vietnamese run French laboratory that provides stool and sputum exams as well as some blood work.

Regarding community health and hygiene, generally there is no knowledge of the cause of disease or treatment. Hygiene is incredibly poor. Superstitions run rampant as to cause and treatment. Chinese medicines are used widely. The wealthy use French medicine in which all meds are given intramuscular (IM) or intravenous (IV). Doses and drugs used are not in agreement with American medical practice. General health of the population is borderline—almost 1000:0 [everybody] have parasitic infestation. Hemoglobin and blood pressure register low. People are small and thin.

Common illnesses and diseases include abscesses and infections, TB pulmonary and extra pulmonary, pneumonia, eye infections, dermatitis, often infected, chronic liver and heart diseases resulting from hepatitis and malaria, kidney diseases, gastritis, parasitic and amoebic infections (hookworm), and tropical diseases such as typhoid fever, dysentery, and cholera, etc. Any disease found in the States is found here, usually in its most advanced form.

Wow! The list was overwhelming! And to think that my practical medical experience in training was limited to the psychiatric ward that had the overflow from the medical ward of the hospital.

Then I read the nurses' responsibilities:

1. *Screening daily clinics (interviewing each patient, prescribing treatment for the less seriously ill, sending the others to the Dr.).*
2. *Assisting the Dr. with special procedures, eg. minor surgery, spinal taps, etc.*
3. *Supervising and assisting with eye surgery, setting up O.R., care and sterilization of instruments.*
4. *Nursing care of patients requiring special attention.*
5. *Nursing care of labor patients and assisting with delivery.*
6. *Supervision of staff workers—teaching, daily assignments, overseeing work.*

7. *Basic lab procedures (can be learned here).*
8. *Transport and errands, taking patients to Nhatrang for X-rays, surgery, and buying local supplies.*

Then a comment that "a background in public health nursing would be good." Too late! I would have to do my best!

The information also included a section on "Problems of Medical Staff" that read:

1. *Professional practice and ethics: There is a general lowering of standards because of the habits of the people—open ward, minimal isolation, communal equipment such as bedpans, minimal diet supervision, no morning care, and clean and dirty areas poorly differ.*
2. *Cultural: Communication is the most frustrating factor because of the language barrier and the vast difference between Western and Eastern methods. Preferential treatment is expected to be given to some, which runs counter to Western medical thought.*
3. *Staff training: Again, communication is difficult. Staff has no background in this type of work. Inclination is not to help sick people. Physical assistance is not done outside one's own family. Keeping trained workers is a problem. Interpreters usually find better paying jobs soon. In the last month one of the best male workers was drafted, and a girl trained to do nursing here had to quit because she felt the workload was too heavy, even though she was only working mornings.*
4. *Administration: The biggest problem concerns maintaining an adequate supply of medication and equipment. Even after equipment is obtained it is often poorly cared for— such as the two-month period in which fifty thermometers were broken. The staff does not assume any responsibility for the care of equipment. Syringes and certain medications have at times disappeared.*

5. *The large numbers at the clinic for the size of the staff and facilities have posed some organizational problems (We found some people "scalping" their numbers which gives the holder a place in the examining line).*

This information proved very helpful and true!

There was also a daily schedule, subject to changes made by the doctor.

Monday - Friday 8:00 a.m. to 1:00 p.m. (or until done):
General clinic
Monday and Tuesday p.m.:
Doctor or nurse takes patients for X-rays and consultations to the American Army Hospital
Nursing care of inpatients
TB clinic at 2:30 p.m.
General rounds when Dr. returns
Wednesday p.m.
Eye surgery or special procedures
Thursday p.m.
Dr. attends TB clinic to check patients
Friday p.m.
Hospital rounds
Saturday a.m.
Eye surgery and special procedures

It was clear that I did not need to think about free time: the information forwarded was very comprehensive.

Orientation for Vietnam

Early on May 26, I said goodbye to the village of Conestogo and my five siblings, and my parents and I began our drive to Akron, Pennsylvania: in the evening I said goodbye to my parents, not knowing when I would see them again. Much could happen in three years to them as well as me.

According to schedule, I appeared in the MCC office for orientation the morning of May 27, 1965. Because MCC wanted to send me to Vietnam as soon as possible, orientation was tailored for me personally. It included spiritual preparation, general orientation to total MCC programs and administration, acquaintance with overseas administration and policy, and an introduction to my particular assignment and country of service. My term of service was to be three years, with a personal allowance of $15 a month, a vacation of two weeks the first year, three weeks the second year, and four weeks the third year. Vacation allowance was $4.50 per day.

I could take forty-four pounds of baggage with me by air: the remainder of my personal effects would be repacked in Akron, in a metal barrel to be shipped to Saigon.

Because my departure for Vietnam was hanging on the issuance of my visa, Urbane Peachey, MCC Secretary of Personnel Services, decided that I should have a tutor to study French for one and a half hours, three times a week: Menno Travel Service thought that it could take eight weeks for my visa to be issued; Urbane was hoping for mid-June.

Meanwhile, MCC kept me privy to correspondence between the Saigon and Akron offices so I would have a better understanding of where I was to be serving. They were seeking effective ways of expanding their projects.

On May 11, 1965, a preliminary report on expansion projects from Paul Longacre in the Saigon office stated:

> *Many people have urged that any expansion be done among the Montagnards (tribal). This by far constitutes the most needy and neglected group of people in the country.*
>
> *I recommend we establish a medical program at one of three places, preferably in Pleiku, with a coordinated material aid program working out of it.*
>
> *The Vietnamese government has generally done little for these minority groups who refuse to be amalgamated into the general stream of Vietnamese life. The tribes are the predominant group in at least seven provinces. Their population numbers about 600,000, but the land area they cover*

is proportionately larger because it is the mountainous area of Vietnam.

The church has been quite successful among these people and has mission work and churches located in all the provinces. I am convinced that we can do the most service to the Vietnamese people in a medical project.

Dr. Yoder at the Nhatrang hospital readily agrees with me that a really effective medical program in this country needs to be localized in one place. Mobile clinics are impractical due to security and the difficulty of giving careful and quality treatment to anyone over a period of time. I feel that if we bring over persons with quality training, we should also put them to work in a situation where they can contribute in proportion to their capabilities. The needs are great enough that patients will storm the doors of places where they can get help.

Pleiku, one of the neediest areas in Vietnam, has a large tribal concentration plus 10,000 Vietnamese who are poorer than in other areas: medical services are almost nonexistent. The church and mission are located there with good national pastors: it is a large town with security, transportation, and communication, and is the best of three options. It had a limited school feeding program in several boarding schools, supervised by an International Voluntary Service (IVS) person which could be expanded; air transportation between Nhatrang-Saigon-Pleiku is quite good. The Christian and Missionary Alliance (C & M A) has a small program with two nurses, one trained in leprosy, and their personnel are enthusiastic about the possibility of a MCC program entering.

The advantages of a project here: it has the greatest possibility for material aid outgrowth, and it is the neediest area medically with good C & M A and church cooperation.

Personnel needs in Vietnam should be one doctor, two nurses, and one Paxman in Nhatrang, and one doctor, one nurse, and one Paxman in Pleiku. (A Paxman is a young man that is a conscientious objector to war due to his religious beliefs and volunteers to serve in another capacity.)

This report was compiled because Church World Service (CWS) wanted to work with MCC in Vietnam. Paul Longacre went on to say that he realized that a medical project comprised a substantial commitment on the part of MCC and CWS, but he felt that the needs seemed to demand such a commitment.

Further correspondence by MCC, dated June 4, 1965, confirmed their plans.

> *... Concerned with the growing medical and relief needs in South Vietnam, the MCC executive committee on May 22 moved to expand its present efforts and to accept the offer of Church World Service (CWS) to cooperate in an emergency relief program on behalf of the war refugees.*
>
> *Although it is growing more difficult and dangerous to carry on with food distribution and other assistance, MCC plans to remain in Vietnam and increase its work simply because there is much work to be done. In the words of a staff member, "Human suffering endured by God's people compels us to be there." Many innocent civilians have been maimed and killed by both sides.*
>
> *Expansion of relief efforts would include distribution of selected material aid items, feeding operations, and medical care to be carried out conjointly with the Evangelical Church of Vietnam.*
>
> *CWS would send four registered nurses to work for ten weeks: two assigned to Nhatrang, one to the Seventh Day Adventist Hospital in Saigon, and one to community services in Saigon.*
>
> *Robert Miller, director of MCC's Overseas Service Department, returned from a visit to review the Vietnam program in light of increased tensions. Of the 300,000*

refugees, 200,000 are in the eight coastal provinces of Central Vietnam.

Refugees are caused by the Viet Cong pushing people out of the interior to embarrass the government. And many thousands more are made refugees by Vietnamese and American military action. In areas considered prime Viet Cong strongholds, leaflets are dropped urging the general populace to evacuate because of planned bombings. It is estimated that the number of refugees will eventually swell to 600,000.

Medical workers will provide health care in clinics in cities and popular centres. The needs are so great that patients will hurry to any place they can receive treatment. The program of expansion is adaptable to both short term and long-range needs. If peace should come, there will be a vast array of rehabilitative opportunities.

The report went on to summarize the history of MCC work in Vietnam that began in 1954.

After nine years of fighting, the French were pushed out of Indo China in 1954. Late in the same year, MCC dispatched its first worker to Vietnam to bring material aid to the war weary and suffering people.

Since 1941, the beginning of a four-year Japanese occupation up to the present, Vietnam has been exposed to twenty-five years of almost uninterrupted warfare. The Vietnamese people who were in need in 1954 have been reduced to greater need in greater numbers in 1965.

From 1965 onward, MCC has sent thirty-six workers to Vietnam and $2 million worth of food, blankets, clothing, medicines, and other supplies. All this time, MCC has been the only Protestant relief agency functioning in Vietnam. It has maintained close ties with the Evangelical Church of Vietnam. Presently, two doctors, two nurses, two material *aid workers, and a Paxman are there. The Paxman, Daniel Gerber, has been a captive of the Viet Cong for the past three years.*

The Evangelical Church of Vietnam and MCC operate a medical clinic in a thirty-five-bed hospital at Nhatrang on the coast of the South China Sea. During 1964, it saw over 36,000 outpatients in the clinic and gave hospital care to about 650 medical and surgical cases.

A large amount of material aid such as MCC food and clothing is distributed by pastors of the Evangelical Church to needy persons in their areas. It's also made available to institutions operated by the government and private groups. One aspect of the support is the Bread Feeding Program in Saigon in which 162,000 loaves of baked bread are distributed monthly to schools, orphanages, and families. The most recent project about to be undertaken by MCC is that of Family-Child Assistance, a counselling program that goes beyond the mere meeting of physical need through material assistance. This effort will be centred in a designated area of Saigon deemed needy by the Ministry of Social Action and will involve casework with a child and his family.

In my mind, Vietnam was becoming more complex than I had foreseen possible.

A powerful letter written by Urbane Peachey to US president Lyndon B. Johnson regarding peace in Vietnam, dated June 4, 1965, read:

MCC decided to write to you of our deep concern over the enlarging war in Vietnam with its consequent toll of human suffering . . . The program of International Voluntary Services has also been supported by Mennonite leaders, and some of our young men are now active in the work in Vietnam. These men work with the village people and are very conscious of the real needs of the people. They would agree wholeheartedly with your words at Baltimore on

April 7, "Neither independence nor human dignity will ever be won by arms alone. It also requires the works of peace."

In the same speech you said that 'now there must be a much more massive effort to improve the life of man in that conflict-torn corner of our world.' That is one of the reasons that we went to Vietnam and why we are increasing our help there. We agree with you that 'we cannot wait for peace to begin the job.'

We share with you the conviction that 'the guns and the bombs, the rockets and the warships, are all symbols of human failure.' We also concur with your observation that 'this generation of the world must choose: destroy or build, kill or aid, hate or understand.'

We are deeply convinced that an expanded war would not be in the interests of the American people in their relationship to the people of Asia, and we also believe that a cessation of bombing in North Vietnam should be an urgent objective of our government. Let us move in the direction of peace by an escalation of compassion rather than an escalation of conflict.

May God's blessing be upon you as you seek His will for peace and righteousness among the nations.

I thought that letter was well said!

Meanwhile, my orientation continued, which included French language study, and my barrel of personal effects was packed as of June 6. Then, I had to wait for my visa.

On Monday, June 14, Bob Miller called me to his office saying MCC had been notified that my visa was issued and travel plans needed to be made as soon as possible: he gave me a choice between going with four registered nurses being sent by CWS to Vietnam, who would be leaving on Thursday, or going alone. I needed to decide by the next morning. If I chose to go with the four nurses it would necessitate an extra trip to New York by myself to get another visa because the nurses were planning to visit Japan. I couldn't imagine navigating such a large city on my own to apply for a visa and getting it within two days.

The next morning, I thanked Bob Miller for giving me an option, but I told him I would prefer to travel alone, which meant that my departure would be from Philadelphia, and MCC staff would drive me to the airport.

CHAPTER 2

Steps to Vietnam

I explained the trip to Vietnam to my family like this:

Thursday morning, I flew from Philadelphia to Honolulu via Los Angeles. It was intimidating to check in at the airport alone, having never flown before: my luggage was checked through to Honolulu directly, so I just needed to navigate around the Los Angeles Airport from one terminal to the other. Menno Travel Service did their best to book me to my destination as soon as possible. Because I had to change airlines in Honolulu, which required an overnight stay, Menno Travel suggested that I ask the airlines if they would put me up for the night. The answer was no, so I booked myself at a motel near the airport due to my early morning flight the next day. While eating my evening meal, a young gentleman at the next table wondered if I wanted to go into town with him that evening because he was planning to take a taxi to the International Market Square. I took advantage of his offer to do some sightseeing. The international marketplace was so alive with many tourists milling around. We enjoyed a fresh coconut drink sitting under a banyan tree where Robert Louis Stevenson supposedly wrote poetry in 1889. The palm trees, flowers, lei, and the bright colourful clothing were absolutely beautiful.

My Pan American flight left for Hong Kong the next morning, with an hour stopover in Tokyo. We crossed the International Date Line, which got me to Hong Kong on Friday evening. The runway in Hong Kong extends into the ocean, so the landing was really frightening because all you could see was water on both sides!

MCC staff met me on arrival, much to my relief. Before checking me into a hotel, we drove up the mountainside. What an experience to look down on Hong Kong. There were many bones in urns scattered on the mountainside because there was no other space for burial. Exhausted, I fell into bed that night.

The next morning, Carl Kauffman, a Paxman with MCC, and their Chinese secretary invited me to go to a kindergarten class in one of the poorest sections of town to distribute "family bundles." The kids' eyes really lit up as each one received his or her bundle. It was not possible to capture the emotion of the moment on camera. Those bright, bright eyes and smiles!

Hugo Friesen's family (MCC director in Hong Kong) invited me for lunch and dinner and a tour around Hong Kong: I saw the large kitchen where MCC prepared and distributed 4,000 meals on school days. They took me to see the small "shacks" built on ledges on very narrow hillsides. Some shacks, not larger than ten by twelve feet, housed a whole family. There were dozens of government resettlement houses, which were seven storeys high, built in the shape of an H: each family had one room, and the washrooms were in the middle. Poles with washed clothing were hanging out of windows to dry. What a sight! Approximately 2,500-3,000 persons lived in each building.

Dinner was Chinese food that had to be eaten with chopsticks! In the evening, I went with three Paxmen and a Chinese female friend over mountainous roads for approximately twenty miles to an English class in a village near the Chinese border. After the English lesson, the pastor extended a welcome to me followed by a testimony by one of the young people. Then they wanted the three Paxmen and I to sing in a quartet. It went alright because Carl sang the melody with me, as he had the same problem that I did of keeping the melody when another part was being sung. They must have been impressed because then they wanted Duane, one of the Paxmen, and me to sing a duet! We tried, let's put it that way. After several games, we took most of the students back to their homes. What an exciting and enlightening day!

I flew to Saigon on Sunday morning. The news said that the Saigon airport had been bombed three days before, so I wasn't sure what to expect. I was beginning to get nervous, wondering what I had agreed to. From the air, the city looked like a massive congestion of buildings.

A Mennonite missionary family and a MCC Vietnamese staff person met me at the airport. I assumed this was my final destination because the Akron office had said that I would be having one month of language study before beginning my work in Nhatrang; but not so.

James [a missionary who met me at the airport] said, "You probably think that you are done travelling for the day, but I've got news for you. Your plane leaves for Nhatrang in two and a half hours," which turned out to be two and a half hours late because one flight had been cancelled to Dalat, as it was shot at, so I got the next flight. This situation was beginning to make me apprehensive. What was awaiting me?

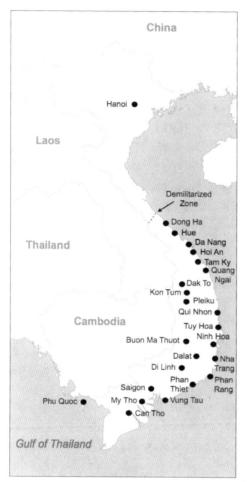

Map of Vietnam.
Courtesy of Dr. Matthew Maher.

My Destination: Nhatrang

What was awaiting me was breathtaking.

From the air I looked down on Nhatrang to see vibrant green rice fields between the azure blue South China Sea and the mountains. Paul Longacre, MCC director for Vietnam, was waving a welcome as I disembarked. As I wrote home:

I immediately felt connected to him because his sister was the wife of my pastor back home in St. Jacobs.

We drove through the town of Nhatrang, crossed a bridge, drove the length of a small island, crossed another bridge guarded by Vietnamese soldiers and, after less than three kilometres, found our vehicle driving up a laneway to the unit house beside coconut palm trees and the hospital.

I was introduced to the medical unit members, Dr. Carl and Phyllis Yoder, Dr. Linford Gehman, Nurse Marva Hasselblad, and Doris Longacre, Paul's wife. The team lived together in a unit house next door to the clinic and hospital.

On Monday morning, Phyllis gave me a tour of the Evangelical Clinic, called Chan-y-Vien Tin Lanh, which

*includes the hospital, clinic, two small buildings for tuber-
culosis patients, and some staff housing beside the MCC
unit house. It is surrounded by mountains in a cove with
coconut trees: patients access the clinic by a lane of 500 feet
from the South China Sea. To the right is a steep hill that
leads to huge rocks jutting into the sea. On top of the hill
is a seminary run by the Evangelical Church of Vietnam
[known as Tin Lanh in Vietnamese], established by the C
& M A. On the left side of the unit house is an orphanage
for approximately 235 children from birth up to the age of
sixteen, also run by Tin Lanh. Our hospital is primarily to
serve the farming and fishing community that cannot afford
medical services elsewhere.*

*As we approached the hospital, I saw that the front porch
was crowded with people. Apparently, it absorbs the overflow of inpatients, and they were on cots or just a straw mat
on the floor. I was feeling sorry for them until I went inside
the hospital. I soon realized that they were the lucky ones
because they got a breeze from the sea, whereas indoors the
heat was stifling. The beds have a basic metal frame with
wooden slats and a straw mat on top. The ceiling fans at
least move the air. Although the cleaning lady did her best to
keep the hospital hygienic, it is apparently a real challenge.
Flies were everywhere, and patients had family members
providing care and meals for them. Patients ate any time of
day, and the remaining food was left on bedside tables—no
wonder the fly population excelled!*

*The O.R. appears adequate for basic surgery done under
local anesthetic. The clinic was a shocker. Patients everywhere. To be seen, patients are required to buy a number
for ten piasters (currency) after claiming a numbered seat
on a bench or tree stump on the porch outside the clinic by
morning clinic hours. Some patients come the day before
or very early in the morning to ensure they can be seen.
Staff give out one hundred numbers each morning, and*

one number covers all family members, so more than one hundred patients are actually seen per day. They are called into the clinic by five numbers at a time to avoid bedlam.

I am so grateful for the information MCC provided me in Akron [about the situation] because that is exactly how it is. It is difficult for people to wait their turn, so "scalping" is not unusual. The fastest and most effective way to be seen is to feign being critically ill and enter the clinic in a hammock slung on a bamboo pole.

Tuesday, Dr. Yoder kindly took me under his wing and gave me helpful orientation for working in the clinic. I watched him diagnosing and prescribing medications in the outpatient clinic: my job will be screening the outpatients while a doctor treats the more seriously ill.

I knew everything would be a challenge, but surely God would give me the grace and wisdom to do the job because I had felt led to come to Nhatrang. My mother had always said that if anything was easy, it likely wasn't worth doing. I sensed that the nurse I was replacing saw me as too young and inexperienced, but I was determined that my age of twenty-one was not going to impede my ability to cope with what seemed insurmountable at the time. I would not give up!

The same evening Pastor Tin, chairman of the hospital board, invited the medical team for a delicious Vietnamese meal of five courses as a farewell to the Yoders and a welcome for me. I would have to become more adept in using chopsticks!

The Vietnamese culture was fascinating. The women's national costume, called an ao dai, was a tight-fitting top with a high collar and long sleeves with two loose flowing panels from the waist down, worn with silk pants. Most commonly seen at the hospital, though, were blouses that extended below the waist, also tight fitting at the top with long sleeves, worn with baggy long legged pants. The men wore similar looser fitting shirts along with loose-fitting pants known as ao baba, similar to western pajamas. They wore conical hats made from bamboo as protection from the sun. Little children ran around the hospital compound with just a little johnny shirt on. Mothers had a small towel around their neck that was multipurpose: to wipe a sweaty brow and/or wipe little bare bottoms.

I saw women carrying bamboo poles across their shoulders, balancing heavy weight in large woven baskets, suspended at either end.

Transportation was incredible. Small three-wheeled vehicles, called Xe lam or Lambretta, with the steering wheel at the front in the centre, and a small cab behind with narrow benches along both sides, could be seen bringing patients to the hospital and providing taxi service. People jam packed in the back, the bicycles got piled on top, as many as four, and the women hung their poles and baskets out back. The buses were more of the same. Then there were the pedicabs that resembled bicycles, with the driver sitting high behind the passenger and peddling as the passenger sat in a comfortable seat with a canopy to protect themselves from the sun. Of course, there were all kinds of bicycles and scooters too. If you wanted to get any place, you just had to sit on the horn!

We met many types of people there. They came to our hospital from all over South Vietnam because it was well known for eye surgery and caring doctors and nurses. Many different tribespeople also came.

I described my life in some detail in a letter home.

Sunday, June 27, was a big day for our medical team, as Dr. Carl and Phyllis Yoder officially completed their three-year term. The airport was crowded with people who came to say goodbye and see them off.

The next day, Barb and Helen, two CWS nurses, arrived for a short ten-week service stint. Dr. Gehman felt that they should focus more on the hospital, while much of my day was to be in the outpatient clinic. Without fluency in the language, I had to be very observant and develop my own sign language to be understood. Not one of us could speak Vietnamese at this point. It became obvious that I needed to focus on language study too.

Because my working day in the clinic began at seven forty-five a.m. and didn't end until everyone was seen—which could be anywhere from one to two p.m.—I needed to find a time when I still had energy to concentrate. I found a seminarian studying at the seminary on the hill, and he surprisingly agreed to teach me from six to seven a.m., before our regular days began. I assumed he was in need of finances to agree to teach a foreign female alone in a room, especially at a time when there were still some arranged marriages for persons pursuing the ministry. I had my first lesson on July first.

My first lesson included the phrase, "How are you today?" I tried repeating it several times, and, at one point, my teacher's face became very red, and I couldn't understand what had happened.

I discovered that the Vietnamese language has six tones. Initially, I could not hear these variations, try as I would. My head would go in the direction of the tone I was trying to say. A tone totally changed the meaning of a word. After I learned to hear the tones, I understood why the Vietnamese did not understand what I was attempting to communicate. At my farewell party three years later, my teacher was married and not as shy as when we first studied together. It was then that he told me my pronunciation of "How are you today?" translated to "How are you to kiss?" Now I turned red!

I soon had to learn to drive into town for errands. It required crossing two bridges, only wide enough for one-way traffic, so the traffic needed to wait until all was clear. Vietnamese soldiers were stationed at both ends, around the clock, directing traffic. When you looked out on either side of the bridge, you could see many fishing boats ready to go out fishing at night. Children were busy rowing in bamboo tubs. We had a Volkswagen van, open at the back, a dilapidated Land Rover and an old Vespa scooter, which I hadn't learned to drive yet.

After two weeks in Nhatrang, Paul and Doris assumed that I needed a few days in Saigon because I had jumped into the work headfirst after arriving in Vietnam, without any real orientation. We drove around Saigon and saw the floating restaurant that had recently been bombed: Americans were using it again. Because MCC was expanding, Doris and I did some scouting for larger living quarters. We used taxis, except once we used a pedicab. Two Vietnamese could easily fit into the seat of one, but, generally, just one Western person. Because Doris and I thought we didn't have far to travel, we decided both of us would hop into the same one. I ended up holding Doris. Unfortunately, the place was considerably further than expected, much to our chagrin. My correspondence to my parents said:

> *Vietnamese just about broke their rubber necks and died laughing at us. It certainly must have looked funny. The poor guy peddled for all he was worth, and whenever someone got in his way he'd holler because if he had to stop, he could hardly get started again.*

My week in Saigon culminated in an invitation to a birthday party celebration for the seventy-year-old father of a MCC staff member. The Chinese restaurant served us nine courses: the last one was a soup I will never forget. Having grown up on a turkey farm and seeing what their feet walked in, imagine my shock and horror to see that the soup bowl placed in front of me was filled with chicken feet, duck feet, and brain floating in the broth!

In my letter home, dated July 10, I was back in Nhatrang.

> *I'm adjusting to this place a little better as time goes on. When our lone turkey starts gobbling, I especially feel at home . . . What I wouldn't do to have some young people from home do something in the voluntary service line. They don't know what they are missing. Before I left home, I found people felt sorry for me, but now it's the reverse. I find myself feeling sorry for them because they have to miss an experience like this. The people you meet here are tremendous.*

With Phyllis gone, Marva was the only nurse with experience and the Vietnamese language. Barb, Helen, and I were eager to do as much as possible, but it became obvious that Marva was having difficulty sharing the work, so we nurses decided that it would be a good time for me to focus on language study on top of working in the outpatient clinic.

Word came that Carl Kauffman (the Paxman I had met in Hong Kong) was being transferred to Nhatrang; Dr. Luez and his wife were also expected in early August to start a clinic in Pleiku, but security was too poor to do so at the present time.

When two of the CWS nurses assigned to Saigon came to Nhatrang for a visit, we had a short swim, then decided to drive into town in the evening. It was the best time because everyone was out on the street. As we neared the main square there was a mob of people blocking the street. We discovered the attraction was an ordinary size movie screen in the open on the main street, with an English show that no one understood.

In town you invariably met up with beggars: often children looked sickly and dressed poorly: they used a snapper (a handheld noisemaker) to get your attention and shoved a hat in front of you, begging for money. Initially, I gave them one piaster each but not more. Marva said people did this as a business, and, generally, the beggars were not poor. For example, we had a very ill baby in our hospital, and the child's mother went into town and told everyone that her baby had died, which wasn't so, but she raised 1,000 piasters for the baby's "funeral!"

August 9, 1965 made the headlines when a loaded plane crashed on the main street with fourteen unexploded bombs. The area was blocked off because buildings were demolished, and they were still finding survivors. Dr. Gehman drove the scooter into town to provide medical assistance, and he ended up suturing a bar girl's face.

I had been having a Vietnamese lesson when we heard a plane that sounded like it was getting lower: we didn't think anything of it circling three times because it was routine for military planes to buzz the town three times, but then we saw it go straight down.

Our cook was in town at the Air Vietnam office when it happened. He saw it come down, ran for his bicycle, and beat it home. When he got here, he was all out of breath, and he talked so quickly that nobody could understand a word he said for the first five minutes. He said that he was sure that the Viet Cong were attacking, and that it was a terrible sight to see people burning. Thankfully, we were not affected or harmed.

Carl arrived on August 13, and he was our jack-of-all-trades, relieving the medical team of tasks that we did not have time to do.

In my letter home, dated August 22, I wrote:

> *Very early this morning the Vietnamese hospital staff on night duty called me: a young girl was in cardiac failure, and then passed away at five a.m. Because her mother had no money or transportation, we were required to drive the body and family home, which was approximately thirty-five km from Nhatrang. Barb and I decided we had best wait until six thirty when it would be light enough because we had to travel through VC (Viet Cong) territory knowing they are usually out early in the morning. We instructed our young Vietnamese interpreter not to tell anyone that we were medical people if we were stopped. We passed some American soldiers at the roadside with their machine guns and helmets. They instructed us never to stop: we passed through a village that the VC had controlled three days earlier, but we made it back safely!*
>
> *Marva leaves today for Saigon. Barb will leave tomorrow. Dr. and Mrs. Luez are arriving on Tuesday, August 31. Because Helen will stay on, there are now three nurses with Lois Luez and responsibilities needed to be designated. Dr. Gehman clearly wants me in the clinic and the O.R., so Helen and Lois will oversee the hospital during the day, and then we would rotate covering the hospital evenings and being on call for the night.*

There was so much to learn and absorb that at times it seemed overwhelming. I felt a bit like a sponge, using all my senses: limited language skills forced me to fully use my eyes and ears.

With the proximity of the hospital so close to our unit house and patients' families milling around outside the hospital, cooking meals, or just chatting, we had access to a language school just outside our gate. Thankfully, I was beginning to hear the tones more easily and understand how critical it was to say things in the proper tone. For example, the word for blood and colour was the same, but the tone totally changed the meaning. The rising tone for "mau" meant blood; the sliding down tone meant colour. I began to understand why I received puzzled looks when I thought I had communicated something clearly. Good thing I never found out what I had actually said sometimes!

I soon learned, too, how we maximized our resources by recycling. In the outpatient clinic we dispensed medications in empty pill containers when available. In the hospital, we used bottle caps to dispense patients' medications and cut up the pill box cartons to make patients' medicine cards. Large cardboard boxes were claimed as soon as they were emptied. When our cook returned from market, vegetables and fruit were generally wrapped with newspaper or pages from children's filled notebooks: meat was often wrapped in a banana leaf. This would make my mother happy because she was a staunch advocate for recycling. Garbage here was truly garbage that nobody could possibly use.

With so little free time, we tried to make the most of it. One Sunday afternoon, Helen, Carl, Doc (Dr. Gehman), and myself packed a picnic lunch and decided to climb a nearby mountain on the left side of the cove.

Doc said it well in an article he wrote about our escapade:

> Wise men take care of themselves. Only God takes care of fools.
>
> The fools in this story are very much like MCC workers anywhere. The man at the head of the expedition wasn't old enough to vote in the States. But already he had climbed mountains in Kansas and Hong Kong. Half of the crew was female, and all Vietnamese boys know that a girl can't climb their mountains. What they didn't know was that one of these girls shot an elephant many years before she saw her first milkshake. The other girl carried a haversack loaded with cheese sandwiches and bananas. The fourth member

of the party had some first aid knowledge but was well up in years.

It was blistering hot when we jockeyed with the Vietnamese soldiers on the lookout guard post for permission to take a hike up their mountain. First, they said "No," then "Khong duoc," which means about the same thing. But the guards got their heads together and came out of the huddle grinning. "Ok," they shouted, proud of their ability to say such a first-rate American word. And we took off.

We advanced about forty-six feet, the distance from the pitcher's mound to home plate in softball, and then turned away from a wall of matted briers. Next, we tried a steep rain-washed gully, ascended ten feet and slid back five, a mathematical progression that eventually got us to the top—and another thick brush line. We had worked hard to get where we were, too hard, in fact, to turn back, and coming down would be harder than going up.

A volley of shouts and "Hellos" burst from the guards on a little knoll far below when we emerged from the brush into a clearing on the first peak. The soldiers had given us the "go" signal strictly for amusement, assuming that the height we attained was only possible by helicopter. We pretended the wind was blowing in the other direction, ate our lunch in peace, and kept going.

The view of Nhatrang was tremendous. Neat homes surrounded by coconut trees flashed cleanly in the tropical sunlight. The South China Sea rolled onto the white sand near a small hospital with a medical cross on the roof. Away up the long fertile plain a winding river phased out between two misty hills hanging in the clouds.

What we saw in the distance was enchanting. What our eyes beheld at the foot of the hill was disturbing. Was it a swarm of ants trying to drag a breadcrumb over a mole hill, or was it a group of soldiers pulling the wraps off guns? A minute later we knew. The cannon's roar in the middle of *a quiet afternoon was unmistakably a vociferous protest to our presence on the ridge above a Vietnamese military academy.*

The noise of the artillery below called for a meeting of the minds. The unanimous decision in favour of descent was prompted by a few big drops of water followed by a driving sheet of rain. We met a messenger in arms at the foot of the mountain, and apologized for our drowned rat appearance. That's the way we were marched before the captain of the compound.

"Yes, captain, we know there are Viet Cong in the area. But surely they stay away from the bare mountain." Bullets flew all over the hill when the soldiers took shooting practice most evenings.

"Ah, but Americans, you ask us next time you climb, no one ever walk this hill before—no one in the two years we plant mine fields all over the top of this mountain."

Mine fields! Did he say mine fields?

On a lighter note, several days later, Doc and Carl confessed that their wallets were mouldy from Sunday's downpour. Doc said, "This is the first time my money has ever gotten mouldy!"

Letter to Mennonite Youth Fellowship

In my correspondence to my Mennonite Youth Fellowship group on September 14, I wrote,

> *Four months ago, I was vacillating on one of the biggest decisions I have had to make; should I go to Vietnam or not? Due to the newspaper headlines, I had never felt more apprehensive of the unknown involved in coming nor had I ever felt more excited at the possibilities which might be*

involved in the same unknown. You must be wondering what life is really like in this country of action.

The hospital and unit house are side by side: looking straight out from our front porch there is a coral reef and, in the distance, several small islands can be clearly seen. The sunrise is beautiful. Our peaceful calm setting is interrupted by military activity at a Vietnamese non-commissioned officers' academy on the left side of the cove, with their training exercises during the day and evenings until ten p.m. They have artillery practice, tracer bullets and flares, parachute practice, troop landings on our swimming beach, and other activities.

Our small hospital has sixty beds, a busy outpatient clinic serving 150-200 patients four mornings per week, and surgery on Wednesdays and Saturdays. I have not yet found the refugee camps I had envisioned encamped along the sea coast. Generally, life seems to carry on as it always has. In our unit discussions we have come to the conclusion that the people really wouldn't care if they were under communist rule. In fact, the majority of the population might be better off economically because of what communism has to offer. The average Vietnamese isn't fighting this war—they just want peace: they are innocent bystanders. A good example of this would be several weeks ago: as we stood on the front porch, we could see bombs dropping only three-quarters of a mile away, then helicopter after helicopter parachuted troops in the same area. Meanwhile, hospital patients that were not bedridden were squatting on our front lawn thinking this was the best performance they had seen in a long time. At the same time, we were wondering how much closer they would have to be before we must be evacuated. After being here three months, I find myself becoming somewhat immune to the majority of military action. Maybe this accounts for the Vietnamese' complete lack of concern because their country has been at war as long as they can remember.

When I first arrived, I was afraid to wander out alone at night, but now I sometimes decide to take a scooter ride into town just to get away, even though we supposedly live in VC controlled territory that is out of bounds for the military. (More than three km outside of town is off limits to the American military.) We do not consider ourselves to have a curfew unless the Vietnamese do. The American military cannot understand this and would never venture out beyond the two bridges.

What does my average week look like? Four mornings a week I screen the outpatients, treating the less seriously ill and sending the others to see the doctor. We finish around two p.m., eat lunch, and then return to the hospital, where Helen assumes primary responsibility. We have three afternoon clinics: tuberculosis, Foster Parent Plan, and the orphanage. Surgery on Wednesday and Saturday mornings include many eye cases, eg. cataracts, entropion (scarring of eyelids causing eyelashes to turn in, rubbing on the cornea), and many other minor cases. Helen and I rotate working evenings so we can have a little time to ourselves.

All patients requiring X-rays or major surgery get taken to the Provincial Hospital or the American Army Hospital. Two temporary houses for TB patients, with siding and roofs made from flattened beer cans, are situated behind the main hospital. They house approximately fifty patients.

What do we do in our free time, besides writing letters, studying medicine, and keeping up monthly reports? Because we can no longer climb mountains, we go swimming (midnight dips) and sometimes go sailing in our sailboat, named Buu Tin, meaning Faith, which is an appropriate name. At the nearest island there is a beautiful coral reef, with shells of every shape and colour washed on a sandy shore. When snorkeling, one can see tropical fish, starfish, and jellyfish in season. Truly beautiful. We have slept on the island even though it is not the best policy due to VC activity not far away. Doc, the name we have given Dr. Gehman, plays the guitar and mouth organ, which provides entertainment along with our singing.

Besides our V-W van and Vespa scooter we have an outdated Land Rover like an army truck that looks like it has lived its life, with the steering wheel on the right side, a speck of power, and a tremendous ability to create a noise. It does give you a feeling that you have accomplished something if you manage to get to town and back without getting a flat tire and running out of gas, even though you left home with a full tank. So far, I have accomplished both!

Then there is the Vespa scooter that we girls have learned to ride. The first time I tried to ride it, I just about ran into a group of Vietnamese soldiers walking along the road. After making a U-turn, the soldiers saw me coming again and quickly lined themselves up along the side of the road— good thinking!

I have much to learn about the Vietnamese people and their beautiful country being torn apart by a long drawn-out war. It is hard for you to imagine the situation here. Your letters and prayer support are so appreciated. Keep them coming! Canada seems far away to me now.

I am learning more and more about the differences in our cultures, such as attitudes toward older persons, display of emotion, manual labour, "intellectual" labour, and punctuality; maybe half of our patients show up for surgery. Highly educated persons avoid using their hands for tasks they consider below their dignity. It must seem most unusual for them to see us working so hard physically. Patients regard us with much respect, which is evidenced by their attitude and the many gifts of food, especially seafood and tropical fruit.

Vietnamese also avoid looking you in the eye when addressing you, which is a polite way to address a superior. When first meeting a Vietnamese, they are most likely to ask, "How much money do you make?" or "Are you married?" or "How old are you?" which signifies that they are merely interested in you as a person. It proves rather embarrassing at first when you are caught off guard.

Public display of emotion is almost always considered in bad taste, so seeing American military walking down the street arm-in-arm with Vietnamese girls is frowned upon.

It hardly seems possible that four months have passed since leaving home. My world here is so foreign to my previous life in Canada that I can already sense in three years it will be culture shock re-entering. One doesn't recognize the energy needed to make the cultural adjustments in the first several months, but I am beginning to feel it now.

Emma Lenzmann, a Canadian nurse from British Columbia, who arrived on October 7, has been told that she will likely be assigned to Pleiku, pending security, along with Dr. and Lois Luez. Currently, many scenarios are being discussed by the MCC Saigon office.

Church World Service has emergency funding for Vietnam that they would like to have channeled through MCC for medical needs. MCC is recommending temporary projects because they would not be able to maintain more permanent medical projects. Two mobile clinics to work with refugees, in addition to the Pleiku hospital, are being considered. Dr. Gehman suggested that the Nhatrang clinic be a second priority on the proposed list.

Helen and I have been doing all the work in the hospital and clinic and have not had time for study in medicine or language. After putting in fourteen- or fifteen-hour days, I don't have the energy to study. We are suggesting that Emma help in the hospital until she goes to Pleiku.

Because our hospital uses the 8th Field American Army Hospital for X-rays, lab services, and consultation, they are aware of three Western nurses at our hospital. It is such a rarity to see young Western girls that we find military personnel wanting to visit frequently and befriend us. We discourage this because our security pends on not associating with the military. We do occasionally attend the chapel on the American army base, though, just to hear an English service.

The morning of October 31, Dr. Luez and his wife Lois left for Pleiku: Emma was going to stay in Nhatrang for another two months, which gave us nurses a chance to organize ourselves better before she left.

A patient came in the previous evening with acute appendicitis that required immediate surgery; Doc gave a spinal anesthetic and, with Emma's O.R. experience, she circulated, and I had the privilege of being the scrub nurse. I loved working in surgery!

Two weeks later, Helen became ill with malaria—because she had previously had it in Africa, she immediately recognized the symptoms. Thankfully, with Doc's care she improved quickly. At the same time, I became ill with dengue fever—a mosquito-borne illness causing high fever and flu-like symptoms: the severe form, called dengue hemorrhagic fever, can cause bleeding, shock, and death. Even though we used mosquito nets to sleep at night, we had no way to protect ourselves around the clock. Fortunately, after a week both Helen and I were working full time again.

In my letter to family in early December, I shared with them an eye-opening experience.

In late November, I was given a rare opportunity to accompany our next-door neighbour, Max Cobbey, a Wycliffe Bible translator, to a tribal village where they had lived until security forced them to move to Nhatrang. He still travels there thirty-five to forty-five km south of Nhatrang several times a week. He said that because many people are very ill and will not go to the hospital, he would appreciate my going with him to provide treatment. Carl and I accompanied him in his Xe-lam (Lambretta) and took one tribal family back to their village. (A Lambretta is a three-wheeled vehicle with two narrow benches on both sides in the back.) Most people here reside in thatched roof shelters, with no walls or just woven reeds.

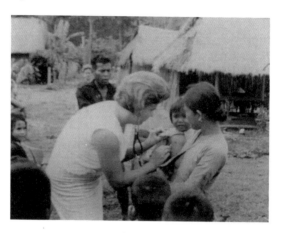

Public Health in Raglai tribal village.

We proceeded to another village further south and walked one km in from the road. Here we saw tribespeople sitting in a circle, gibbering away as they looked in this basin of water, saying, "The dog ate it all. He ate it all!" They knew there was an eclipse! This amazed me. We considered them uneducated but, in reality, they were so attuned to nature and the universe that they were aware of the eclipse and that they should not look at the sun directly. To them, the eclipse equated to the "dog eating the sun." These tribespeople were forced to leave their nomadic mountainous way of life and relocate to the hot coastal area. With no access to clean drinking water, a subsistent diet and limited protection from the elements, many villagers became ill. We took as many patients with us as we could get in the back of the Xe lam after visiting three villages.

That evening, on a visit to 8th Field Hospital, we dis-
covered that three American soldiers who had travelled the
same road the same day had been ambushed by VCs just a
little further down the road at a village where we had been.
(We had checked about security before going.)

My First Christmas and New Year in Vietnam

Days ran into each other with the heavy workload. We three nurses scheduled time so we could alternate having Sundays off in the hospital, but we
had to do the cooking for our unit because our cook was off on Sundays.
Doc seemed to think we couldn't cook, but we showed him! After eating
a delicious dinner, Emma convinced Doc and Carl to do the dishes. Doc
made the comment, "Dinner must have been good if you can get us guys
to do the dishes."

It was hard to believe that Christmas was only six days away. My first
Christmas in Vietnam! Monday evening, Emma and I went to the church
on top of the hill where the seminarians gave a beautiful program. Tuesday,
on my day off, I baked cookies for our staff Christmas party on Thursday
evening. Wednesday evening was the Christmas program for the hospital
patients on the outpatient clinic porch, which was beautifully decorated.
Our chaplain related the Christmas story, followed by Doc and myself
giving our testimonies. Then Doc, Emma, Helen, and I gave out cookies
and candy to all the patients.

One of the first persons to receive a bag of these treats was Em Lieng,
a five-year-old girl. ("Em" denotes a child in Vietnamese.) She had been
around the hospital since late October when her twenty-five-year-old
mother had been admitted with TB in both lungs. Since her father had
been killed three years earlier and she had no other family, she stayed at
the hospital with her mother. She shared her mother's bed in D ward which
had three other TB patients. Em Lieng soon became a favourite of the staff.
Her mother did some sewing for other patients to support themselves: she
often read for other patients who could not read, and she taught Em Lieng
how to read because she could not go to school.

As Christmas was approaching, Em Lieng had been wondering whether she would be getting some candy. The French had introduced Christmas, which Vietnamese didn't celebrate; but Em Lieng had always been given a little candy by her mother for Christmas. Her mother did not disappoint her this year either. But, much to Em Lieng's delight, she received a dress and a small doll from the hospital staff and a Christmas bundle from the Western staff, made available through MCC, that included a dress, sweater, toothbrush, soap, and a small doll. Em Lieng was overjoyed with her gifts. This was also the first time she had heard the story about baby Jesus. Her mother's health had significantly improved by January, so the doctor was preparing to discharge her, when Em Lieng developed a cough. An X-ray confirmed that it was only pneumonia, so two weeks later they returned to Banmethuot. It was unlikely that her mother could afford the injections she required three times a week, but she was determined to return home. You wonder if the Christian message, delivered every morning by the chaplain, heard by Em Lieng and her mother, who had been in our hospital setting for several months, had made a difference in their lives.

After the Christmas program, Carl and I had to take several people back to Nhatrang. Because the night was still young and driving in areas of flooded Nhatrang was a real challenge, we decided to do some exploring. Many homes had been flooded and the water level was too high on some roads to drive. Carl and I decided to drive down some streets just for the fun of it. It was at least two days since we had had much rain so the water level had gone down considerably, but some roads still couldn't be used by the average vehicle. We proceeded down one road in the Land Rover: houses were partly under water on both sides, but we kept on going. Then the water level rose as high as the lights and the car just about stalled—this was about all I could take, but there was no turning around and there was a lot of water ahead. At this point the Land Rover just about stalled again, but we managed to get through, only to discover that it was a dead-end street. We had to go back the same way we had come! Thankfully, we made it back home but didn't share the escapade with the rest of the unit.

Gary and Chris, two VNCSers, came up from Saigon to spend Christmas with us. The orphanage held their Christmas program on the Thursday evening, and the children belted out the Christmas songs with such gusto and volume! After their inspiring and entertaining show, we returned home for our own staff Christmas party. Carl and I had made two batches of ice cream to go with the cookies I had made on Tuesday.

On the Friday evening, the Vietnamese young people had a program at their church in town. The decorations and the children's singing were out of this world! Afterward, we were invited to a C & M A missionaries' home for cookies and coffee. Then, after returning home, we decided that we'd like to go Christmas caroling. So, at eleven-fifty p.m., seven of us started up the hill and sang at various missionaries' and pastors' homes and for hospital workers, who had never heard of Christmas caroling before.

At that point it was one a.m. on Christmas Day. Before retiring, I had to cut up the turkey to prepare it for the pressure cooker the next day. The next morning I was up early to get the gobbler on. (He came from Saigon and was ten pounds, as big as they ever get there.) Thinking of making the Christmas dinner worried me to death, but it had to be done because I was the one voted in to prepare the dinner. We eventually had turkey, gravy, stuffing, baked potatoes, jellied salad, and instant pudding with bananas and fresh grated coconut, along with assorted cookies, and it was all delicious, but it was a very difficult process.

In the kitchen we had one gas plate with two burners that were temperamental: it was impossible to properly regulate the gas flow. There was no stove with an oven, but we did have an oven box to set on top of the two burners. Other than that, there were four built-in charcoal pits, but I couldn't build a fire worth mentioning. Amongst all the turmoil, dinner was finally served and enjoyed. After the dishes were done, everyone except Emma and I went swimming. The two of us opted to take the scooter into town to a Baptist missionary's home, where we enjoyed a piece of Christmas cake.

I guess our caroling was so impressive the night before that we were asked to sing at the local Tin Lanh church the next evening. After the program we went swimming, then came back and played Rook and talked until three-thirty a.m. when we decided we had better get some sleep. It was a memorable first Christmas in Vietnam!

Doc was to take the organist in town for a service the following Sunday, but unfortunately, the rainy season had caused considerable damage to the roads. The road at the end of our lane was washed out in two places, so he decided to turn right and go up the hill. Deep gullies had formed in the road: Doc was almost at the top when he got stuck. After digging for thirty minutes or so and using a crowbar, he made it to church in time for the doxology! He came back via the orphanage and parked the Land Rover at the end of a lane on the other side of the washout. We all hoped to go into town for a restaurant meal that evening. One could say that we lived life to its fullest.

Thursday, December 30 proved to be a routine day until four-thirty p.m., when Helen came rushing to the front of the hospital to ask me if I'd like to give an injection to a "cow." Thinking she was joking, I said sure. As it turned out, she was serious. A Vietnamese farmer had come to the TB clinic with a filled prescription of penicillin for his sick cow, but he had no one to give the injection. Helen was not inclined to go, so I decided to do it because the farmer was standing there waiting for a response. I had given injections to turkeys on the farm at home, so this was no big deal. I grabbed a syringe, a large needle, and a handful of alcohol swabs, and then quickly got changed.

The farmer hopped on the back of my scooter, much to my chagrin: a Vietnamese farmer riding on the back of a scooter driven by a Western female!? We travelled north on the main road two or three kilometres, then turned off on a side road that was partly washed out, so we ended up pushing the scooter through a shallow stream and continued on our way. We then proceeded to walk along narrow paths and through fields to a thatched mud home where he motioned for me to sit down, then rattled something off in Vietnamese that I assumed was equivalent to "Wait here until I get it in the field and tie it up."

Another reason I readily accepted to do this was that cows in Vietnam are small and thin. When he came back and said, "duoc" (okay), I proceeded to follow him, dodging trees and bushes, until, in a clearing, I could see an object tied to a tree. A big grey water buffalo! There was no way I could back out now. After wiping caked mud from its rear end with soaked alcohol swabs, I rammed the needle through his thick hide into his buttock. It jumped around wildly, the syringe with the penicillin still stuck in the buttock, bobbing in every direction. I prayed it would not fall off! When the water buffalo finally calmed down, I was able to inject the penicillin. Then I heard loud cheering and clapping. Vietnamese soldiers hanging out of the second-floor windows of their army barracks had watched this whole performance! Hardly embarrassing!

I wish this was the end of the story, but it isn't. The farmer then told me that his water buffalo needed an injection three days in a row, which meant tomorrow and on New Year's Day! When I got home and told Carl, he said he wanted to go along the next day and take a picture. Well, when we were eating our noon meal the next day, the farmer appeared at our front door. He came to inform me that I need not come to give the second injection because his water buffalo had died. This was a great loss to the farmer, but, truthfully, I was relieved, although I was ribbed by unit members for killing a water buffalo!

The Christmas meal must have impressed the unit because I was asked to make the main meal for New Year's Day too. It had to be a Western meal because I didn't have the skill to cook Vietnamese food. I made a potato salad, tossed salad, jellied salad, devilled eggs, and unbaked chocolate cookies for dessert. We discovered that January first was not a big celebration for the Vietnamese; rather the Lunar (Chinese) New Year in several weeks.

After the holidays, I was feeling ready for a break. Work was heavy and living and working together as a team twenty-four hours a day, seven days a week, was proving to be a challenge. Always being one to avoid confrontation, back in September I had agreed to let one nurse take my position in the outpatient clinic on a monthly rotation basis because she really wanted that position. That also meant I had to forfeit the O.R. too because surgery was scheduled for days when there was no clinic. That hurt! Now it was mid-January, and I was still working in the hospital full time. After we nurses and Doc discussed the situation, Doc made it clear that he wanted me in the clinic and O.R., so the matter was settled.

I was due to have a vacation, so I went to the Air America office where one could make reservations on all USOM flights (United States Operations Mission) free of charge. Because it was unsafe to travel domestically, one had to fly from city to city within the country. There were no other options. Paul preferred that we not use USOM more than necessary, but the fact was that many of their flights were not full, even though most were small planes such as Beechcraft, Caribous, and helicopters.

Our medical unit discovered that in Vietnam everything stopped for Tet, the Lunar New Year. The hospital was quiet. It was decided that this was a perfect time for my vacation.

In my correspondence home, dated January 27, 1966, I wrote:

Presently, I am in Hue spending a week's vacation. Boy does it feel great! I never realized how exhausted I was. I had intentions of going to Dalat for several days first, but because it was impossible to get a flight from there going north without stopping in Nhatrang, I decided the night before not to go. Friday morning at five-thirty a.m., I got up and went to the US Air Force Port and boarded a C-123 used for transporting troops and went to Qui Nhon where I had to check in for another flight. Fortunately, I got a flight to Danang early afternoon. Finally, I found a hotel that had a room available at three p.m. The room was facing the river and canal, along with the balcony, which sounds great, but the room wasn't clean: it had dirty sheets and a plugged john! The officer on my last flight offered to take me to the Officers' mess hall for dinner because restaurants were closed for Tet, and he booked me on a medical evacuation flight (for casualties) to Hue the next morning. When I arrived, whom should I meet but Doc himself!

We hitched a ride into town and located Chris' home: he was a VNCSer (Church World Service and Lutheran World Relief amalgamated with Mennonite Central Committee to form Vietnam Christian Service). I moved into a house that the boys had just rented but had not moved into yet. Chris took us out to the farm to see the trainee program that WRC (World Relief Commission) was working on with Bob Davis. They planned to train refugees in farming, such as raising chickens, pigs, etc. For example, each trainee could have a pig to raise, then, when it reproduced, they must give one pig back to the farm to hopefully become a self-supporting project. It was in the beginning stage, and they had 200 trainees. Chris was very enthusiastic about it, and I was impressed.

Monday morning, Doc and I planned to ride bicycles to see various tourist attractions. Doc got up early to rent two bicycles but could only find one boy's bike at a rental shop, so he told me to hop on the back of his bike (all Vietnamese bikes have a small "tin seat" on the back for a passenger or parcels). Well, we were all set for the grand take off—I really felt sorry for Doc because I was bigger than he was—but he insisted that I hop on. He tried so hard to take off that the front wheel went straight into the air, and I was literally dumped into a water puddle. It must have been comical to see. If that wasn't enough, we weren't able to get another bicycle before dinner so we decided to eat at a restaurant first. After eating, we were ready to leave. Doc couldn't steer properly and we veered to the left, hit a curb, and he dumped me again! Fortunately, there were no injuries, and we laughed along with the many spectators. One cannot make up stories about these ridiculous incidents that happened, and they are all true.

In the afternoon the next day, we got another bicycle and rode out of town to see an ancient Buddhist pagoda, one of the six tombs of the Emperor, and the Imperial City. The countryside appeared peaceful and beautiful, with little military presence compared to Nhatrang. The Perfume River flowed through Hue with many sampans plying the river. What a fun, relaxing vacation.

Em Thuc and His Request for Prayer

Several parcels from home arrived for me in early February. One from VJ, a nursing classmate, with honey from Ellie's Dad, strawberry jam, puddings, and Jell-O: it was better than Christmas! Another two arrived from Dr. Yoder and his family with candy, chocolate chips, vanilla, cinnamon, and books.

In correspondence to my parents early in March 1966, I wrote:

> *Emma has been gone for two weeks already for language study in Saigon, making it very busy with just two nurses. Sunday afternoon Helen and I decided to travel thirty-three km north up the coast to Ninh Hoa with our old Vespa scooter just to get away for a change. Although the area is considered controlled by the VC, the province sector advisor said they have not had any casualties but recommended not to travel beyond Ninh Hoa. Carl and Doc chose not to go because they could be taken for military personnel. A family that had been patients at our hospital saw us going into Ninh Hoa and flagged us down. They had sweetened rice cooked for us, which I tried to eat to be polite. We stopped at two fishing villages on the way back. One village gave me a little puppy we nicknamed Talofa, a Swahili name meaning "my best friend." We got back in time for me to go to work in the hospital.*

Nhatrang was definitely on the MCC map for most visitors coming to Vietnam. On March 11, Frank Epp, editor of the *Canadian Mennonite* came on a world tour sponsored by four organizations. He interviewed us and took many photos. He went to India to meet Ken Shantz from my home church, who was serving with MCC. The people that we got to meet were amazing!

Work had been really heavy and stressful, and it continued to be so. Helen was scheduled to leave for home in two weeks. I had two new orphans from the orphanage next door that needed to be trained as staff. (We were expected to provide employment for them when they turn sixteen.) They had no previous medical training. Staff in general were very young, fifteen to twenty years old, and they did not readily take responsibility for treatments and medications, due partly to the fact that they had no concept of medicine or the anatomy and physiology of the body. A seven-to-eight-week course had been given previously, but we did not have the time to continue the teaching program due to our hospital work and language study.

Initially, I was able to study Vietnamese for an average of two hours daily, five days a week, but since August there had been too much nursing to do to really concentrate on it. It would have been helpful to have had language study before beginning my assignment, just to learn the basic fundamentals. The medical terms commonly used could be learned while working in the clinic. When working in the hospital, the staff said they appreciated working with me and that my pronunciation in Vietnamese was good, which made me feel that there was hope yet.

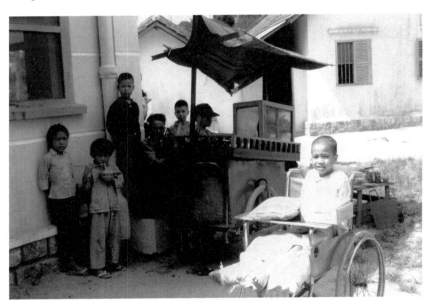

Em Thuc with severe burns to his legs.

One person who stands out in my mind is Em Thuc, a boy, age twelve, who came to our clinic having sustained serious burns to both legs, one leg much more than the other. He had been treated for several weeks at a hospital in Banmethuot, 185 km from Nhatrang. When he had been told that he would lose one leg, his mother decided to come to our clinic. The bandages that had been on his legs for two weeks had to be removed. Em Thuc cried and had reason to! He begged to be put to sleep. Under the bandages was dead grass and maggots in the one leg! I wanted to cry with him! Doc helped me initially so he could assess the extent of the burns. The first challenge was to clean up the infection. Doc felt that it was best for the same nurse to do the daily dressings, so Em Thuc became my responsibility. It wasn't just doing the dressings but also doing minor exercises so his muscles would not atrophy. When he was admitted, he could not even move the toes in his left foot. Two weeks later, he was able to wiggle them a little. He began to trust me, and we had some interesting conversations with my limited Vietnamese.

One day he asked me if I would pray for him. I said I would, and then asked him if he wanted me to pray in English or Vietnamese? His answer was, "Please pray in Vietnamese so God can understand." His request was so sincere and touching. I said a very elementary prayer, but I think God understood, and Em Thuc seemed happy about it. He gradually had the confidence to do some exercises himself.

I tried to have conversations with Em Thuc to distract him while changing his dressings. Although I did not ask specific questions about the cause of the burns, he said that a can of gas was overturned, but one doesn't know for sure. It could have been napalm or terrorist activity. He lived in an area that was controlled by the VC at night and South Vietnamese Army (ARVN) by day. We heard stories of villagers being forced by the VC to dig all night to block roads or plant land mines, and then the next day forced by the government troops to undo what they had just finished. Our job was not to ask questions, only to provide medical care for anyone coming to the clinic or hospital.

After several weeks, Em Thuc had a smile: he tried not to cry when the dressings were changed. We told him that he would not lose his left leg, and he began to believe it. He only weighed forty pounds on admission, but when he began to think he would get better, he began to eat. In two months, he gained twenty pounds! He needed to have extensive skin grafts on both legs, but we did not have a dermatome. We had to transfer him to the provincial hospital in Nhatrang where a team of American surgeons agreed to do the skin grafts. It was a long process, but the story ends with

Em Thuc being able to go home—walking on both legs! He had been hospitalized for over a year. His beautiful smile on discharge warmed my heart, and he will always be remembered for the trust he put in me.

I guess the fact that I gave a water buffalo an injection did not escape the memory of people in our small Christian community, namely the orphanage next door, even though it had died. Having grown up on the farm and vaccinated turkeys put me in good stead. They had some pigs that needed to be immunized, so guess who was asked to immunize six squealing pigs? The scene provided free entertainment for many excited children as staff cornered the pigs one by one, and I plunged the needle through some thick hide. Thankfully they all lived, as did I to tell the tale.

On my day off, I rode the scooter (no muffler now) into town and sat on the beach. As a Westerner, I attracted attention here too. One child stood in front of me staring at my white skin. She had a runny nose, so the girl looking after her squeezed the discharge out of the nose, wiped it on the sole of her rubber thong, then on the trunk of a palm tree. It seems impossible to have privacy away from my own bedroom!

On March 25, Emma returned from language study in Saigon with two visiting nurses. When Helen left a week later, Emma and I had the responsibility of the hospital, clinic, and surgery. Having Dr. Brenneman there with his positive attitude was wonderful.

When Carl took his two-week vacation, we realized what his job entailed. It was agreed that I would drive the scooter into town at six a.m. to buy the sixty mini baguettes for the TB patients. The bakery was in front of the local market. It took a little skill to ride the scooter with the baguettes in a bag between my legs. I had just picked up some speed when a large Vietnamese army truck pulled out of a side street and cut me off. I slammed on the brakes and was pinned under the scooter, the bread scattered on the road: women came running out of the market, hollering, "Ba Bac si, Ba Bac si." (Mrs. Doctor, Mrs. Doctor.) They recognized me and quickly got the scooter off me. Fortunately, I wasn't injured. We collected the bread, and on I went. The experience did rattle me though.

One day in early April, after getting work done in the hospital, Emma and I decided it was our chance to go to Cam Ranh Bay, about forty-five km south, on the scooter. We got to the second bridge, just inside Nhatrang, where there were demonstrators who would not let us through. A bus driver had been dragged from his bus, held for fifteen minutes, and then shot. There were armed guards at all the government buildings, and the main square was completely blocked off by coils of barbed wire two heights high. It was at times like that we were reminded that we were in a country at war. Thankfully, we were stationed just beyond the city of Nhatrang.

There had been many demonstrations lately, and the town had been off limits for several weeks. Political unrest had been widespread, and the two most politically influential groups—the students and the Buddhists—had taken to street demonstrations again in cities throughout the country. They were demanding the ousting of Premier Nguyen Cao Ky's military government. Some Vietnamese military were defiantly parading with anti-government banners.

We didn't know how long this unrest would last because of the variety and validity of the complaints. However, from all we could learn from firsthand accounts, the most common and general feeling among the Vietnamese people was that they were tired of the war, and all they wanted was peace and quiet. We'd had strict curfews and no trips into town at night, but things quieted down considerably with a curfew from midnight to four a.m. again.

With all the political disruptions, there was really no point in writing letters because mail service had stopped. Then, on April 17, we finally got mail for the first time in three weeks. I got four Christmas cards. Funny getting them after Easter.

Another reason I didn't write letters during this time was that with Helen gone and Emma off with a very sore foot and leg and unable to walk, I had been holding the fort day and night for more than a week, and two doctors created more work than one. Emma sent a note with Dr. Brenneman to Saigon requesting nurses SOS. It was not humanly possible for me to keep functioning on three to four hours' sleep per night, with only an occasional meal. Dr. Brenneman was to return from Saigon the next day, hopefully with two nurses. It turned out that the earliest they could come was when Dr. Brenneman would leave in two weeks.

On April 23, Paul Longacre and Dr. Beechy, VNCS interim director, arrived from Saigon to have a unit meeting to evaluate our situation. Ruth, a nurse, had just arrived from Saigon for a month, and was scheduled to return to Saigon to organize a nursing program for Nhatrang and have more language study— did I ever envy her! Another nurse, who had come through CWS (Church World Service) and still had one more month of language study, had only a one-year term of service. So, basically, it was just going to be Emma and I until Dr. Brenneman left. The most discouraging part was that it took about nine to ten months to be really effective and know everything that was going on, given the communication barrier, so this eliminated language study for me at this time. Emma felt depressed and, frankly, I was feeling low too. Oh, to get away for just a few days.

On May 6, Mary Sue arrived from Saigon. She was a twenty-six-year-old from Ohio; a thin, tall, and outspoken gal who played the ukulele and had a good sense of humour. She was sponsored by the Disciples of Christ Church to serve one year at our hospital. Emma and I decided to break her in the next day and have Sunday off before working in the hospital on Monday.

The next Sunday, Emma and I decided to go for a little scooter ride north through the mountain pass toward Ninh Hoa. When we got to the other side of the mountains we had a flat tire near a resettlement village. We had several spectators that soon developed into a congregation, but no one was able to help us. We needed a wrench: of course, there wasn't one on our scooter, so I proceeded to flag everyone down who was travelling on the road. Not many people bicycled past: scooters and army jeeps were few. Finally, after about an hour, a scooter with two Vietnamese stopped, and they proceeded to help us. After a strenuous job, they finally got the old tire off, but the spare tire was flat too! They drove off and came back twenty minutes later, with the tire blown up. Emma and I were getting concerned because we didn't have one piaster between us, so the option of hopping on a bus to Nhatrang was nil. It would have meant standing on the back runner and holding on for dear life anyway. Thankfully, good Samaritans were there!

In my letter to family the end of May, I shared my vacation experiences. In Vietnam it was not safe to use local transportation. This necessitated taking advantage of the American military presence; they were more than willing to fly women from place to place.

Soon after Mary Sue came, I took a week's vacation. I had made reservations for Co Ly [Co, in Vietnamese, indicates an unmarried young lady], my interpreter, to accompany me to Kontum, north of Pleiku in the central highlands, to visit a hospital run by Project Concern, another NGO (non-governmental organization) that provides medical services for various ethnic tribespeople who are so different than the Vietnamese. Many women wear skirts but no tops, with their babies strapped around their backs; the men wear loincloths. Everyone squats to do their work. Because they live a nomadic life, they weave baskets that they carry on their backs. Drinking water is carried in a dried gourd.

We toured the hospital that had patients and families everywhere: the leprosarium was depressing . . . dark, dirty, and isolated.

On Sunday, we had a twenty-minute flight by helicopter to Pleiku where we stayed with Dr. and Mrs. Luez and met Mary Pauls, another Canadian nurse, and Rufus, who was to work on an agricultural project. The hospital building was progressing well.

We enjoyed just looking around the small market and bargaining for the best price. On Thursday, Co Ly returned to Nhatrang, and I flew on to Saigon and hitched a ride into town where, unexpectedly, I ran into Rufus, who was en route to the VNCS headquarters.

On Saturday afternoon, three of the guys in language study and I rode two scooters to Bien Hoa, about thirty km northwest of Saigon, to meet a doctor friend of mine. In the evening we went to see the annual Vietnamese opera, which was fascinating. Early Sunday morning, when I returned to Nhatrang, I had a chance to co-pilot a plane on my vacation. I got back in time to get everyone out of bed! It was great to get back.

When I returned, Emma was on a week's vacation, and she was due back soon. I couldn't wait to hear her stories because she also wanted to go to Pleiku and Kontum. Dr. Gehman wanted to go to the Christian and Missionary Alliance Conference again because he had enjoyed it, and their baseball games, so much the previous year. He decided at the last minute to go and left Friday, leaving me with the remainder of clinic: he left the hospital in my hands and told the other nurses that I was in charge. I resented this a little and was uncomfortable and uneasy about it all because Carl and I had just had a long talk the night before in which I discovered that I had caused hard feelings just before going on vacation.

It was this way: I had worked all day and in the evening on Thursday before going on vacation on Friday at noon. There had been at least three people I was expecting to pass away on my shift. One was a young girl with advanced TB, who was hemorrhaging to death. I knew that I wouldn't get much sleep but didn't really care because this girl meant so much to me. It was obvious she would not last long.

At eleven-thirty p.m., the Bible School bus drove in with a student with a medical emergency. Doc did a white blood count, and it confirmed acute appendicitis. Doc asked the student if he wanted surgery here or at the provincial hospital because we could only give a spinal anesthetic. He wanted surgery at our hospital, so Doc decided to do it as soon as I could get set up and call Anh Tin to come and assist him. We managed to finish at three a.m. I never did get to bed because of the other dying patients.

Apparently, Emma felt hurt, thinking that I should have had some sleep before going on vacation. Frankly, I enjoyed doing surgery again and never thought that I had been unfair to Emma and Mary Sue.

On June 29, 1966, I wrote home to my parents. I was back to a regular routine, on night duty.

Presently I'm taking a thirty- to forty-five-minute break; I probably will spend most of the night sitting up with four kids in the hospital with temperatures of over 104, diagnosed with typhoid or possible meningitis. Tomorrow night won't come too soon because Thursday is a heavy clinic day. Presently I am getting a little bogged down with all the responsibility and all so I'm trying to get a flight to Pleiku for Saturday morning, and then come back on Sunday evening. We girls have arranged to have a day off and then take turns on Sundays: it turns out that we have every third one off. It sounds terrific, but other days you put in such long hours and usually you work the evening before your day off, and you might have been up all night, so what happens is you end up sleeping your day off away. Then on Sunday we have to make dinner and wash dishes which takes a while because you don't have the commodities you have at home. This weekend will be a release of tension.

Dr. Gehman's article published in the *Youth Christian Companion* on July 10 vividly describes the situation at our hospital. He entitled it, "Maybe War is an Accident?"

A thin dark-skinned mother with scarred eyes feels her way into the crowded office with one arm and clutches her screaming baby in the other. She tells the doctor's interpreter that her little child, besides having an infected scalp, has been coughing for a month and cannot eat.

Above the hacking noise of helicopters, the doctor hears telltale rattles from the baby's congested lungs. A brief three-way discussion reveals the discouraging fact that the child cannot stay for nursing care and medical treatment. His mother must go back over 100 km of rugged terrain, hot sandy plains, and Viet Cong hideouts to Phan Rang to care for her children.

The doctor scribbles a few orders on a small dog-eared card, and mother and child leave as another patient from the long line outside launches his aching frame through the open door.

On the ward, an old man, with a bandage covering one eye and a cataract in the other, sits in bed and tries to look around a room he cannot see.

On the floor in the hallway, a young man coughs, moans a little, turns on his good side and tries to get the sleep that he missed the previous night because of an emaciated infant on the next mat.

In the courtyard, a Lambretta rolls to a stop and four people unceremoniously pile out, leaving only a prostrate, feverish grandmother stretched out on the short seat. A long gray dog, a coconut gripped tightly in his powerful jaws, saunters passed a roll of sprawling patients on the front porch.

Out across the bay a pointed sail poised smoothly on the dim horizon. The sun goes down as a group of patients cooks rice over charcoal fires.

And, silently, the first red tracer bullets spray against the faraway hill. The diffuse noise of artillery fire breaks the air, and you remember that this is Vietnam, and there's a war going on.

Rarely is the routine of Vietnamese life broken—the routine of eat a little, sleep a little, cough a lot, and wonder where your next bowl of rice is going to come from. But a war is being fought right on their soil.

The army is everywhere. Tall, confident American advisers and native boys in fatigues and boots, bogged down with guns, sacks, and clipboards stand prepared. There is the expected attack, which is far less devastating than the threat of attack.

And there is the usual accident of war. The afternoon is balmy as usual. Children scream and splash on the

Nhatrang beach. A mission nurse sips a cool drink at a beach house while on a downtown errand. Her attention is diverted from the breaking waves on the shore to two jet bombers as they roar through a swarm of helicopters, sky raiders, and beavers. One of the bombers holds an eccentric course, much like a crow that has had its pinions clipped on one wing. Out over the bay, two small figures fall from the circling plane and two parachutes open.

"Bac si, met qua," (Doctor, I'm so tired.) sighs a weary Vietnamese lady. The usual sound of planes intensifies overhead. Gently the doctor injects a long, thin needle into her fluid-filled abdomen. Somewhere, a motor drones in the sky, followed by a sound that resembles a sonic boom.

A clear yellow fluid begins to flow into the syringe.

In a cloud of dust, an MCC cook frantically appears in the driveway. He had fled the main business street of Nhatrang on bicycle while the bombs were blasting and the bricks were still flying.

Dreadful minutes pass and bits of information begin to accumulate. Half of the townspeople have witnessed the calamity, have seen the bomber bank sharply, complete a half circle, lose altitude at full tilt, and dive into the business district with bombs bursting.

People have fled their homes while flames engulfed their favourite restaurants and tailor shops. Casualties and corpses have been removed from the burning scene. Before the last fiery explosion, lacerations have already been stitched. What unit on earth is prepared for disaster like the US Army?

A crowd gapes in suspense at a live bomb hanging dizzily on a ledge three storeys up. Several blocks away, another crowd watches a doctor sew up a hole on a bar girl's face.

It was an accident of war, they say—only twenty-two lives. Twice that number die in sneak attacks on slumbering villages. Maybe war is an accident.

The fortune of man is such that disaster is usually of short duration. The smoke diffuses into the clouds. The flames diminish, smolder, and die. Traffic moves again in the streets. Trucks rumble across the bridges.

Toward evening, a thin dark-skinned woman carries a sleeping boy child on her right hip as she feels her way across the bridges.

The above article captures how fragile life can be in a war-torn country. Lives are disrupted but we just carried on treating patients as needed.

Language Study in Saigon

On July 15, I began one month's language study in Saigon. It was so hard sitting and studying all day after being in the routine of putting in a long day's work. At first it was just review and sharpening up my pronunciation, which had become a little rusty.

In Dr. Atlee Beechy's farewell letter as interim director, dated August 8, 1966, he wrote:

Dear VNCS Co-Workers:

In my final word to you, I want to say a few things about our vocation–the work of Vietnam Christian Service.

I know many of you are out there on the firing line where the going is tough. Others are here in Saigon where sometimes the going gets tough also. There are many in supportive roles at home where this would be true as well. The problems related to "doing good" seem so complex and difficult that you begin to question the validity of your work. You become weary of the fabric of obstacles that stretch your toleration ability to the breaking point.

There is real possibility that you may be overwhelmed by the needs. You begin to wonder where to get hold of something specific, something manageable. Perhaps compassion *fatigue is setting in and you are tempted to turn away from the ugly sores around you, but something pulls you back to the task. Also, you'll become aware again that **being** precedes the **doing**.*

What is our task? In one real sense we are the church at work in this situation, this place with all its suffering, it's dislocation and its chaotic confusion. In the midst of this we are called to be the "fellowship of the caring."

Acts of service must emerge out of a real sense of caring, out of a deep response to God's care.

This caring must be genuine.

This caring must be personal.

This caring must be sensitive to human aspirations.

This caring must be free from condescension.

This caring must not be used to make others feel obligated, but rather to help others discover again a sense of self-respect.

This caring is not deterred by hostility, by rejection, or lack of appreciation.

This caring opens the way for hope to emerge and for the one cared for to start caring again.

To live means to care, and

To care means to live.

This is our vocation.

"I thank my God upon every remembrance of you, always in every prayer of mine for you all making request with joy, for your fellowship in the gospel from the first day until now; being confident of this very thing, that he which hath begun a good work in you will perform it until the day of Jesus Christ." Philippians 1: 3-6.

The month went by quickly. I would have loved to have stayed and studied for one more month for the sake of learning more Vietnamese, but it was difficult to study all day when I was used to active work. I also really missed Nhatrang and the hospital staff. I knew it would be hard to leave in three years.

August 6 was my last Sunday in Saigon. Barb and I had a car (Peugeot) to go to church—there were honest to goodness cars in Saigon, which reminded me of home.

On August 10, I was back in Nhatrang and working in the clinic. I was invited to one of the C & M A missionaries' home for supper and had my first apple pie with cheese since leaving home! It delicious! There were no apples in Vietnam, so they got them and a lot of other food from the US.

Dr. Harold and Esther Kraybill soon arrived in Nhatrang. They were a friendly young couple and a real asset to our Nhatrang medical unit.

There was such a tremendous influx of new workers coming in that it was impossible to keep up-to-date on the latest. When I came to Vietnam there were seven of us; and at this point there were forty-nine—and they were still coming.

The Cobbey family, Wycliffe Bible translators, were leaving for one year, so VNCS agreed to rent their residence because there were now eight of us, with four bedrooms and a makeshift one next to the storeroom, where Carl slept.

Mary Sue and I volunteered to move into the Cobbey's home the next day. The house did not have water on tap—a well was just beside the house—or a fridge or stove, but it did have a regular Vietnamese squat john. There were three rooms in a row with cinder block steps into the rooms: there were no ceilings, just a tin roof, and the walls were concrete. We planned to get them painted or whitewashed in the near future. The front of the house was screened in, with bricks laid in the sand for the floor, and that was our dining and living area.

In my letter to my parents on September 1, 1966 I wrote:

Barb arrived in Nhatrang from Saigon for a week's vacation, and she said that she would like me to go with her to Hue for a week's vacation next month. (The Imperial City of Hue, built in 1362, was the capital of Vietnam from 1802 until 1945 during the reign of the Nguyen dynasty.) When Ken and Chris, VNCSers from Hue, had been down to Saigon, they had asked Barb to have me accompany her there in September. Because Emma and Mary Sue had talked about going together some time, I decided that I would go with Barb.

September 10 found Barb and I on our way up to Hue. Everyone had been warning us not to go there because it was not secure, but we wanted to go so badly. Others said it was impossible to get there until after elections. The vice president of USOM in Nhatrang had been on our flight to Danang, and he was not allowed to travel beyond Danang to Hue for security reasons. We weren't even in Danang for an hour before we were on our next plane en route to Hue.

Ken and Chris welcomed us to their animal husbandry project. They had just received 700 baby chicks shipped in from the US. It was like feeding the poults on the farm back home. Were they ever cute! Barb and I even helped the guys and their Vietnamese refugees build a pig pen, smashing the ground and packing it to put in a layer of concrete. It was lots of hard work and fun.

Chris and Ken allowed Barb and I to use their scooter to do a little sightseeing on our own, so we rode out to the Hue Imperial City (The Citadel), the former capital, which had a moat and ten ornate gates guarding a palace, temples, gardens, and tombs. Unfortunately, we were only able to see the seven-tier pagoda because many of the places were off-limits due to the election the next day. The atmosphere was rather tense. Most of the people were afraid to vote for fear they would be killed. The last two nights two Vietnamese policemen had been murdered not very far from our house.

Barb and I thoroughly enjoyed our week in Hue. We booked ourselves a helicopter ride from Hue to Danang, 100 kilometres south. Then Barb had to find a return flight to Saigon and I to Nhatrang. (This was an easy feat for anyone wearing a skirt.)

Work was waiting for me as soon as I returned to Nhatrang. Each day presented challenges reminding me that I was not living in a stable country and there were constant demands on my time. This became apparent in my correspondence home in September.

I was just getting out of the Land Rover from a trip into Nhatrang tonight and grabbed for my shopping bag only to discover it wasn't where I had left it. I had asked a baker to watch the Land Rover while I went to a restaurant just several yards away. He readily consented, so I left all my belongings on the Land Rover seat because it was impossible to lock it. I had left my raincoat, one sandal each from three different pairs to get fixed, plus several important letters, one from MCC (a business reply) and one that I had just finished writing to you. When I returned everything was missing. The shoes were really good still—it was just that they had been made in Saigon due to my big feet. No matter which country I live in, my "understanding" has always been problematic. Maybe I have to resort to wearing rubber thongs!

I worked in the hospital today and had three babies come in with fevers and mild convulsions. We did a cut down (surgery on a leg to start an IV) and one hour later, the baby died. Just when I was ready to go eat dinner, an eight-month-old baby came in with exactly the same symptoms. We did another IV cut down immediately: the infant just about died twice when we were doing the cut down. Then a third baby came in with exactly the same symptoms. If the second baby would have died, I don't know what I'd have done because all three of the babies were such cute well-nourished infants—no scabies or boils. God, what's happening?

We loved having guests. Nhatrang was a highlight for tourists with its pristine beaches. However, guests meant extra work and less free time.

This weekend a couple from Saigon will arrive and the Neufeld family from Quang Ngai. We enjoy the company but it is difficult due to the time spent running to and from airports and waiting for their arrival. To top it off, we have no cook or maid on Sunday so we have the cooking to do. We don't have the conveniences of back home. Dr. and Mrs. Kraybill and Ruth Yoder went to Pleiku for the weekend for the dedication of their hospital.

Mary Sue and I entertained our first company this weekend when a couple was up from Saigon. Doc and his guitar and a ukulele that was passed around made for a fine sing song. We bought two reed mats for the floor to cover the bricks and found four old couch type cushions and put new covers on them. They are our main chairs. So we sat on the floor and sang folk songs, made some Vietnamese tea that we served in our Vietnamese tea cups, and nibbled on some popcorn that Doc had gotten in a care package.

Our company came and went but there was no such thing as a regular schedule. On September 25, I wrote:

Emma leaves for a break next week, then Doc takes one week's vacation, followed by the Kraybills who leave for two months of language study in Saigon. Change, change, adjust, change. One vicious circle. I'm dreading the time when I have to return home because it will all be so different. So much has changed here in sixteen months.

Change was a constant as were security concerns. On September 30th I wrote to my parents saying:

Security continues to be a major concern. There is no such thing as a secure place here. The places that are considered insecure by the US Army have guards placed everywhere. That's where many terrorist acts occur. But out in a place like we are, I personally feel quite secure. Reports are that Nhatrang is very infiltrated with VC. Some of the missionaries are surprised when they find out that I come home alone two evenings a week after nine p.m. on the scooter. I don't worry about it because many people in this district know me from my work in the outpatient clinic: no doubt we look after many VCs at the hospital. (The Viet Cong known as VC by the American military called themselves NLF, National Liberation Front fighting for independence from Western colonization.)

In the same letter, I reflected on how the constant demands of the work were felt by everybody. Each person coped in their own way which impacted our functioning as a team.

I have been feeling very discouraged the last one to two weeks. Every clinic day we are scheduled to start devotions with the staff at seven-fifty a.m., with the clinic beginning at eight a.m.; but, if the head person doesn't come on time regularly, it has a domino effect. Now the staff are not coming for devotions as well as coming late for clinic hour. I feel so discouraged. Emma also. I don't know what I'd do without her. Nothing seems to get done on time around here.

On Thursday, October 8, I started to feel sick but managed to work until Saturday, even though I could hardly crawl: I was so tired by Tuesday, when Doc left for vacation. I developed nausea and vomiting, yellow eyes, and urine the colour of tea! Hepatitis! Doc came back from vacation on the eighteenth, surprised to find me in bed. The next day, my bed felt like a prison, but I was too weak to even sit up in bed. Recovery was painfully slow but eventually I could write home that I was making a steady recovery.

By October 23, I was feeling better but not well enough to work: still sick with hepatitis. Paul Longacre asked me if I was well enough to go to Saigon at the beginning of the month because on November 6, the Vietnamese government wants to give out two awards for the medical work that VNCS has done for their country. Dr. Gehman and I were nominated, so we would go early the next week.

I still felt weak, though, so it was decided that I would stay in Saigon for a week to recuperate before going back to work at the hospital. Finally feeling better, I was able to help in small ways, as I wrote in this letter home.

> *Jerry and Judy (two VNCSers), who are setting up a house-hold in Di Linh, south of Dalat, sent a list of items to be purchased in Saigon. Doug and I went shopping for them. What a riot! There was an art to bargaining, and I was still learning. If you couldn't get the price down and thought it was too high, you just walked away, and then you'd hear the merchant calling you back, deciding to sell it to you for your price.*
>
> *The last item on the shopping list was two big tubs! We piled everything we had bought in them and proceeded to walk down main street to the office, when it started to pour. Doug said, "We might as well put the tubs on our heads. We wouldn't be any more conspicuous than we are now." So we did, and we made it to the office.*

Life in Nhatrang

My morale was really boosted on November 14, when packages arrived from home with Jell-O, chocolates, popcorn, and toiletries. The boxes of my clothing from Akron also finally arrived after seventeen months.

It was a time of confusion for us in the unit because I wasn't sure who belonged where. Doc wanted me in the outpatient clinic, and Carl wanted me to start a mobile clinic, and in the end, I was tasked with setting up the TB hospital, which we dedicated that day. I would have loved to do both jobs, but I knew I couldn't do everything. To top it off, I felt terribly fatigued and was hoping it was not a relapse of hepatitis.

My reflections to family on November 18 include my frustrations:

I am feeling very negative about so many things. One is the frustrations of being unable to start the clinic on time due to consistent tardiness. It wastes everybody's time waiting. Medicines are being stolen. My interpreter wants to quit in two weeks, even though it is required to give one month's notice. Vietnamese staff can go to the US army and get a much better salary. Then there's the provincial hospital that has expanded tremendously and is very well equipped: US Agency for International Development (USAID) has a very good surgical team and a nursing education team there. They will be starting a fabulous one-year nursing program next year and have all kinds of equipment and experience. We live just five to six km away and also want to begin a one-year nursing program but do not have the equipment or experience, no major surgery, and little obstetrics, too, so I question whether we should be setting up such a program ourselves, especially because we affiliate with them. If we can't provide X-ray and lab facilities like the Provincial Hospital, are we being fair? If we have two doctors here, we only need one clinic nurse, which eliminates Emma or me, more likely Emma because everyone feels that that is where I belong, and one nurse in the hospital who could take surgery too. All this is only feasible if there are enough competent and conscientious staff. At the present time we are doing much of the work they should be capable of doing; but, instead, one of us nurses is on duty every evening and required to stay up all night if necessary. We should pay more and try to get registered, capable staff (easier said than done because nurses just aren't available here) but the doctor doesn't impress this on the board members.

I question whether we are really fulfilling a desperate need here. There are many more needy areas without a nurse or doctor— couldn't we serve there? Here we look after the orphanage. All the Bible School students and surrounding Christian community tend to think that they have priority because this is their hospital: they usually aren't very sick and use up much of the doctors' precious time. Are we really fulfilling a need? We are looking after sick people, yes, but there's other medical help available. Regarding interpersonal relations, I had a long talk with Mary Sue until three a.m. Mary Sue's words were "No matter what you do, you do it well and with self-confidence: you speak the language: no matter what has to be done in the hospital, you are capable of doing it. No matter what medical problem is brought up or questions regarding the hospital, if there's a doubt, your word is what counts: you know where everything is."

Dr. Stoffel, a Swiss doctor with VNCS, came for a one-week visit. He had twelve years' experience in Africa. His comments were, "What a crime to have so much American staff here—train native staff!" Wow! Today I had to bury myself in the storeroom organizing medications because Emma preferred to work in the clinic. Dr. Stoffel says the place could run on one doctor and two nurses if it was organized and set up properly: just how I feel. Then everyone would be doing work that is a challenge and wouldn't be stepping on others' toes.

I decided to talk with Doc as unit leader because unit members are not working together as a team: I discussed my frustrations and later felt bad because he looked crestfallen. He definitely wants me to work in the clinic. If I choose to transfer, perhaps it will ease the tension, but Doc was very clear where he wants me working.

Carl also confided in me that he wants to start a mobile clinic on the condition that I'd be the one going with him. He'd like to go out to surrounding refugee areas and toward Cam Ranh Bay. He said if something like this developed, perhaps we could go out four to five days per week and make it a full-time job: that I could teach him how to take temperatures, blood pressures, and give injections. Co Ly suggested to Carl that after she quits, I could work without an interpreter. Well, that is overestimating my Vietnamese ability, but with this future in mind, a mobile clinic or transfer, I want to study more again—starting this Monday evening! There are many dialects but knowledge never hurts anyone!

What does the future hold? Emma feels like returning to Canada in the spring—so—the answer is to live one day at a time and put my trust in someone who is higher than I am. One thing I have learned since coming here is how difficult interpersonal relations can be, especially living and working together twenty-four hours a day, seven days a week. One also has to consider the stress of war and adjusting to a new culture. Not everyone has the same level of coping skills, which creates unneeded stress.

Many interesting things have happened since last week. Three VNCSers arrived Wednesday morning, stranded on their way to Quang Ngai. Then Thursday, the Hope family arrived with their three children, so we had eight extra persons. The poor cook! Thursday, we celebrated the American Thanksgiving with a big beautiful turkey that was donated. It was delicious. Emma and I were planning to go out and enjoy the Canadian Thanksgiving but that was the time when I was in bed with hepatitis. In the evening, we were asked to sing at the Christian Servicemen's Center. There were many testimonies and then Rev. Revelle, a Baptist missionary, gave a sermon. Getting to know so many fine Christians since coming to Vietnam has been a source of renewal for me.

It's only Friday night but I can't sleep in tomorrow morning on December 6, on my day off, because 3000 pounds of relief and canned beef supplies for TB patients are to arrive at the airport from Saigon in the morning. Waves can be heard distinctly washing in on shore: our road is in the process of being washed out due to the tail end of a typhoon. Maybe we won't get into town tomorrow morning.

Emma left on vacation today for a week. Supposedly, in less than two weeks, the TB hospital is to be opened—if the beds come! My interpreter is quitting, and we've got no one to replace her. This weekend I also want to write a personal report to Saigon. We are supposed to write monthly reports, and mine for this month will consist of my ideas for this place, etc. Presently, I am back to my Vietnamese studies again—I don't speak enough. My comprehension is much farther advanced than my speaking. Well, I must get to bed. I guess I have just been pushing myself further than I should. Tomorrow morning, a Vietnamese family is taking me out for some pho, Vietnamese noodle soup, at eight-thirty a.m., then I have another family to visit, business and correspondence plus having four IVSers out for supper—that's if the roads aren't washed out.

Correspondence to my family a few weeks later on December 20 read:

Merry Christmas family! All of your parcels have arrived to date, and it sure is fun getting them. Thanks ever so much for all the treats, toiletries, and cosmetics. I haven't been quite feeling up to par—hepatitis probably. I work really hard one day, and then I'm not worth a wooden nickel the next day. Christmas definitely centres around the church here in Vietnam. Our schedule starting tomorrow evening is: our hospital program followed by a staff party at our house; the Seminary's Christmas program on the twenty-second; the orphanage's Christmas program on the twenty-third—but, instead, that evening I am having supper with Billy Graham at the American Air Base—the twenty-fourth is the Christmas program at the church in Nhatrang with our staff singing; and Christmas morning the Vinh Phuoc Tin Lanh Church near our hospital has their program with our staff singing; at one-twenty p.m. our staff will be singing at the Korean military hospital!

I don't really know where to begin to update you. Co Thanh, Doc's interpreter, is quitting in February to study (she worked here for three to four years); Co Ly, my interpreter, has quit; Co Trang, an excellent nurse (in clinic with me) quits in two weeks due to travelling issues (worked here three years); Co Huong, hospital head nurse, wants to quit in one month; Kim Anh is going to Pleiku! That leaves us with two men and three young girls with no training who show little potential. When Dr. Kraybill and his wife return from language study all we will have are three people to work in the clinic and two interpreters. I toss and turn all night wondering what'll happen. Staff just isn't readily available. At the same time, I struggle with my relationship with one Western nurse: working and living together is difficult. I don't know what I would do without Carl. He understands and is a good listener and brother! Helen sent a letter that she will be coming back to Nhatrang in early 1967 as a photographer and freelance writer.

The TB hospital was dedicated on November 14, but no patients have been admitted yet due to the beds being too long; they were supposedly made to order! They are two metres long and need to be shortened and painted. This has been a learning curve. After the building was completed, it was painted; then they remembered that they forgot to put in the air vents at the top of the wall so they knocked out bricks and plaster to make vents, then plaster had to be filled in around the vents and then another paint job! The electrical wiring was then added on the wall, which meant painting again! Seeing is believing!

Carl wants the song "The Canadian Christmas Carol." He heard it one time in Hong Kong and liked it so much and couldn't believe that I didn't know the song.

This being my second Christmas in Nhatrang, I was prepared for all seasonal activities. In my letter to family on December 30, 1966 I wrote:

The year 1966 is almost history! Your Christmas card arrived yesterday, and so did two other big parcels. What a prize! About thirteen of my nursing classmates went together and bought scads of things, mostly treats, cake mixes, puddings, pizza mixes, some candy, soap and powder, a song book, gum, and several toiletries. It sure was fun! Ron Sutherland, a C & M A missionary living on the hill above us, came and said he had two parcels for me at his house, so I went bounding up the hill. Well, they were huge, and I slid down the hill on them. We all had Christmas together. The Kraybills barrels arrived from Pennsylvania, so we are well-stocked for the next coming months regarding cake mixes, etc.

For New Year's Eve, I made up one cake mix for some friends. Well, Ken, one of our guests, came into the house and in a joking manner, said that someone ate half the cake. I went out to the kitchen to see and, sure enough, the dog had eaten half of it! So I spent the next ten minutes chasing the dog around the house. The others just laughed about it because they got to eat the other half of the cake. Today I'm very fatigued. The TB hospital is still not open, although the beds are now shortened.

I hope you had a lovely Christmas in Canada. We did, except our formally invited guests were unable to come, so we invited several of our close friends from around here. We had ham, yams, jellied salad, and fruit salad with Vietnamese fruits and cookies for dessert. I am so relieved Christmas is over because of all the singing appointments and programs. Emma was bitten by a snake on Christmas Eve, which was rather serious, but she is able to be back working half time on duty now.

Oh, and if you recall I told you previously that I was going to have dinner with the Reverend Billy Graham at the American Air Base just before Christmas? Well, it was a wonderful evening and I even got to shake his hand.

On January 7, 1967, I wrote:

A lot has happened since last week. My interpreter is finished and I have been trying to function without one, getting the histories, then sending the more seriously ill to see the doctor. It has worked out all right because the clinic hasn't been so busy now due to the weather. I did have a long talk with Paul Leatherman, VNCS personnel director, regarding the current situation. He said, "Marcy, you are doing a job that not too many other nurses would care to do," referring to the clinic. True. Reflecting on the ongoing stress with one nurse, I kept thinking that if both of us felt led to come here, surely, we can work things out. It is energy draining. Mobile clinic is still being considered and Carl would like to see it materialize. I will likely be setting up the TB hospital and developing a mobile clinic according to Paul Longacre. Paul Leatherman also mentioned that when Barb retires in the spring, they'll need a new nurse at Pleiku. An ophthalmologist will be coming here in the middle of February, so it'll take a nurse in the operating room much of the time: it'll be mass confusion. Mrs. Kraybill is expecting the end of January, so another addition to the family.

Today I went to the Nhatrang market with Ba Ba. It was fun listening to a Vietnamese bargain for things for a change. Then we drove to Cau Da to buy some pho, the delicious Vietnamese noodle soup, but they were sold out. Unexpectedly, we met a recovered TB patient in Nhatrang who insisted on treating us to pho noodle soup. We were just ready to go home when we heard someone call, "Co Marcy." Here was Anh Tin, hospital staff, who had just returned from Qui Nhon. We finally made it home by noon. It sure was fun. I slept this afternoon away. Monday, Mary Sue should be coming back from vacation.

Christmas has passed and so has half of January, would you believe it? This morning the Christmas cake,

Artex textile paints, and the St. Jacobs Mennonite Church's Sunday School class' box of greeting cards arrived. What a surprise! Everyone enjoyed the cake! It was delicious! Carl's mouth was practically drooling! I took two slivers to two different Vietnamese families, and they loved it. Some of my Vietnamese friends go so out-of-the-way to prepare food for me, so it's the least I can do. I was going to make a chocolate cake to share with Miss Minh's family. Because the dog ate half of the first one three days ago, I made another one. Well, I had baked it in two-layer cake pans; it wasn't a layer cake mix, though, so, after it was baked, it was only about a third of an inch high. We all laughed. The unit will never let me forget the cake mix experiences.

Miracle of miracles! We finally admitted patients in the new TB hospital on Tuesday. Still no cupboards or water. What confusion! Dr. Kraybill and I are pushing for an additional TB hospital to be built but it must be talked over at the unit meeting on Tuesday evening. As it works out there's a lot more involved in setting up the hospital than was previously anticipated. It will be another hospital. In the TB houses and the TB hospital we now have thirty-seven patients.

There's so much to do: an X-ray machine will be coming so we have to organize and set it up as well as a filing system; we also need to set up a lab for a lab technician; an eye specialist is scheduled to come in one month; staff problems plus interpreters; checking out mobile clinic possibilities, plus a nursing school (will it materialize or not?). I'd like to take the outpatient clinic and TB hospital now, plus the medicines. Carl feels that the mobile clinic will develop too which means that I will need to give up some of my responsibilities.

Regarding the mobile clinic, a memo was received on January 25 from the Saigon office regarding the discussion of one as well as health education work out in Nhatrang. Negative factors to be considered were, first, the hospital board may not be too excited about this kind of activity and, second, such a program may take some additional competent Vietnamese staff who are difficult to get. They asked us to please discuss the matter and respond.

The last week of January, Paul Longacre came for several days to discuss the direction of our work in light of the memo. Carl had been pushing to have a mobile clinic. Paul interviewed various people, including some USOM officials and Vietnamese doctors. Paul suggested that I start planning, and that I would be the one designated to run the mobile clinic. He wondered what my ideas would be: just teaching or diagnosing and prescribing medicine or just what had I envisioned? He said the other public health nurses were mostly working on teaching preventive medicine and not giving out many drugs. Carl and I were both very interested in working with tribespeople. There were several villages within thirty to ninety minutes' drive toward Cam Ranh Bay. I also wanted to continue to work with TB patients at the TB hospital which had been operating for almost two weeks.

I received a letter from Barb in Pleiku, and she asked me to go to Malaysia with her before she went home after retiring in March. I wanted to, but I didn't think I should because there were so many proposed changes which could make my being away difficult.

It was looking like only one doctor would be staying in Nhatrang and that would mean two nurses would be required in the clinic, and I wouldn't be able to start a mobile clinic unless VNCS dropped the idea of starting a nursing school, which wasn't too likely. So, the future was undecided.

The Dalat VNCS retreat was only two weeks away and all of our medical team were attending except for those needed to cover the hospital and clinic. I was staying behind with the Kraybills for the first half of the event because Esther was going to deliver her baby soon and also so I could be in Nhatrang for Tet, the Lunar New Year. It was a big celebration, and I had been invited to two Vietnamese families' homes; I didn't want to turn down the offers because it was considered a great honour to be invited to their homes on the first day of Tet. I was going to try to get a helicopter flight up for the tail end of the retreat.

We weren't terribly busy in the clinic due to the rainy season and the Lunar New Year. Patients wanted so badly to be at home for the celebrations, no matter how sick they were, so they would rather not come to the hospital in case they would have to be admitted.

Our X-ray machine arrived plus fourteen barrels of medicines, so, with all that in the clinic plus my work at the TB hospital, I was kept busy.

The TB patients enjoyed working on a jigsaw puzzle that my mother sent. They had never seen anything like it. It was interesting to watch them try to fit the pieces together. They couldn't believe that when the pieces were put together they would have a picture. After the first puzzle was finished, they were so excited at what they had made, and they began working on a second one.

In mid-February, I wrote home.

In early February we celebrated the Lunar New Year, known as Tet in Vietnam. I thought we had a big celebration in Canada on New Year's Eve, but it's nothing compared to the way these Eastern people celebrate their New Year. They have open shops set up along the main street, which are blocked off for traffic. Tet New Year feasts last three days. For the well-to-do people their feasting lasts longer. Today at noon we were invited up to the Bible School for a feast to welcome the Year of the Goat. Last year was the Year of the Horse.

Our rainy season has come to an end, and we're enjoying the best time of the year. It's very warm during the day but gets cool enough at night that you can sleep like a baby. There's enough of a breeze to still have whitecaps. It's beautiful!

As for excitement, well, it's always here and probably always will be. I was taking eight patients to the American Army Hospital for X-rays on Wednesday when, suddenly, flames shot out from under the hood of the Land Rover. I had smelt gasoline when we left home but nothing else appeared wrong. I came to a dead stop and tore around to the back of the Land Rover: everyone was getting off, except the old man from the bed in A13, sitting in the passenger's seat. I got on one side of him and a TB patient on the other side, and boy did we move! I don't think his feet touched the ground until we were about twenty feet from the vehicle. I was expecting the Land Rover to explode any minute. Before I had all the patients out, a bunch of American and Vietnamese men had ripped the hood open and were shoveling sand all over the engine. We were still quite far away from the military hospital, so a kind American soldier drove us there in an army truck. After X-rays were taken, the chief of the X-ray department got an ambulance to take us home. It sure was a life saver, but it doesn't help our image as conscientious objectors too much! In all the excitement, I forgot to get my own X-ray done. All I need to do is get TB myself examining all these far advanced cases who cough in my face and spit up sputum.

Keeping in Touch

I needed to write home frequently to keep them aware of all the activities in my life. We always were a close family. Friends also would inquire of my family about my wellbeing.

Last week, the unit members left for the retreat at Dalat, and I stayed back for a week to "hold the fort." Then, on Saturday, I was able to get a flight booked to join them. There were seventy of us at the retreat. It was great sharing our joys and frustrations. It went too fast. We returned on a C123 military cargo plane on Monday evening.

We were very busy after we returned. So much was happening since our X-ray machine had arrived: we needed to train an X-ray technician, and we have a lab technician scheduled to come in the future. We also have several very sick patients with typhoid fever and plague.

We have an eye specialist coming soon. Our best interpreter quit last week, and they are just not available because the American military absorbs them.

At the end of the month, I will be going back to Saigon for a three- to four-day conference for public health nurses because of my work with the TB hospital. Paul thinks that I should be included because the mobile clinic could develop after my out of country vacation, which I will be taking at the end of March and two weeks into April—Barb is retiring then, and she wants me to join her on a trip before she heads home. [Earlier I had not thought that the doctors would agree to my taking vacation at this time. However, the schedule opened up.] She is planning the trip—which will include Cambodia, Thailand, Malaysia, and Singapore— because it is difficult for both of us to coordinate it. It will be great to get out of a war zone for three weeks: no military jeeps, trucks, or soldiers. Fortunately, MCC is covering the cost of a round trip to Bangkok due to the war situation in Vietnam. One cannot really relax in Vietnam.

In the middle of the night once when I was on call in early March, a patient came in panting like a dog: he was a terrible cyanotic colour. I called Dr. Kraybill. We tried everything, oxygen, IV, a cut down on one leg, external cardiac massage; but he died anyway, due to cholera. He had become sick three days earlier and traveled all the way from Phan Thiet (175 km away) by bus to the clinic: it took him two days to get to a fishing village after he hadn't been drinking for two days, had diarrhea, vomiting, and a fever. The village was on the left side of the bay from us and the road was terribly rough for persons bringing him on a Honda motorbike. We didn't understand how they ever made it, but vehicles were only available at night, which was so sad.

When I returned from Saigon it was agreed that TB was still a very important issue and that I would continue to work in the outpatient clinic.

Emma had been kept busy in the operating room with Dr. Troyer. Later that month, I was set to begin my three-week vacation: two with Barb out of country and one in Quang Ngai to see the TB hospital run by the Canadian government.

I was very happy that Emma decided not to terminate after two years. She had come to Nhatrang three months after I did, so I thought that maybe I would extend my term a few months and go home with her. I found out that if an MCCer wanted to extend, you could extend three months through the field director, but, if more, it needed to be cleared through Akron, to a maximum of six months. There was also a chance that we could all be shipped home before then because USA International Aid (USAID) was on a six-month trial basis, and if it failed, all civilians in South Vietnam would be under military jurisdiction.

It was discouraging to discover that many people were not getting the letters that I had written. The postage had gone up to twenty-one piasters per letter, so the Vietnamese were probably taking the stamps off and throwing the letters away. Many times, I also received letters without the stamps!

On Saturday, March 25, I wrote home sharing about my trip:

> Barb and I left Saigon via Air Cambodage for Phnom Penh, the capital city of Cambodia. We had a brief stopover, then flew to Siem Reap, which is the nearest town to the famous Angkor Wat, the big tourist attraction with many ancient temples. We did not have reservations for accommodation so, after mass confusion, we managed to squeeze into this ancient bus which puttered into town, stopped at the Grand Hotel, then promptly demanded fifty-nine riel (Cambodian currency). We only had traveler's cheques, so we quickly ran into the hotel and they kindly cashed our cheques.
>
> We checked the rate for staying there and discovered it was way beyond our budget. In the process of discussing a solution, we were given the name of a less expensive accommodation and bombarded by cyclo (pedicab) drivers, one pulling one arm, another the other arm, someone else

with our baggage to take us to the recommended hotel. We hopped into a cyclo with our luggage (what a laugh!). The cyclos were different than in Vietnam. In Cambodia, the passenger sat behind the driver; in Vietnam, it was reversed.

We proceeded to go down a street when, suddenly, we were dumped at "a hole in the wall." Because we couldn't communicate with the lady at the desk, she wrote down some figures and we finally agreed to sleep there. It was basic: we had to share the toilet and shower with other guests on the second floor. We got cleaned up and decided to go out on the town for a bite to eat.

We met some interesting people staying at another hotel who told us about a Cambodian dance performance at Angkor Wat in the evening, so we quickly purchased tickets. A rickety bus got us there late, but the performance was amazing! When we returned to our hotel, the lady at the front desk told her staff, in Vietnamese, to get the key for Room #1! She became so friendly with us when she discovered that we spoke Vietnamese. She arranged for us to rent two bicycles early the next morning: we quickly went to the market, bought the regular little five-riel loaf of bread, some bananas and tangerines, and then set out for Angkor Wat, about four miles to the first temple. The steep stairs and height were staggering. When we reached the top and looked below, we hardly had the courage to climb down. At one point, we hung on for dear life and slowly made our descent, much to the amusement and delight of several Cambodians at the foot of the stairs (the steps were much narrower than my foot!).

The temples were spaced three-quarters of a mile to a mile apart, and we peddled for all we were worth for a total of close to twenty-five miles. Our bottoms were sore from cycling, and we were physically exhausted. After a brief rest, we decided that it would be more fun to go to Bangkok by local transportation, so we cancelled our plane reservations *because the Vietnamese lady at the hotel desk said that it was possible to take two buses to the Cambodian/Thai border, and then catch a train to Bangkok. We got up at four-thirty a.m., packed, and boarded the five o'clock bus.*

We had been warned that we'd have to change buses about two-thirds of the way. The bus did not have front or back doors but rather rows of seats the width of the bus with a door on the right side for each row: we had to climb about three feet to get on the bus. Our luggage was piled on top of the bus with everything else imaginable.

We travelled at a slow rate, stopping frequently to pick up more passengers and, if passengers wanted to go to the john, get water from a nearby stream, or buy something, we stopped again. Each time we came to a regular stop, girls would come out with trays of food and drink in plastic bags on their heads to sell. We travelled in and out of towns, but it was mostly miles and miles of perfectly flat land. The population centred in towns and cities with just a few homes scattered along the road. The sound of the language, dress of the people, and homes reminded me of the tribespeople in Vietnam. Houses were built on stilts—many made of beautifully carved wood. As the only Westerners on the bus, we found ourselves the centre of attention and conversation.

At one point, the bus driver stopped at what we thought was a hospital and chattered away to us. We sat there because we didn't know what else to do. A doctor appeared and wanted to give us an injection—what, we didn't know, so we promptly showed him our immunization cards. He browsed through them and nodded his head as if to say, "I don't know what this book says but let it go anyway." It was almost ten o'clock when we arrived at Sisophon and had to change buses. We were immediately marched off to the office of the Police Nationale, where we signed our names on some kind of declaration form: the officer informed us, in English, that the road to Poipet was "very dangerous, with Thai plant mines in the road that recently blew up some of the railroad tracks." Barb and I looked at each other and wondered what we should do. We decided to continue on our way and boarded the second bus and arrived incident free.

Barb and I didn't worry about time because the Vietnamese lady at our hotel in Siem Reap had said that we'd have lots of time to catch the one o'clock train going to Bangkok at the border. Well, at twelve-thirty, the bus driver pulled up to a building and motioned for us to get out again. We did. Guess where? Police Nationale again! Men started running in and out and motioned us to just sit and wait a minute. We did so, impatiently, because one o'clock was drawing near. Finally, at twelve forty-five, we had completed umpteen more papers and were turned loose by the police, who pointed to the left in the direction of Thailand. There was no transportation of course, because Cambodia and Thailand do not have a diplomatic relationship, so we started walking with our suitcases down the path running parallel with the train tracks, hopefully to lead us to Thailand.

After half a mile of walking, we came to an immigration customs office and Police Nationale again! We filled out more papers. It was twelve fifty-five at this point, and there was no train station in sight. We were told that the train station was in town, eight km away; the next train wasn't due to leave for Bangkok until six the next morning, so we hopped into the back of a Peugeot taxi (a little like a small pickup truck back home) with several elderly ladies and their tubs of live eel swimming in water, splashing us and our suitcases as we hit every pothole. It really didn't matter because we were already grimy and dusty from our bus trip on gravel roads with wide open windows with no glass! The immigration officer at the border—who could speak some English—had told the taxi driver to take us to the hotel by the train station. Of course, we didn't have any Thai money, just travellers' cheques, so the poor driver had to wait until we had cashed one illegally because there was no bank in this little town.

After we got cleaned up, we met a Thai tour guide staying at the same hotel. He had just returned from four years in Germany and was working as a tour guide for a German tourist company in Bangkok. His tourist group had come from Bangkok by bus to this hotel, and then gone on to Angkor Wat with their own chartered bus. He couldn't accompany them because he was Thai. He gave us a tour of the town and took us out to supper in a little restaurant for Thai food. It was delicious!

The next morning, we were up at five a.m. to catch the six o'clock train. Originally, we had reservations for air travel to Bangkok but thought this was more exciting by saving $64. Bus plus train tickets from Siem Reap to Bangkok were only $4.75 whereas plane travel would have cost us $67.50 per person. One person recommended that we take second class on the train because third class pays your way but you might not get a seat. It was reasonably comfortable and had open windows: we arrived at the big city of Bangkok at three p.m. It had been a long journey. It felt great to be in the "Venice of the East" with big buildings, two to three lane highways, and real taxis and cars! No cyclos! The first real civilized city I have seen since leaving home almost two years ago.

We stayed at the Bangkok Christian Guesthouse, went shopping in the evening and had some real ice cream. A city with no army trucks, Jeeps, or soldiers anywhere. We couldn't believe it: and no curfew or restrictions. We booked ourselves for a tour of the floating market the next morning.

In the morning, we boarded a boat that wove through the canals, and we got to see much of Bangkok from the water. The tour boat stopped at several interesting places, such as a Thai silk factory and store, a precious gem shop, the Temple of Dawn, and a large Buddhist temple. Many small boats plied their fruit, vegetables, and market goods in the canals. Apparently, 2,000 families live in the canals in sampans. It reminded me somewhat of Saigon and Hue. The next day, we toured the Grand Palace and the Temple of the Emerald Buddha.

Afterward, Barb and I bought second class train tickets to Penang and Kuala Lumpur for Saturday. From there we would take a taxi to Singapore. The whole trip only came to $140 minus $95.50 that MCC covered, round trip from Saigon to Bangkok, plus the $5 per diem, so it has been a fun and economical holiday thus far.

Barb and I had been in Bangkok from Tuesday afternoon to Saturday afternoon, when we boarded the train for Penang, Malaysia: twenty-eight hours in second class: no berth, but we met several fascinating people: Malay, Thai, American, and Australian worldwide travellers. It was spring break for university students, so they kept us entertained all night with their singing and guitar music. We were rather fatigued when we arrived in Penang. Because it's an island, we had to take the eight-p.m. ferry. We stayed at the YWCA and toured the town the next day, taking the cable car up the mountainside—what a spectacular view—and we had a delicious high tea at the summit! Barb was a great travelling companion: our interests were very similar, with about the same exercise tolerance.

The next evening, we took the train from the mainland to Kuala Lumpur, arriving there the next morning. We stayed with a young missionary gal, an acquaintance of Barb's who was struggling to learn the Chinese language. She kindly showed us the area. The next afternoon, we went to the market place where you can get a taxi to Singapore. You wait until there are six passengers to fill the taxi. We had Chinese, Malay, Indian, American, and Canadian passengers on our ride. I prayed that we would reach our destination alive, as our taxi was travelling at breakneck speed, winding around curves and rubber plantations. A ride never to be forgotten! Fortunately, we had reservations at the Methodist Guesthouse in Singapore.

Our two days' sightseeing in Singapore went by quickly. Singapore officially consists of a small main island and many smaller offshore islands, a total of 279 square miles, at the southern tip of the Malay Peninsula. It is a multi-ethnic city that just gained independence from Britain in 1965. People spoke Mandarin Chinese and English primarily. What a fun time we had exploring the city. Everything worked out beautifully, no mishaps, just humorous incidents all the time. The bus and train took longer, but we got to see the countryside.

Sunday, April 9, Barb and I parted ways at the Singapore airport; Barb flew to the States, and I flew to Saigon. What a wonderful feeling to be in a big commercial plane again—airline stewardesses and all, no roaring engines and soldiers. I got immune to the war and things that go with it, but after being in other Asian countries without war, I realized the tensions we lived with in Vietnam.

Monday morning, I arrived safely in Nhatrang. It was great to be back, and everyone was glad to see me too.

In my absence, Anne Falk, a fellow Canadian nurse, had helped Ruth in the outpatient clinic. Anne had been assigned to Tam Ky, which is north of Quang Ngai, and she lived with a home economist. They were evacuated due to mounting tension caused by a rumour that the Viet Cong were going to attack. She had just been at Nhatrang two days when a radio broadcasted that there had been an attack there and, apparently, by word of mouth from USAID staff, the Viet Cong were shooting on their front lawn. They had been caught in the midst of an attack once before when their house was in the middle of three USAID military homes, and theirs was the only one without much damage. Paul Longacre had been there and they spent the night under their beds, and then were evacuated at four a.m. They found two bullet holes in the house and one hole in the roof. One of the other houses had a mortar land in the front living room. I think we in Nhatrang were in one of the most secure areas in Vietnam, even more than Saigon.

Getting responsible and reliable staff and interpreters continued to be a major problem for us. The latest shock was that our cook, Anh Ba, was quitting after eleven years!

In the midst of all this, there were still times where we could laugh, as I wrote to my parents:

Last night was a full moon: the sky was clear and bright, and the water was calm–it was great for a midnight dip. When I splashed in the water there were all kinds of phosphorus particles that glimmered in the water. When I looked toward town, yellow flares could be seen dropping, lighting up the whole sky. That is as near to our Victoria Day as we get here.

Recently my friend, Chi Hue, and her family bought a TV. The Americans have a station at Cam Ranh Bay, seventy km away, so reception was good. They invited me to watch it last Sunday evening, so we watched The Ed Sullivan Show and Bonanza. I couldn't believe it! What really amused me were their comments, because only two of the family spoke some English.

We got a new motorbike. Emma took it through the fence the first day we had it, and then Mary Sue was in a car accident with it several days later. As it turned out she was hurt more badly than the motorbike. We're just minus a mirror—lucky enough.

Recently we have invited a young man from New Zealand, who came to Vietnam on his own to teach English. Because Tony lived alone, he joined us for dinner every Tuesday. Being a jovial person, we enjoyed his company and he enjoyed being with us. We had three different nationalities that spoke English, but, oh my, we did use different vocabulary at times. Like last evening, I asked Doc to reach for a serviette on the buffet behind him. He looked at me, like what is a serviette? Then, "Oh, you mean a napkin?" Then Tony burst out laughing. "A napkin? That's what babies wear." We needed that laugh.

If one cannot get away from here, we do get to meet other people from other units.

Nonetheless, the reality of our situation seemed to be changing with tension building up. On May 20, 1967, I wrote:

> *I'm not sure what the newspapers all say back home, but things are getting serious here. USAID, American aid to underdeveloped countries, run by the US State Department, was responsible for the pacification program for civilians in Vietnam. Then, in February, it became known as OCO which stands for Overseas Contingency Operations. At our retreat in Dalat in February, we had an OCO representative speak to us about the new structure in the organization. He mentioned, rather casually, that, because the US is escalating the war effort in six months, there is a possibility that OCO will be turned over to the military, but that it is very unlikely. We, as a group, discussed what an organization such as ours, representing pacifism, would do in these circumstances because we would be crippled regarding transportation, supplies, etc. It's happening already.*
>
> *Has anything been in the newspapers back home? We're not under any strict contract, but if conditions get critical and the military orders us out, it means out. He said that the US is currently significantly escalating and everything is in the hands of the military—the US is aware that anything could happen at any time. I might not be spending three years here after all. I'm not apprehensive about the situation here at Nhatrang, but one gets the feeling that some agreement will have to be made in the near future. The US Army has had forces at the DMZ (demilitarized zone) for one week. News reports say that Russia is going to supply North Vietnam with missiles. So—World War III? Maybe at present I'm just a little pessimistic. It would certainly be interesting though to read up on the current events back home and hear what they have to say, including Dr. Frank Epp's perspective. I'm dreading my return home because*

*everyone will want to know about Vietnam, and the longer
one stays here the more complex it seems to become.*

*This Friday, Paul Longacre, Paul Leatherman, and Mr.
Ninh will come to discuss a project evaluation and proposed
planning, war or no war. I doubt that the mobile clinic will
ever develop. Sad to say but maybe it's wise.*

The evaluation committee report about our project came out at the end of
the May. It stated that they'd had a lengthy discussion concerning the TB
work connected with the hospital. It was felt that a second TB ward was
badly needed. There were twenty-seven beds in the new TB hospital and
the census had been running around sixty-four. We were continuing to
use two old buildings and at least one of them needed to be destroyed after
another TB ward was built. They also talked about beginning a TB control
program in Bao Long village. The committee strongly encouraged this
type of preventive TB work. The possibility of implementing a one-year
nursing training program to start in August was also discussed at length.
That would require some classrooms, a dormitory, and a library.

Work and an Unexpected Visit

I received a letter in early June that was really exciting! Two Kens, friends
from home, had completed their three-year terms with MCC: Ken Shantz
in India, Ken Martin in Pakistan, and they were coming to see me for a few
days in July. It was exciting that someone from home was coming to visit.
I planned to go to Saigon with them, and then stay there for two weeks
to study about the BCG vaccine at Hong Bang Hospital, which was being
used to fight tuberculosis.

The more I thought about extending my term in Vietnam, the more I
thought it was less likely. Things were changing there so much all the time,
both with the war and at the hospital. A lot would also depend on what
staff was going to be staying on and what my duties would be in the future.
At that time, I was still responsible for the outpatient clinic as well as the
TB hospital and its houses.

The Vietnamese nurse assigned to the TB hospital has been exceptional in the way she relates to the patients. She sincerely cares about them, besides providing their daily medications of oral INH and PAS, as well as their intramuscular injections of Streptomycin. One must note that we do not have disposable needles: needles are sterilized and used so many times that occasionally we have to sharpen them. Giving an intramuscular injection with a dull needle into a thin buttock is painful for the patient and nurse alike. Giving injections daily over a period of several months means there is scarring, which makes it even more painful. The nurse also provides injections for out-patients who come three times per week on Monday, Wednesday and Friday afternoons.

One Sunday in June, our unit took a trip by car to Phan Rang, about 110 km south, to attend the dedication of a tribal centre. Our party of six—myself, Carl, Doc, Ruth, Emma, and Jim Bowman, who was visiting from Saigon—was excited to go somewhere. Carl did the driving, and what a chore that proved to be. The road threaded mostly through a valley between two ridges of mountains, excellent VC territory. Small tribal or Vietnamese villages were scattered here and there at the roadside. There were large rubber plantations started by the French and likely deserted since. There were acres and acres of tall stately coconut palms, row on row waving gently in the breeze with the blue waters of the bay shimmering through. Numerous gardens of bananas and mangoes could be seen: there were rice fields, some flooded and ready for planting, some a verdant green, the tender sprouts of the new plants and others with the newly transplanted rice in neat straight rows. Other fields were being worked by oxen or water buffalo.

The road itself was really something. As Jim said, it would be impossible to make folks back home understand what it was like. It took us about three hours each way, and we drove as fast as possible, with just a few interruptions. It was so bumpy and narrow at places that we kept going on and off the road. I thought even the VC wouldn't consider them worth their dynamite to blow up: usually they were crumbling away with little repair jobs plastered over top now and then. There was a good deal of traffic too: military, cars, buses, scooters, bicycles, ox, and pony carts, as well as pedestrians.

When we arrived in Phan Rang, we were pleasantly surprised to find a clean, well-kept little town. The flame trees were literally "aflame" with their blaze of orange blossoms.

The tribal centre had been erected by the Vietnamese church, I believe, with the help of American military personnel, as an elementary and Bible school for tribal people. The building was small and modest but adequate. The service was conducted in the open under some trees, and it was attended by a fairly large group. Choir selections were given by Vietnamese, Roglai, Koho, and US Air Force choirs. The American military was well represented with their cameras and video and audio recorders. It was an impressive sight!

Because we preferred to travel by daylight, we began our homeward trip about four p.m. before the refreshments were served. En route, we made a small detour at Ba Ngai to say hello to our Baptist missionary friends, who were surprised to see us. We arrived home safely at dusk, tired, hungry, and dirty after three more hours of being bounced about in the back of the VW. All in all, we considered it a challenging, worthwhile and enjoyable trip.

My vacations and language study had been accidentally well spaced, and it allowed me to meet new personnel coming into Saigon with VNCS. Paul Longacre's family was soon leaving, and I was sorry to see them go.

We were expecting a lab technician from India soon, coming to work through MCC for two years. We had been using the old lab as a second doctor's office, so I wasn't sure what we would do now. There were so many changes, and people coming and going. There was no such thing as a normal routine, and it was increasingly more so since the organization was no longer just MCC.

On June 9, 1967, I replied to my parents' letter rejoicing with them over the Leafs' win.

The Toronto Maple Leafs took the cup this year? Yay, three cheers for the Leafs! I wish I could talk hockey with someone here. The guys here don't know anything about it. Doc says he recognizes the name Gordie Howe, though.

A parcel from home has just arrived with goodies, news, church papers, and scrapbooks. I immediately took the scrapbooks out to the TB patients to look at. They are fascinated with the beautiful North American scenery.

Our lab technician hasn't come yet, so who knows when—he's been coming for over a year now: visa is the issue.

Work has been very heavy: only one doctor in the clinic for the last two weeks: we have seen over 200 patients per day in the clinic.

Our six-month medical report showed that we had treated 15,283 patients in the regular clinic, plus 2,424 patients in the TB clinic. There were 827 hospital admissions, of which 189 were TB patients, and 174 were eye patients, the two primary areas we had been focusing on.

I had been looking forward to the days when the Kens would come. They arrived in Saigon on July 12. No one met them at the airport, so they had quite a time until they got to the VNCS office. The centre was full with people who had come in for orientation and language study, so they decided to fly to Nhatrang one day early. Thursday morning, who should walk into the clinic but Ken Shantz and Ken Martin! I couldn't believe it! How they ever found our place, having never been to Nhatrang and not knowing a word of Vietnamese, was beyond my comprehension. They had come all the way from the airport by cyclo, paying an outrageous price.

We went swimming in the afternoon in the sea directly in front of the hospital where the tropical fish and coral were exquisite. On Friday, the guys spent some time with Carl in town. In the afternoon, Emma, the two Kens, and I drove out into the countryside, saw the big Buddha, and had some Vietnamese food. It was fun watching them struggle with chopsticks. We took for granted that everyone could eat with them. Then we tried to see a movie. Saturday was spent running around: in the evening we played Rook and had popcorn, which everyone enjoyed immensely. On Sunday, we started to go to the Military Assistance Command Vietnam (MACV) church service but ran out of gas (the gas metre had long been broken), so we decided to rent a boat to go to an island, where we had a picnic, swam, snorkelled, etc., and got home in time to get cleaned up and go back into town to eat supper. Then the two Kens showed their slides of their work in

India and Pakistan with MCC, which reminded us somewhat of Vietnam, so similar and yet so different. Carl and Doc really enjoyed having them around. Ken Martin's humour matched Doc's spot on!

Monday afternoon, Carl took the two Kens and me to the airport, where we waited three hours for our Air Vietnam flight to Saigon. It was a lovely flight and gave me a chance to talk with the Kens a little more. That evening, we hunted down a friend of Ken Martin's who was working in Saigon, whom Ken had first met in West Pakistan. Tuesday was spent running around in time to get to the airport. It hurt to see them go home. I was also sad that Carl was leaving in less than a month. It would be like losing my big brother.

In my letter of July 21, I wrote my parents from Saigon where I was studying for two weeks.

> *I've been in Saigon for one week now. My efforts have been concentrated at Hong Bang Hospital and studying more about TB. Getting there has been the challenge! VNCS has given me a scooter to drive, with Anne Falk sitting on the back. We are living in Gia Dinh, a suburb of Saigon, and the hospital is all the way across Saigon to Cholon, the Chinese section of Saigon. The traffic jams have been unbelievable! Scooters, cyclos, army trucks, convoys, taxis, cars, bicycles, etc. We had to leave one hour early to get there in time. Now, I need to start working on plans for work related to TB.*
>
> *The Nhatrang mobile clinic idea has been thrown out the window, but it sounds like the nursing program will go through later this year. I am to start a village extension program whereby patients' families and their villages get skin tested for TB: persons testing negative will get the BCG vaccine. I can't wait to get started. Today, I went outside of Saigon with a VNCS team into an insecure area and gave BCG to about 300 to 400 children.*

On Monday, July 31, I returned to Nhatrang after spending two weeks in Saigon. I was hopeful that in a couple of weeks this program would begin. It was exciting to be the one elected for the job, with the added responsibility to start a new faucet of work. I prayed that I would not have to give up the outpatient clinic.

Paul Leatherman, recently appointed as VNCS director, came for the dedication ceremony for the X-ray machine, which was donated by a Vietnamese bakery in Saigon. Paul said that they had asked for another nurse for Nhatrang, and their request had been granted. She would be coming to Vietnam at the end of September, but she would have two months of language study before being assigned. Mary Sue was scheduled to leave at the end of February, which left only three months of overlapping: Doc was also supposed to leave in April, and I was next in line!

Rocky Moquin, an IVSer in Nhatrang, would be working with me to get the TB program started, going out into the nearby villages to find out where and how many public schools there were. Dr. Wong had suggested we start in schools before going out into the villages. I said we would try that, but in two weeks we would be facing another crisis—no staff!

Co Liddie, who was the hospital head nurse when I first came, studied at the Bible School since the previous fall and had come back for the summer, but she was due to leave again in two weeks for her second year: our current head nurse was leaving to study too. Since May, they had also both been serving as interpreters in the clinic. We always managed to survive, so there was no point in getting all upset about it.

Carl's Departure

It was really difficult when Carl began packing to leave. He was like a big brother to me, and I knew I was going to miss him a lot because we did many things together: like one night just before he left, we were recording music tapes on the American military base. He was trying to get a real collection to take home with him.

As a farewell gift, I decided to buy him a sky-blue sweater that matched the colour of his eyes. Watching him pack his barrel was too good an opportunity to pass up playing a prank on him. One of Carl's most disliked jobs was to bury unclaimed bodies from the hospital because it meant he had to make a coffin. I made a miniature coffin, lined it with red paper, made a mummy, added some uncooked rice, and closed the top. I succeeded in burying it in the bottom of his barrel without him knowing. (Unfortunately, he never discovered it since he was killed in Singapore.)

Before Carl left, he gave me an autographed photo: 'Keep up the good nursing, Marcy. See you in Canada sometime?'

The hospital census was down that week, and there were numerous empty beds because of the upcoming election. Everyone was expecting all kinds of politically motivated action/violence, but we thought Nhatrang would be one of the quieter and safer places.

On election day, Lambretta's were making their rounds with their loudspeakers on full volume with all kinds of propaganda. I do not recall the results of the election. Clearly it did not impact my life.

By the middle of September, Carl had gone and it was like a family member was missing. It was hard for him to leave, farewell parties everywhere. For my own departure, I thought I might do it the coward's way and just tell people a couple of days before leaving to eliminate farewell tea parties and speeches.

On rereading my parents' letter, I discovered that the Canadian government was building a TB centre in Quang Ngai. My parents had mailed me a feature article from the Toronto Star about Dr. Venima in Quang Ngai. They had two French speaking nurses and two lab technicians, and they were looking for another nurse. They would have one-year terms which could be extended if they wanted; I was interested and wanted to visit and find out more about their program and look into future possibilities of working there. On the other hand, I could change my mind and settle down back home. I did not have any idea what was in store for me, but I still had another nine months in Nhatrang. It wouldn't be hard to get a job back home at KW Hospital because they were always short staffed.

With all of this percolating in my mind, I had to get away for a little while. In a letter to my parents, I wrote:

Last week I was really down and out, probably because of Carl's leaving, so Emma and I went to Pleiku together. We left Saturday morning on a very comfortable Beechcraft passenger plane. We stopped at Banmethuot before arriving in Pleiku. It was raining, and the red clay mud stuck to everything. Jessie, my friend, and I went to the market and literally waded through mud and water. I had Mary's rubber farm boots on and almost thought I was back home again slipping in my mother's boots to go into the garden.

We left on Sunday afternoon on a military flight, a big C130, a four-engine job for transporting troops. The first stop was at An Khe. When we wanted to take off, the engines wouldn't turn over, so we had to wait for two and a half hours until another plane landed. We were getting a bit nervous because it was getting late and security was poor. The plane backed its tail end toward our nose and revved up its engines to get ours started. Emma and I watched as the metal sheets on the airstrip flapped from the force of the engines until, finally, our engines turned over. We reached Nhatrang at eight-thirty p.m., then, between hitching rides and walking, we finally made it home at nine-thirty p.m. Emma and I decided that we are not meant to travel together—we are hexed or something!

Regarding a project for the MYF: if they are interested in doing some fundraising, maybe a blood pressure cuff, a Vietnamese typewriter, etc., would be good ideas, and they can communicate about it with the MCC Akron office.

Yesterday, I went through more red tape regarding the TB screening program in the schools. I must wait for public health officials and the district chief to come and see me. Hopefully, I can start the beginning of October.

On September 20, we received the saddest news. I was in the middle of the TB clinic when Emma came to get all the doctors and nurses to come to the house. Sam Hope (our personnel director) was bringing bad news. Shivers went up and down my spine. Somehow, I sensed that it was about Carl. When we were all assembled, sure enough, Sam said, "I don't bring good news with me. Monday morning our office in Saigon was notified by the US Embassy that Carl was killed in a motorcycle accident in Singapore." This terrible news dropped like a bomb out of the sky, and somehow it didn't seem real.

In a letter home, I wrote my parents about Carl's death:

> We don't have all the details, except that he was killed on the fifteenth. Today Helen will leave for Singapore to find out more. In the afternoon, Sam Hope and I stopped at various places in town and told them about the memorial service we were having at Vinh Phuoc Church that evening.
>
> Most of the service was in Vietnamese, except for Dr. Gehman's speech and Dr. Kraybill's reading of the verses of the song, 'Lift Your Glad Voices,' which was one of Carl's favourite hymns. Carl and I got along so well and did many things together. Carl was such a great guy: his personality plus always eager to help someone out. It just doesn't seem right that he's gone. Two weeks ago, we were having tea parties celebrating his departure and now, his memorial service.
>
> Carl's parents had pleaded with him not to go home this way. He gave it serious thought. In the end, he reasoned that he was a good driver and not reckless, that he hadn't taken any chances before going. He purposely didn't go to Dong Ha, which is near the North-South Vietnamese border at the 17th parallel because, he said, 'I don't want to press my chances any farther: I've just completed my three years and I want to get home again.' He did too, but not the way he had planned.
>
> After we came back from the memorial service, we learned more bad news. Apparently Mary Sue's family had sent a telegram to Saigon earlier regarding her father, who was critically ill, but the telegram had not arrived. Soon

after, they sent another one saying that they had sent a telegram earlier, and they requested that Mary Sue come home immediately.

Two days later, Mary Sue left for good. With so many things happening here, we are living one day at a time. They say things happen in threes: right now, I don't have the strength to weather the third if it comes: we live one day at a time.

I really missed Carl. It wasn't the same without him. We were the closest in the unit—if there were any problems, Carl was always there: a sympathetic ear, words of wisdom, encouragement, or understanding, and a contagious smile on his face. It made me realize how short life was and that one must be a good steward of time.

We received a letter from Paul Longacre saying that Carl's body had been sent home and his funeral held. Apparently, over 500 people had attended. His life impacted many people. I prayed that my life would be as much of a witness as his was. He had mailed all his slides home, which Paul showed while he talked about Carl's work in Vietnam. It was so sad to hear that Carl's mother was not able to attend the service because she was in the hospital with cancer.

Emma and I had to hold the fort until Katy Peters, a Canadian nurse in language study in Saigon, would come to replace Mary Sue in two months.

Fred Gregory, a VNCS worker from Quang Ngai, was still with us, recovering from hepatitis. We were thinking of starting a club called Heppies.

Recent events involving unit members made me aware of how important it was for my parents to understand my wishes should anything happen to me while I was serving in Vietnam. I wrote my parents about this on October 15:

Today is exactly one month since Carl's accident. Time is a good healer, and I was doing well until we got the mail today and there was a beautiful letter for me from Carl's parents to share with the unit. Sadly, they wrote that the death certificate said Carl died of a skull fracture and cerebral hemorrhage. If only he had bought a helmet, like so many people had suggested to him?

The church magazine, the Beacon, arrived and I saw the prayer requests. Including me in Vietnam is much appreciated. We do need the prayers and support of the people back home. We are not capable of doing this work on our own strength. If any such thing would happen to me as did to Carl, I trust you as a family could accept it as well as Carl's family did.

Tomorrow I will be twenty-four! Wow! I'm getting old!

The doctors have received a letter from Carl's parents that they are setting up a memorial fund and will be sending the money to our project. We are considering using it to build a warehouse because that was Carl's line of work. I'll have to write his parents a letter today because they have various questions about Carl's articles, and the farewell gifts he received.

Regarding the TB skin testing project in the schools, it's getting nearer. There's just so much red tape to go through. Patience is a virtue! But we're getting there slowly, one step at a time.

One day in late October, I spent the greater part of it sitting at the airport waiting for a shipment to come, which gave me time to reflect. I thought about how it hadn't been too difficult to say goodbye to people when I had left Canada because we would most likely see each other again. But the friends I had made in Vietnam and so highly valued in my life, I would probably never see them again.

The TB skin testing was finally going to start at the end of October, Lord willing.

Thinking about My Termination

In mid-November Sam Hope, our personnel director from Saigon, arrived and spent some time interviewing Doc and myself. Many thoughts passed through my mind at that time and since, which left me even more uncertain about my future in Nhatrang. It had begun with Paul Longacre writing a letter asking if Dr. Gehman and I would consider extending our term because they were unable to get replacements in time. Sam wanted an answer the day he met with us, but I told him I needed to think about it, so I was given until January to decide.

There were so few options that I had to work out in my mind:

1. Should I go home the next summer, and then come back again?
2. Should I go home and never return.
3. Should I stay on one more year because communism could take over, and then nobody in VNCS would be allowed in Vietnam?

Some of the pros of staying were:

1. I could see an addition to the TB hospital and probably have the privilege of setting it up, as well as seeing the nursing school develop.
2. I could serve as a stabilizer because there would be considerable staff turnover, both international and Vietnamese
3. I enjoyed my work in Nhatrang.

Some of the cons for staying were:

1. The workload and division of duties could change my responsibilities.
2. The stress and strain of war could become too much.
3. I could enjoy nursing in a hospital back home again more.
4. It could have been better to take an MCC assignment elsewhere.

I would have to take a lot of time to think about my options.

Work was going great out in the schools in the villages, and I was enjoying it immensely. When you get out into the community, you see places you would otherwise never see and meet new people. It was quite funny to observe the reactions of the kids lining up to get their injections, and then when they did get them. Some kicked and screamed, some had blank expressions, others just said "dau lam" which meant "that hurts a lot," and some just made fun of others after they'd had theirs.

Correspondence to my family dated November 27 read:

> *Ruth and Doc left today: Katy is here and will probably work out great. Another Canadian! Since starting this letter, I have received yours. It was good to hear from all of you again. I often wondered what you were all doing. Rob, you're really fortunate not to have been seriously injured in your car accident. After hearing about yours and Brenda's accidents this summer, I think I'm safer here in Vietnam!*
>
> *Security in our immediate area is still 'secure'—whatever that means. The Korean army camp just two to three km north of us is suffering tremendous losses. One company was completely wiped out in one and a half days. The road to Thanh, just ten km south of Nhatrang, was hit hard. The NLF killed many civilians, and the road was closed even for Vietnamese. That has never happened in my time here. They also blew out a bridge below Thanh. Our next-door missionary neighbour says that the police have just discovered a plan in Nhatrang that the NLF devised to take over the end of this month. Last Saturday night, the Nhatrang air base was mortared—twenty-eight mm rounds: several were injured. A big C130 plane was destroyed. Security here is worse than it's been in a long time, actually, since the spring of 1965, just prior to my coming.*
>
> *The hospital board is clamping down on our regulations at the hospital. We don't have the nursing staff, so we require family members to stay with patients. We have families*

with kids, some come from long distances, and some are refugees, so their whole families are here. Some people just hang around regardless of orders or threats from the director. We recently discovered where some of our cardboard boxes get used. Families use them for 'temporary housing' in the cemetery beyond the hospital compound.

The latest rumour is that we are harbouring NLF at our hospital, which could very easily be true because we do not ask for any identification: we are sent to Vietnam with the idea that we are to help anyone in need of medical attention. We have been having regular midnight prowlers in Vietnamese army uniform—possibly NLF suspects? I guess I'll start locking my bedroom door at night, although, if kidnapping was their goal, they could still easily get away with it because a national worker always sleeps in the hospital at night and calls us as needed.

Work has been getting me down with so much responsibility involved. The question regarding to extend or not, how to go home, new personalities here, etc., and I'm having so many sleepless nights. I'm planning on taking two weeks' vacation in January between Christmas and Tet around the end of January. Then, hopefully, after that the nursing school will start.

Correspondence from Paul Longacre on December 6, 1967 indicated that MCC welcomed me to extend my scheduled termination of June 1968 by three to six months or serve a three- to five-year term.

I was still somewhat undecided about my future at this point.

We received a telegram from Saigon letting us know that the Ministry of Health had approved the School of Nursing. Ruth was ecstatic. However, she would have to search for a Vietnamese counterpart; it would prove to be difficult to find a qualified person who was bilingual.

Katy, the latest addition to our unit family, 26-27 years old, was from Winnipeg and was just great to have around. She worked out well. After the Kraybills left for Saigon there were only five of us: Emma, Katy, Jim,

Doc and I at the supper table. Emma committed the unpardonable sin of mentioning one night that the Canadians outnumbered the Americans. Doc didn't miss a beat and said, 'Yea, but you're all women!'

Now that all the Christmas festivities and programs were history, I took time to write my general newsletter to family and friends in early January 1968:

> *I want to let you know that the support you have given me, the letters and prayers, are appreciated very much. There is no way to describe the good a letter can do when you are rather alone and miss home. So, thank you.*
>
> *If I had one wish, it would be for each of you to share my privilege of living in Vietnam. It is indescribable on paper. I have had too many experiences to explain well. After two and a half years in Vietnam, I look back on the challenging and difficult times, as well as on many worthwhile experiences. The more time one spends in this war-torn country, the more complex the situation seems to be. As a Christian and as a pacifist, I cannot help but disagree with the US policy, but, at the same time, I feel helpless because I cannot offer a better approach or solution to the problem. Each of us has an obligation to do anything the Lord asks, and so our work at Chan-y-Vien Tin Lanh, the name of our hospital, continues, for the most part unaffected by the war that is being fought around us each day.*
>
> *Our Western staff has doubled in size since my arrival in June 1965, due to the heavy workload and because MCC has intentions of expanding the clinic and hospital facilities, developing two new areas to meet the increasing demand. One area is related to tuberculosis. TB runs rampant and claims many lives every year here. In the summer of 1965, on my arrival, we had approximately 100 to 150 patients on TB therapy, and we were becoming known as the TB hospital in Nhatrang, even though we only had two scanty "TB houses" to accommodate twenty-six patients. The*

houses would compare to shacks back home. So, in the fall of 1966, the hospital board approved the construction of a twenty-eight-bed facility to provide better accommodation and more bed space.

One of my most frustrating experiences in Vietnam has been watching the construction of this building. The fun began after the four walls and roof were completed and the walls were painted. It was then unanimously agreed that vents had to be put in near the top of the walls. The crew knocked out the bricks and concrete, filled in the spaces around the vents, and proceeded to paint again! Then electrical wiring and outlets had to be installed. The wiring is never done in the wall, rather on the wall. This meant another paint job. At this point, we assumed the majority of our problems had been solved because the beds and several pieces of furniture were being made to order—or so we thought until they all arrived! The metal bed frames were too long and had to be shortened. When the desk arrived for the nurse's station, we had to tear out half of the wall to get it in because the sink had already been installed. As it turned out, we had to take the sink out anyway to get the cupboard in. And on top of all this, the sink was stolen before it was installed the first time. Now the plan is to build another TB hospital within the next month, and I sure hope it goes more smoothly!

As you may have gathered, TB work is one of my major responsibilities. Last July, I was able to spend two weeks at Hong Bang Hospital in Saigon, observing their TB program and public health work of skin testing in public schools and villages. At the end of October, plans and dreams for our program materialized. I had trained the clinic staff and organized a team to go out to several of our surrounding schools in the district. In the beginning, it required two Western personnel to go along, but now the team is going out on their own. Since the end of October, the team has skin tested about 4,275 persons. Including the new cases, we've picked up with this program and the clinic patients, the grand total of registered TB patients is 1,350 persons. It is a joy to be involved in a work that you can see expand every month and meet the medical needs of so many people.

The sad part of it is, up until recently, the majority of the patients did not come for treatment until they themselves realized they had TB, which invariably meant bilateral far advanced TB with cavities.

Working mornings in the outpatient clinic one cannot complain of boredom. Each day is so unlike the previous day. One thing that does not change is the number of patients to be screened.

The second new area of work is the nursing school. Ruth Yoder came in February 1966 with high hopes of starting a nursing school. She, and everyone else, had not realized all the red tape that was required. On December 14, 1967, she finally received official permission from the Ministry of Health to open the school. At present, we are completing the construction of the building and tentatively plan on beginning classes for a one-year program in mid February for eight students. We had about given up hope.

Our major problem at this point is staff. The army claims all men from the ages of nineteen to thirty-three. Most girls who have command of the English language are employed by the army because of the fantastic salaries. As long as there is war, we will undoubtedly have this problem. We employ three interpreters: Co Thanh is scheduled to leave for Eastern Mennonite College (EMC) in Pennsylvania to study theology; Anh Quang was accepted to study at Goshen College, also in the US, but decided he would rather go to EMC with Co Thanh. It turns out that Quang had to leave on the twenty-seventh otherwise he would have been drafted by the Vietnamese army the next day, so they left together. Then Anh Huong was drafted at the same time. Now, we do not have any *interpreters! We pray that our needs will be met. In the past, we had many trying times too, but our needs and supplies were always met. We have learned to go one day at a time.*

Doc continues to specialize in ophthalmology, doing surgery three mornings a week. The main hospital is usually filled, including the front porch.

This gives you a glimpse of what we are doing and trying to accomplish as a medical team. I pray that the work will continue to grow and be as effective in 1968 as it was in 1967. Wishing you good health and happiness in the new year.

On January 9, 1968, Paul Longacre accepted my decision not to return with MCC for a second term and acknowledged my willingness to extend until September if necessary. I was relieved to receive an understanding response from Paul regarding my difficult decision. I had really struggled with it. However, it seemed to be the right time for me to return to Canada. My letters home continued as usual; I did not include my decision at this time.

Today finds me in Saigon helping Anh Tin get settled for his studies at Hong Bang Hospital, then I will begin my vacation tomorrow. My hope is that he will assume responsibility for the TB extension work out in the villages when I leave.

Saturday morning, I boarded a C130 with combat troops for Can Tho in the Mekong Delta, where I caught a helicopter to Sa Dec to stay with Johanna, an IVSer and Doc's sister. Sa Dec is a beautiful prosperous town with rich farmland: everything was available at the market. When I arrived, Johanna shared that the town had been attacked two nights before, but I need not worry about it because it is now considered safe.

Wednesday, I flew back to Can Tho by helicopter, where I stayed with Dick Pandel and his C & M A missionary family I had gotten to know when his wife had her baby at our hospital in September. They informed me that a refugee place where they had been working, and quite near their home, had been attacked the night before.

Thursday, I flew to Saigon for one night before flying to Pleiku on Friday morning. I was able to go out to some tribespeoples' homes and into villages with VNCS staff. That night the air base was attacked and the military hospital was hit. Many Americans were seriously injured. One Vietnamese worker died of a heart attack and two Viet Cong prisoners who were patients there were killed. I decided to stay until Tuesday, but Saturday night Engineer Hill was attacked. There were all kinds of bombing and flares: bomber jets and rockets that we didn't have in Nhatrang.

Tuesday, I flew to Danang and stayed with another C & M A missionary family and discovered that Bob Miller and his family, Wycliffe Bible Translators in Khe Sanh, had been asked to leave their place two weeks ago. They were translating the book of Acts into the Bru language. Bob had just gone into their village on Saturday morning to get his translator so they could continue working at Kontum. They had left their home at five p.m., flew out at five-thirty, and, at six, the North Vietnamese attacked the village: one of the biggest battles yet.

On Sunday, there was still a lot of fighting there so Vietnamese were being evacuated: that's how it was when I arrived at the airport in Danang on Tuesday morning. There were Vietnamese everywhere being evacuated to Quang Tri at the 17th parallel, but they wanted to stay in Danang or go to relatives in Hue.

I also wanted to go to Hue. I went to the airport early in the morning, hoping to get a flight. There were Vietnamese captured at Khe Sanh with paper bags over their heads and hands tied behind their backs: they were treated inhumanely, loaded onto buses to be flown somewhere. I couldn't wait to get out of there, but couldn't, no matter how hard I tried, *so I returned to the missionary's home for another night. I met a Vietnamese pastor from Khe Sanh, who had just been evacuated. He shared that his church in Khe Sanh and Miller's home had been flattened by American bombing.*

Thursday, I was finally able to fly to Hue. I planned to stay with June, a VNCSer. We enjoyed riding bicycles around town when we ran into Premier Thieu: he was so close that I could have shaken his hand! I enjoyed visiting the farm that the VNCS guys had developed with their pigs, chickens, and gardening.

My vacation was coming to an end on Saturday, so I had booked myself on a Beechcraft leaving from the walled city in Hue. In the morning, an American came to June's house to say that no flights would be leaving that day. If I had to fly to Nhatrang then, he recommended that I go to Phu Bai airport, eighteen km away, which functioned as a military and commercial airport. Apparently, there had been an attack during the night as well as at Danang, but the guys and June agreed to take me there.

At the airport, I checked with the American military to see if there was anything flying to Danang and was told that they weren't taking any civilians that day. I decided to check with Air Vietnam in the same airport to see if they had a flight to Nhatrang that day because it appeared to be my only chance. Miracle of miracles! They had a direct flight to Nhatrang once a week, which happened to be that afternoon with one seat available! This had to be a miracle because Vietnamese always rush to make reservations more than a month in advance of Tet.

I told the guys and June that I could wait alone until the flight came. I was sitting on a balcony watching all the activity and everything going on, when someone from the American military personnel appeared and asked me if anything was bothering me. I responded, "Yes." He said, "Well, lady, you haven't seen anything. We've got ninety flights coming in today, with just the Air Force." C130s were being unloaded and loading non-stop, with five planes lined up: vehicles, ammunition, and soldiers in and out! The troops from the 1st Cavalry and 101st Airborne from Anh Khe were just marching out, so many young soldiers looked like they were in a state of shock. Injured soldiers were being carried out on stretchers, one after another. Helicopters were coming in from Khe Sanh and Dong Ha: One man walked out with his whole head bandaged and couldn't see where he was going. Another man hobbled on one leg to a nearby hospital. There was not enough help for the injured.

The C130s continued to load with forty to fifty military personnel and all kinds of vehicles and equipment. There were jets, bombers, helicopters, Air America, and Air Vietnam planes. One ambulance was stationed in front of the airport building with seriously injured patients when I bought my ticket in the morning, and it was still there when I left in the afternoon.

Some American soldiers looked too young to be here— maybe nineteen years old, carrying all kinds of combat equipment, guns just brought over from the US directly to a war zone. You could read their faces—like they felt they were going to their grave. Some were being sent to Khe Sanh. One drunken soldier told a young soldier who looked frightened that if he didn't know how to get there, just come back here. War is horrible and everything that goes with it! There are no winners.

Saturday, I returned safely to Nhatrang from the war zone! What a vacation! I saw too much at the airport in Hue. On Sunday morning, when we went to the military chapel in Nhatrang, they warned us about a possible attack and that the NLF were threatening to take over Nhatrang, but we didn't believe it. These are troubled days and, suddenly, the war has moved very close.

The Tet Offensive

The chaos began around midnight on January 29, as we were celebrating the first day of Tet. I shared what happened in a letter dated January 30, 1968.

There was noise and more noise as firecrackers exploded. We mentioned that this would be an ideal time for the NLF to attack because in the noise and confusion, no one would notice. At three a.m., the fire siren went off at the Vietnamese Military Academy around the bay, and then again two more times. Soon after, the power went off, and we were in darkness. I was so scared that I couldn't move. My bedroom was behind our main house so I was not in the same building as the other unit members. The shelling of mortars, etc. was terrifying.

In the morning, we woke up to South Vietnamese soldiers everywhere: on our front porch, by our back door, and on the front porch of the hospital with their guns set up. They overran our compound. The radio told us that Nhatrang had been attacked during the night, but the news was incomplete. We kept tuned in to the radio to learn more. Then Tony, our friend from New Zealand, came to update us. He was a good friend of the priests at the nearby Franciscan monastery. Apparently the NLF had come into the cathedral during mass and demanded that the village give them all of their boats so they could cross into Nhatrang. They had no choice. Then the NLF added, 'Please be sure to listen to your radio tonight because you will hear us and what we have to say.' Sure enough, they took over the radio station and the province chief's house—the province chief and his wife had dressed in peasant's clothing and escaped through their back door unrecognized.

Dr. Quin, one of doctors we knew personally, was not so fortunate. He was captured and his hospital taken over. Dr.

Quin asked the NLF, "How dare you come and take over our hospital?" For this remark, he was immediately beheaded.

Patients who came from Cu Lao by the first bridge said there had been shooting from the Nhatrang side to our side. We didn't realize that it was so close. We went about our work with some war casualties and gunshot wounds. We were told that there had been many killings and battles along the main road in our area, but we didn't see or know anything because we were along the beach road. We also heard that the NLF controlled both bridges, our only access to Nhatrang. We were told that people were not allowed to go into town, though they were able to get out. We knew that the NLF had been active in the area and that trouble was brewing.

I keep referring to the NLF that was organized around 1960 to overthrow the South Vietnamese government and reunify North and South Vietnam. Then, in 1962, the Communist Party became a central component of the NLF, but the NLF included many non-communists. They were fighting for reunification and independence.

Our Vietnamese staff was very upset because they had relatives in other parts of the country and didn't know whether they were safe. Early in the evening, we had several patients come from Ninh Hoa, about thirty km north of Nhatrang. We wondered if we would be getting more patients from there but no more travel was allowed on the roads.

In the evening, we were frightened because we had heard that many NLF were trapped in Nhatrang and were trying to return north, which meant going through our area and the mountainside. This was the first time we locked all our doors: sleep didn't come. Poor Emma was on call that night and was called twice but still no electricity.

The night was anything but quiet, and we slept little. Most of the time, planes, and helicopters were flying

overhead, strafing, and gunning, etc.: the shelling and mor-
taring sounded uncomfortably close, sometimes five or six
flares illuminated the night at the same time. At five a.m.,
flares were dropped almost directly over us and the activity
sounded even nearer. What a relief when daylight brought a
decrease in noise and fighting.

We were told in the morning that we were surrounded
by the NLF. A few truckloads of South Vietnamese soldiers
were deposited on the road in front of our hospital and soon
marched in different directions. A man appeared at our
house very excited. I finally understood what he was trying
to say. His wife, a patient at our hospital, was missing. He
had dozed off during the night and, when he woke up, she
was gone. His wife had become psychotic as a result of
typhoid two months earlier. He had looked everywhere and
could not find her. He reappeared at our doorstep at ten
a.m. saying that he heard that his wife had been shot at the
military academy, and he wondered if Dr. Kraybill and I
could take the car and go with him. We didn't get very far
when we were stopped by Vietnamese soldiers who wanted
to know where we were going because it was unsafe to travel
the roads. Feeling responsible for our patient, we pleaded
with the soldiers. They refused to let the husband go but
gave Dr. Kraybill and me directions to the military academy.

When we got there and tried to explain who we were
looking for, they said, "Oh, yes, we did have a lady here
who was running around like she was mad." They radioed
several places, including a police station they told us to go
to, because they had seen her. When we got there, they said
two policemen had taken her to the hospital in town. Well,
we got stopped and checked so many times on the way there,
but finally succeeded in getting to the provincial hospital.

The staff checked the admission book and checked all the
wards, but they could not find her. We returned home and
reported this to the husband who was beside himself. We

decided to go to the police station again to check whether they had taken the patient to the provincial or military hospital. They said that they had taken her to the provincial hospital but she had refused to go in, so they just left her there. Very upset, we returned home again.

In the afternoon, I was still upset about the inability to locate our patient so Emma agreed to go with me. We went to the same police station to inquire if there was more news. There wasn't, so we drove into town to the provincial hospital again, when Ruth appeared on the motorbike: our patient had been found between the two bridges, so we finally got her back to our hospital. Meanwhile, our unit was very concerned about us because we had been gone so long.

When Emma and I stopped at the provincial hospital, we were shocked to see all the war casualties: the halls were crowded with patients and their families: people in a state of shock, blood everywhere. What a terrifying experience! They were treating a nineteen-year-old patient whom they wanted to send back with us because of his eye injury. He had returned home and opened the door, which set off a grenade. He will never see again: his fingers were blown off, and he had shrapnel throughout much of his body. He was only at our hospital one day when Vietnamese soldiers came, combing the area and our hospital, searching for NLF. Because he is a suspect, we will have to take him to the military academy when discharged. I cannot help but be sympathetic for him, regardless of his political loyalty.

The doctors and nurses at the provincial hospital told some wild stories about what had transpired at night. Several of them had gone to the rooftop to see what was happening. One male was with them. He was shot and killed instantly, so the nurses ran downstairs and evacuated to the military base. Much shooting had been going on in the streets in Nhatrang. One missionary family said

there had been shooting on their street, with shots whizzing
through their trees.
At home, Katy and I moved into the main house because
we were too frightened to be alone.

Premier Thieu declared martial law and a curfew, so we were under military rule and knew that they were still expecting trouble. Everyone had to stay home, not go out on the streets: no travelling on the roads, no public meetings, no going to market.

We learned that the offensive was countrywide and well-coordinated: more than 80,000 NLF and North Vietnam's Army troops had struck more than 100 towns and cities, including thirty-six of the forty-four provincial capitals. Later we learned that casualties numbered 106,820, with 28,078 civilians and soldiers killed.

We still didn't have electricity, and we carried water from the well, both for the hospital and for us. There were few new patients because people were not allowed to travel with the roads blocked and a curfew. We were thankful for a quiet night until early morning when we could hear bombing again.

The American army eventually brought us two generators, so we had light and water again. Even though this was considered really dangerous territory, a dozen or more men volunteered to come. We appreciated their concern for us, which was a significant risk on their part. Vietnamese soldiers continued to patrol and comb our grounds. Having electricity again enabled us to take an X-ray of a two-year-old's leg that had sustained a bullet wound. Unfortunately, it was so deeply lodged in the bone that we could not remove it.

We were not allowed into town to check for telegrams. We heard that all flights, in and out of Nhatrang, had been cancelled because the air base had been significantly damaged. We also knew that Saigon was also been hit badly in nine places, one near the VNCS home, and we had no idea if all VNCSers were safe: all we could do was listen to reports on the radio and pray for the best.

I wrote home on February 3:

Jim got news this morning from our neighbouring missionary that five C & M A missionaries were killed at Banmethuot. On Sunday morning we got more information at the military chapel. The NLF had launched a surprise attack in the village in the middle of the night, blowing up houses, one at a time. At daylight, two missionaries started digging for casualties. Mr. Griswold, a widower who had come to visit his daughter, was dead; Carolyn, his daughter, whom they dug out of the debris, was injured and unconscious; two missionaries pleaded with the NLF for mercy to take Carolyn to the provincial hospital, but, instead, were killed. Two other missionaries moved Carolyn into the bunker because they heard that there was to be another attack that night. Reverend and Mrs. Thompson came out of the bunker, pleading to be let go and were shot immediately. Then the NLF entered the bunker to kill the rest.

Mrs. Zimmer pretended to be dead. We don't have all the details but understand that she has been evacuated to 8th Field Hospital in Nhatrang, alive, but in a state of shock. Also, someone had taken Carolyn, who was still unconscious, to the servant's quarters at Betty Olsen's home: she was a missionary nurse with the C & M A. Carolyn passed away from her injuries, but Betty was taken captive along with Hank Blood and his family, who were Wycliffe Bible Translators.

Later, Mrs. Blood and the children were released, but Hank and Betty were kept as captives. Ruth Wilting, with the C & M A, fiancé of Dan Gerber, MCC worker who was captured in 1962, was also killed. Those remaining were all evacuated to Nhatrang. Some native pastors were also captured. When it's people you know, it really hits hard. Betty had just been to our hospital a week before for a routine medical checkup.

The pastors who had been released felt that it would be best if all missionaries left the country because the NLF had voiced their hatred of Americans. So now we are giving serious thought to our effectiveness and if we were in more danger than we realized. The Wycliffe Bible Translators' compound in Kontum was also overrun, and all forty of them were evacuated to Camp McDermott in Nhatrang. Since then, the Americans have flattened their village.

On February 4, I continued:

Jim, Katy, and Emma went to town and picked up several cables at the post office. Thankfully, all VNCSers were safe. The Pleiku unit was sent to the 71st Evacuation Hospital. They had a very difficult time: they had to jump their fence six times to escape—just got to one side and then ordered to crawl back again. There were North Vietnamese in the house across from them, but they were finally able to escape. One of their houses was overrun with shooting: the second house was bombed by the Americans and destroyed after they left. The guys were evacuated to Nhatrang, but the medical team stayed to help with medical emergencies at 71st Military Hospital, and the C & M A missionaries were evacuated to Nhatrang.

There has been no word from our Hue unit, but we know that Hue was heavily attacked on the other side of the river.

Every day we heard of incidents happening in our area. When Dr. Kraybill and I drove into town a few days ago, we saw three bodies by the first bridge and two near the post office: we saw two trucks going through town collecting NLF bodies, which they then drove several km north of us near the leprosarium and just dumped; they didn't even bury them! Rumour has it that the NLF were given enough food for one and a half days because they expected to have control of the town in two days.

As to our situation now, we have permission to go into town and Vietnamese are free to walk into town: no vehicles, bicycles, or buses from up country are allowed. They can catch a small Lambretta to the bridge, then walk into town. A few Lambrettas are running in town, but they are not allowed to cross the bridges. They obviously are expecting something to happen again.

Bless Tony: he keeps us informed. He heard that six NLF who were sleeping in Hon Chong on the rocks near us were captured. A man was brought in to our hospital by two other men with stab wounds to his head, inflicted by NLF. My interpreter, Co Ly, who lives nearby, was told by Vietnamese soldiers to close all windows in her home because about fifty men were attacking and stealing money. In Vinh Hai, on the other side of us, the army was catching NLF members. One NLF was dressed in a South Vietnamese military uniform and had entered the orphanage next to us: the children didn't think anything of it because it was not unusual to see soldiers walking through their compound. This 'soldier' exited at the beach gate next to us and was immediately captured. When Jim bought gas at the gas station, they had just caught an NLF member.

People in Thunh Hal are very frightened. Many people are finding NLF in their washrooms and kitchens in the morning. We hear about so many incidents and don't know what to believe or expect, but we hear that many NLF are in the vicinity and another attack is expected because NLF in the city are having a hard time getting out. They say that 200-300 were killed in Nhatrang.

Our unit was the only one in VNCS that was still functioning. During the days of heaviest fighting, a number of VNCSers were in dangerous situations. The most striking was the experience of seven persons in Hue, where for eight days, North Vietnamese troops controlled the area surrounding their house, where the VNCSers were hidden in their bunker. The North Vietnamese had set up a supply base across the street. The Saigon office received a cabled report that American Marines had evacuated the VNCSers by landing craft. They were transferred to Danang.

My TB program came to a halt, and I didn't know if it would get started again. I knew I could never come back to Vietnam again unless there was peace. I was so tired of war and all I had seen.

None of us knew what would happen to VNCS. Bill Snyder from the MCC Akron office and Dr. Atlee Beechy came to Saigon to look into the situation. They were reluctant to pull out staff. Bill said that MCC did that in the Congo and later wished they hadn't. Wycliffe personnel were going to be evacuated, and the C & M A missionaries' future was undecided. My time in Vietnam was getting short and at that point I didn't even know if VNCS would be there until the end of my term.

In my letter to my parents, on February 18, 1968, I wrote:

> *An IVSer joined us for dinner tonight. He said that they are reducing the number of their personnel from 150 to approximately forty in the country, just to work in cities or 'rather secure areas.' Apparently, one person was assassinated in the Mekong Delta and their whole unit in Hue is unaccounted for—likely captured. The Hue IVS unit lived right beside the VNCS house. Fortunately, the VNCS guys were at June's home, where I stayed just less than a week ago, when the North Vietnamese attacked the morning of Tet, January 30. June had invited them for an early breakfast, and at seven a.m. they heard commotion and saw North Vietnamese file out of a warehouse kitty corner across the street, loaded with ammunition, shooting and entering houses, where Western people lived on their street. The unit decided to go into June's bunker and only occasionally came out to look around. A bullet had gone through her house. There was intense and prolonged fighting. They sensed that the North Vietnamese knew they were there but did not enter. They stayed in the bunker for five days and were down to half a cup of water per person when there was a knock on the door. It was an American inquiring if anyone was alive in*

the house. Apparently, all the houses rented by Westerners except for June's had been entered. When I heard this, I said a prayer of thanks that I had been able to leave Hue the day before.

I received a note from my friend Jessie, another VNCSer, formerly in Pleiku, saying she was leaving for the States in two days. I really wanted to meet her again, so I raced to our unit house, where everyone was finishing their lunch, and asked permission to visit Jessie in Saigon. They said yes, so I took a quick shower, packed quickly, and found myself on a plane going to Saigon that afternoon!

Saigon was depressing. Six people had left Vietnam for good the day before, and Jessie and another nurse would be leaving in two days. There are twenty-two VNCSers terminating in June. The Dong Ha and Hue units are definitely closed. The future of Tam Ky, Quang Ngai, Dak To, and Di Linh are in question. The Pleiku and Nhatrang medical projects will work close to a normal schedule.

Regarding personnel, the whole picture of Vietnam has suddenly changed, and we are considering the necessity of cutting programs and personnel to only what is necessary to maintain a presence or holding action until this war changes one way or another. A memo from the VNCS director in the Saigon office said, 'It should be stated again that I believe that anyone who feels that he or she cannot work in this situation for whatever reason should leave. No one should stay in Vietnam at this time who does not have a strong feeling or leaning that this is the place he should be. VNCS will need to urge people in certain selected cases to leave. If a person feels he is not making a contribution at present and cannot have enough patience to wait this phase out, it may be that that person should leave. Those of you who feel you cannot continue to work in this tense situation should report to Sam or me and we will initiate proceedings for your reassignment or termination.'

Most C & M A missionaries' wives and children have left the country. Several have been given permission to stay if they are stationed in Saigon, Nhatrang, or Danang.

On February 24, the Vietnamese nationals were saying that the NLF were passing out pamphlets saying that they planned to attack Nhatrang the next day because they had gotten poor cooperation from the people the first time they came. The American military had heard different dates for an intended attack, and we had heard various reports, but everyone was expecting more trouble

Saigon, Quang Ngai, and Pleiku units began building bunkers. We decided not to build one in Nhatrang because in our situation, a bunker wouldn't save us if they were after us. We were always on call for the hospital. If the enemy wanted to get us, they could simply call us. As medical people, we were of more value alive than dead. Thankfully, at that point, I had decided not to extend my time there. I loved my work and was not sorry that I came; but working under this tension was trying.

Tensions were so high that there was a chance we could be evacuated. With this in mind, I began sending some things home by APO (Army Post Office), the only reliable postal service at that time.

Regarding my trip home, I was thinking of travelling across the States. First stop, Oregon, to visit Jessie; Kansas, to visit Carl's parents; then Co Thanh and Anh Quang at EMC and Akron, Pennsylvania. From there I could take the train home or my family might be interested in coming to the States?

I wrote home in early March:

> *One night, sometime after my last letter, a helicopter sounded very close, hovered, then landed in front of our house. The American military had sent a chopper to evacuate us because they had received an intelligence report that our hospital was going to be attacked fifteen minutes after their arrival. The only thing I could think of to put in my carry-on suitcase was my slides. I ran our keys over to Anh Tin and we all went, except for Ruth, who insisted that she*

would just crawl into bed with a patient and nobody would find her (Ruth was petite and had black hair). We landed at the air base and were put up in the barracks. Well, that night the air base was attacked so we spent the night in the bunker. Our hospital was not attacked!

We got news about Dr. Pat Smith's hospital in Kontum for the tribal people. The German nurse refused to tell the NLF where Dr. Smith was at the time of the attack. Apparently, she was lying flat on her bathroom floor at the hospital when they came and asked for her. Paul Leatherman came up from Saigon last week, upset about the incident, thinking we were in the same situation.

Paul brought Das, our Indian lab technician from Calcutta, who finally got his visa. What a memorable time to arrive! Regarding my replacement, VNCS is thinking about transferring Tharon McConnell from the Quang Ngai unit.

Our security? Well, I don't know what to say. Yesterday the American air base was hit again, and so was Camp McDermott. Apparently, the barracks that we stayed in when we had been evacuated were hit pretty hard by mortar attacks, so we were spared again. The Army of the Republic of Vietnam (ARVN) soldiers are everywhere.

Emma has this prayer by St. Francis of Assisi hanging in her room:

Lord make me an instrument of your peace.
Where there is hatred let me sow love.
Where there is injury, pardon.
Where there is doubt, faith.
Where there is darkness, light.
Where there is sadness, joy.
O Divine Master, grant that I may not so much seek
To be consoled, as to console,
To be understood, as to understand,

To be loved, as to love.
For
It is in giving, that we receive.
It is in pardoning, that we are pardoned.
It is in dying that we are born to eternal life. Amen.

This has become my daily prayer.

Our Nursing School

Ruth's nursing school started in early March, which drained us of five hospital nurses.

On March 10, Ruth had nine students for the one-year nursing program who were required to be eighteen years of age. At the same time, it became mandatory that all girls between ages eighteen and twenty-five have military training, if unmarried, unless they could provide legal documents saying they were exempt. What chaos!

By March 18, things were getting back to normal again. Curfew was extended to eight p.m. for vehicles going into town. I prayed that the Lord would give the faith, wisdom, and strength to carry out our daily tasks with Christian love and not get too upset and involved in rumours. I prayed also that He might guide and direct Paul Leatherman and Paul Longacre, that wise decisions might be made on their part regarding the future of VNCS. There were diversified opinions regarding VNCS remaining in Vietnam. Some felt strongly that we didn't belong there now, but others felt that we were needed there now the most and the people needed our support. The Di Linh project was folding shutting down: Hue and Dak To already had: Pleiku was questionable, and Quang Ngai was restricted.

Katy came back from Saigon with news that Tharon, who was to replace me, was terminating, as was June from Hue: Pauline and Armand Hostettler from Hue would be reassigned, Becky, a nurse from Pleiku, was also terminating, as were Dr. and Mrs. Luez from Pleiku. The two nurses left in Pleiku didn't want to run the hospital without a doctor, so I wondered if they would pull a doctor from Nhatrang when we had such a full program?

Just as I thought things were getting back to normal, we began to hear more rumours about an attack on Nhatrang. Dr. Kraybill met Dr. Hoang at the provincial hospital, who said that USAID was withdrawing all their nurses within six months. Our morale was very low. The ARVN troops had recently pulled out of Hon Chong (on top of our hill) because security was to be better; but they did come back again.

On March 24, Jim, Emma, and Katy went to a different chapel and several people came up to them, one a captain, who said that seventy of his men had volunteered to come out and get us the night we were evacuated. Those guys didn't even know us—they were a new company that had moved into the area just prior to that happening. It made me feel very humble to think that so many were that concerned for us that they volunteered to come out into what could have proven to be a battleground. We obviously were in a lot more danger that night than we ever knew. Apparently, the NLF went through our area and to this day I can't figure out why they didn't attack us.

On March 29, I wrote another letter home:

> *Yesterday, I heard the best news I've heard in a long time. Paul Longacre is coming to Vietnam the middle of next month, and he will be bringing a portfolio of prospective personnel for VNCS. Apparently, all has been at a standstill back in the States regarding recruitment because of the instability of our present programs and the uncertainty about what units could operate and which personnel were staying.*
>
> *Another surprise was that Esther Kraybill and Eugene returned from Saigon with a little Vietnamese girl that they want to adopt. She's two or three years old. Also, Tharon McConnell, who was the nurse at Quang Ngai, came. Previously we had heard that she was going home, but as it stands now, she came to Nhatrang to assess the situation: if she feels she would like to stay in Vietnam and could*

appreciate working here, she would be my replacement. She will be going back to Saigon this weekend, and then, maybe in two weeks, we will know what the outcome will be.

I took Jim, Tharon, and an IVSer to catch their flight to Saigon this morning. I had to drive the IVS Land Rover because all of our vehicles were out of commission. Tharon was going to report her final decision, which, I assume, is to stay. So I'll be able to go when the time comes, but, oh, what mixed feelings. It hurts to think of leaving.

The hospital has been extremely busy. A seven-year-old boy whom we diagnosed with rabies, cute as a button, came in yesterday morning. Such a pathetic sight. The disease has progressed to the stage where he has excess saliva, wants to drink, but has difficulty swallowing: he is so hyper, moving uncontrollably and disoriented. The saddest part is at this stage we cannot help him. There's absolutely no medicine at this stage. It is so painful and heartbreaking to watch.

This is cholera season. Patients pass clear water from their bowels by the litre! We just have to pump IV fluids in as fast as we can. Our supply is so meager now to start with. Our total patient load at present is 112: sixty TB and fifty-two in the main hospital. Work has been very heavy in both the hospitals and clinic. Clinic hits as high as 200 on Mondays and Thursdays, 150 to 180 on Tuesdays and Fridays. Wednesday is strictly for TB. They finally started building the morgue today and the TB kitchen. It was started about seven to eight months ago: it just takes a long time for things to get done around here.

At the beginning of April, I sent congratulations to my brother, Rob, and his fiancé, Helen, on their engagement! I am looking forward to meeting Helen, on my return home.

President Johnson gave a speech over the radio about sending representatives to the Paris Peace talks to discuss a resolution to the Vietnamese conflict. I wondered what would happen in the next several months. Many people sounded dubious about the North Vietnamese and NLF coming to an agreement. At least it was evident that Johnson wanted peace and was making a sincere effort to do his part in bringing it about.

One night in April, there was real heavy firing over our house. It turned out to just be practice, but the American and ARVN forces aren't taking any chances.

We heard a rumour that the Vietnamese were expecting another attack on Nhatrang in early May, and that the NLF had been passing out propaganda. Major Knight, the sector advisor for our area, was visiting and he said that the North Vietnamese and NLF were indeed building up on the west side of Nhatrang. So we were expecting trouble again, we just weren't sure of exactly when. In the meantime, we were free to come and go as we pleased in the daytime, with a seven-thirty p.m. curfew to cross the bridges.

We did not expect much from the proposed peace talks in Paris. Anh Tin said that when they proposed this in Korea it took two years. Premier Thieu had now drafted everyone from ages eighteen to forty-five.

On April 16, we were informed that Paul Longacre, Olgie Neilson, LWR (Lutheran World Relief) representative, and Paul Leatherman would be coming for six days to discuss our project and staff, which included Doc, Emma, and myself with our terms expiring. They had to decide if they should continue with the programs and bring a new doctor in or not. Emma was going to ask to go home earlier than the end of September. If her replacement could come and Paul agreed, she would leave the end of August. If so, I thought I would go with her, so I didn't have to travel alone.

We had our interviews on April 23. Paul Longacre said that five to six nurses had expressed willingness to come to Vietnam, but he wasn't sure anyone could come by June. Emma asked if she could go home earlier, like mid-August or thereabouts, which Paul thought was possible. Knowing this, I planned to stay on past June so I could travel home with her. This would give me a chance to see the village extension work develop, which I couldn't if I left in June. After doing all the schools at the district level the previous year, I didn't want to see the program fall apart.

I wasn't sure when Doc was leaving. His replacement was likely Dr. Smith T (yes, this is her name), a woman who had spent five years in Korea and was an internist, who had already studied language in the States. We were worried about surgery when he left, though, because Dr. Kraybill was not a surgeon. Paul said a Methodist doctor and his wife, a nurse, who had spent ten years in Rhodesia, might be coming. He was a surgeon and had also done some ophthalmic surgery.

One day while making rounds in the TB wards, Dr. Kraybill said that they might be leaving before I did because he didn't want to endanger his family by moving them elsewhere in Vietnam and chances are they'd be assigned elsewhere in the country. Their situation was also complicated by the fact that they were in the process of adopting. I was thankful that I was not one of the few staying because with the Kraybills, Doc, Emma, and I all leaving in a two- to three-month period, we were the backbone of the place.

We learned that the South Vietnamese army had moved into Hong Chong, again on top of our hill, machine guns and all.

Chi Cuc (Ruth's counterpart) and I had a meeting with the district health chief to discuss our village extension work of TB skin testing. This necessitated a trip about eight km south of Nhatrang. It was so beautiful! The women were out in the fields harvesting the rice. It was the first time I had seen it done. Mr. Huu was very obliging: he said he would do the groundwork and notify us on Saturday. We hoped the program would be functioning again in two weeks.

One day, Ruth returned from Saigon with two VNCSers and we had a gabfest until after midnight. Then, at two a.m., there was all kinds of action, like we hadn't seen since Tet! Flares made it seem like broad daylight. Bombings! Mortars occasionally interspersed with small gun fire. Puff, military jargon for a helicopter, was busy with her mini guns too. Then there was a plane flying around with a loudspeaker, and all we could understand was, "Attention all US personnel . . . Attention all US Air Force . . . Attention all US Army . . . don't move . . . of Nhatrang." Finally, at two-thirty, I decided to try to get some sleep because there wasn't too much to be done other than pack a few clothes in a bag with all my important papers, lock my door, and doze off. At one point a chopper flew very low, and I wondered if we were going to be evacuated again.

In the morning, the Vietnamese didn't know what had happened either. News on the radio was poor. We heard enough to know that Saigon was secured very tight again. Work continued; the clinic was very hectic that day with 234 patients.

Suddenly, Dr. Kraybill was assigned to Saigon, and none of us were consulted. Jim, who never got upset, wrote a letter of protest to Saigon administration to send help soon, and we all signed it.

Chi Cuc, Ruth's counterpart, had been helping me get the public health program on its feet again. The district health advisor said that he would contact the necessary people in our area regarding organizing the villages. Then, one Saturday, the local person we were to work with came to see me. He turned out to be a man I enjoyed talking to when I taught English at the Tin Lanh Church in Nhatrang. Small world! He was tremendous to work with. From then on, the program was in Tharon's hands. There were advantages to being well established in a community before starting a program. Tharon could run on my merits for a while because there weren't too many people that I didn't know in the area.

Doc hit the nail on the head one evening at supper when he said that he didn't have the enthusiasm that he used to have anymore. Emma made a similar statement to me too about losing interest in the place. Frankly, I was also finding myself letting go in some areas. I guess going home was becoming more of a reality.

Das was back from Saigon and busy setting up a lab. We were certainly getting an international flavour in the unit. Das from India, Cuc, a Vietnamese, three Canadians and Americans. Emma's replacement was Swiss.

Tharon began the public health program in the villages, going out four afternoons a week. The skin tests needed to be read in thirty-six hours. Those with a positive result needed to have a chest X-ray: if negative, they were given the BCG vaccine.

Katy was going on a two-week vacation, and Emma and Tharon would start teaching O.R. techniques and surgical nursing respectively in early June when she was gone. The book work was picking up too due to lab requisitions. In July, Emma would take nursing students to the provincial hospital for experience in the O.R., surgical nursing and pediatrics until she left in the middle of August.

Jim came back from Saigon to help Emma with our monthly financial reports and to balance the books regarding unit and hospital funds, and he seemed rather depressed. Apparently, Saigon was in worse shape in certain areas than it had been at Tet, especially the area of the VNCS house. It was located in the Gia Dinh area where much bombing happened nearby with bullets bouncing off the wall in front of the house. They discovered that the Buddhist funeral facility was the storehouse for the NLF's ammunition, and one evening, a building less than 500 ft. away went up in flames with small arms fire, which continued throughout the night: at noon, a loud-speaker drove down the street asking everyone to leave in five minutes. Fortunately, only four persons were staying at the centre at the time. It didn't take them long to throw some things together (only one person had an emergency bag packed!) As two of the four were driving vehicles into the street, they saw NLF being caught in front of the house. Jim also said that Saigon shook with bombing all day and into the evening. Since the guys' house next to the centre was raided, the centre likely would be too. Radio reports had left us under the impression that the situation in Saigon was improving. Quite the contrary.

We continued to be 'secure.' The air base had been hit several times with mortar and rocket attacks, though.

Due to our security, Emma really wanted to terminate at least two months early. She had requested this to MCC's head office in Akron. I wrote home at the end of June to say that Emma and I finally got the news we were waiting to hear.

> *Emma's request to terminate one and a half months early was granted in light of Marcella Weber's willingness to extend two months, which meant that we could travel home together! We will start working on our plans so you can also make plans to meet me in the States.*
>
> *Time is flying, and I don't know how I will ever get everything done in time to leave.*

Last week, Paul Leatherman and the office manager from Saigon were here to talk business regarding replacements for Emma, Dr. Gehman, and myself. We were thrilled to hear that the Kraybills would not be going to Pleiku. Emma's replacement, a Swiss nurse, will be coming at the beginning of next week. Regarding Doc's replacement, the Methodist doctor and his wife are not available until the end of August. I'll be leaving before meeting my replacement. Meanwhile, Tharon will have to cover the outpatient clinic. Oh, how it hurts. She has been so kind and considerate, being fully aware of how sensitive I feel about giving up the clinic and the public health in the villages too.

I talked with Tharon and told her that I had better let her start taking the clinic next week, so this will be my last week there. Even though I am happy to be going home, I do love my work and it will be difficult to give it up to Tharon.

Katy and I had originally planned to get away for a couple of days and take a bus trip to Tuy Hoa, about 120 kilometres north of Nhatrang, but we were strongly advised against it. Instead, we decided to drive our new Land Rover to Phanrang, 120 kilometres south of Nhatrang, with three white Thai tribes' girls and a Vietnamese staff nurse. What a beautiful ride, but, oh, how dusty and dirty! If we had not had four-wheel drive, we never would have made it through the deep mud. We arrived at the clean city that had also been disrupted by the Tet offensive. We stayed at an uncle's home of our staff nurse. It challenged my language skills, but what fun: then we drove back on Sunday.

Monday, Tharon started working in the clinic. It's killing me to give it up. It's really hitting me that time's running out here, and it bothers me. I hope it didn't show—but Katy asked me last night whether I am holding something against her because she sensed that I wasn't my usual self. I assured her that I was just finding it extremely difficult to give up my work and not have something to occupy my mind to forget about leaving. TB patients were upset when we returned from Phanrang because someone told them that I was going to Saigon to 'di choi' (to have a fun time) for a month, and I wouldn't be coming back.

I just wrote a letter to KWH inquiring about employment, as well as one to Menno Travel Service about our return plans. Now to write a detailed report for MCC and VNCS regarding my job description, the challenges, etc., then most of the big assignments will be done.

I will not be writing too many more letters from here. Once I get home, my correspondence will mostly be coming here instead. I must remember to buy a Vietnamese dictionary so I can make a feeble attempt to write a letter in Vietnamese.

Today was Co Liddie's engagement party. She was in charge of the hospital when I first came to Nhatrang in June 1965. The whole Tin Lanh hierarchy was there. A rather sober, impressive service, if I must say so myself. The bride and groom must not appear happy or show emotion, and they are not to be seen together: one was on one side of the room, the other on the other side. She may be getting married before I leave.

This Sunday I am invited to an American wedding in Saigon. Two C & M A missionaries will be wed at the International Protestant Church. There are so many activities now. Last night I ate supper at home for the first time in seven days.

Tension seems to be really building up again in Saigon. I hope I can leave before a third offensive happens. Neighbours are saying there is much infiltration again. Jim said that the question is not if, rather when: some say July 20, to coincide with the signing of the Geneva Agreement in 1954. Others say early August, but whenever, everyone is getting ready for a bigger offensive and fear the political implications because the government is not very stable.

*We've been hearing all kinds of rumours too in Nhatrang;
but rumours are rumours: if you pay attention to all of them
you go crazy. We were just talking about how one adjusts to
or accepts the security situation here.*

By the end of July, I realized that my time in Nhatrang was running out, and I would need to buy some clothes and shoes on my way home because my three years' supply was running out. It was cheaper to send parcels to the US than to Canada, using APO, so I sent my belongings to Dr. Kraybill's parents' home in Elizabethtown, Pennsylvania since that area was in my travel plans.

I had received a letter from the director of nursing at KWH a few days before, saying that I was hired for the beginning of November, so I would be able to help around home for a while.

My nursing classmates were having a reunion in Kitchener, Ontario on September 21, and they were giving me ninety minutes to share about my experiences in Vietnam.

Emma and I planned to leave Nhatrang on August 14 and Saigon on August 18. We received a schedule from MTS for our requested flights and would be traveling together to Tokyo, then she was going to fly to Vancouver, and I would head to Portland.

Although I was excited to go home, leaving everyone in Nhatrang was one of the most painful experiences of my life.

My Return Home

Emma and I planned to embark on our return trip to Canada on August 18. Both of us would be travelling to Manila, the Philippines, Seoul, Korea, and Osaka and Tokyo, Japan. There we would part ways. I would fly to Portland, Oregon, to visit Jessie, my friend who had worked in Pleiku. Then to Kansas to visit Carl's parents. My parents would meet me at the Dulles airport, Washington. And then we would go to MCC's head office in Akron, Pennsylvania to meet for debriefing with Paul Longacre.

About our travels in late August and early September, I wrote:

The first lap of our trip is over. Emma and I left Manila today: we changed airlines in Hong Kong en route to Seoul, Korea.

We had a fabulous time in the Philippines. The people are so friendly and outgoing. The tranquility was unbeliev-able—no planes and no military! These modern extravagant commercial flights cannot be compared to the military planes I have travelled in.

Our bus trip to Baguio in the highlands was fun until we were in an accident and had to wait at the roadside for six hours to catch the next bus. When we did get to Baguio, it rained and rained, so we never made it to the famous rice terraces due to landslides. They used jeepneys—a surplus of WWII army jeeps made over for public transportation. They're painted in the gaudiest colours and all "jazzed" up with ornaments, radios blaring, and they charge down the streets at breakneck speeds. We watched students making things with silver, and went to a wood-carving school, and, of course, spent a little money.

It was wonderful to be met at the airport by Jerry Sandoz, former VNCSer, in Seoul, who was a gracious host. He gave us a sightseeing tour and introduced us to his assignment in Korea. Korea was officially divided into North and South in 1948: the US controlled the South and China the North.

On August 30 we flew to Osaka, Japan, where we stayed with Mennonite missionaries doing evangelistic work in the city. We just couldn't believe how clean and orderly it was in Osaka: the trains followed a schedule! No military: no police visible either. A middle-aged Christian Japanese couple invited us to their home for a traditional Japanese meal Sunday after church. We understood this to be a real honour because Japanese homes are so small that they do not usually entertain guests at home, rather they share meals in restaurants. I sat on cushions around a low square table, eating sushi. This was a unique experience because

Vietnamese sat on chairs to eat. I definitely need more practice to sit in the polite Japanese posture.

Kyoto was a highlight: we toured the ancient temples and learned about their history.

September 4, Emma and I took the Shinkansen bullet train from Osaka to Tokyo. What an experience. It could reach the speed of 199 miles an hour. It was so clean and fast, making our ears pop going through the tunnels. It debuted in 1964 for the Tokyo Olympics. We navigated our way to the Mennonite Guesthouse in downtown Tokyo, where we were met by Carl Beck and his family, Mennonite missionaries running a peace centre. We felt overwhelmed by the public transportation system, but succeeded in navigating our way around the city.

Sunday, September 8, Emma and I said our goodbyes and parted ways. Immediately after church, Carl drove me to the airport, at breakneck speed, to catch my two o'clock flight to Seattle: an hour between flights, then on to Portland, Oregon, where Jessie, my dear friend from Pleiku, met me. Jessie wondered if I wanted to go to church with her, and I did, so off we went. I had crossed the international date line in the Pacific so it was Sunday morning in Portland—I went to church on a Sunday morning twice in one day in two different countries!

In Portland, I was able to meet Co Tuyen and her husband: Co Tuyen had been my interpreter for a short time at the Nhatrang clinic. After three days of getting caught up on each other's lives, Jessie drove me to the airport to catch a flight to Wichita, Kansas to visit Carl's parents.

I will never forget this visit. Carl had been a special person to me and his parents seemed to be aware of that. They had many questions because they had not seen Carl after he had left for an assignment with MCC in 1964. His first year had been in Hong Kong, then he was transferred to Nhatrang for his last two years of service.

His parents had not done anything to his room, waiting for closure. They informed me that his barrel had finally arrived, but two-thirds of the contents had been stolen. Then I felt uncomfortable, knowing what I had hidden in the bottom of it when Carl was packing. Embarrassingly, I asked if they found a small crude box in the bottom of the barrel, to which they smiled and replied that they had. I apologized for the insensitivity but their response was they thought that I had put it there.

Apparently, Carl had written home enough about me that they felt they knew me. I discovered that Carl was buried in the blue knit sweater I had given him as a farewell gift. All his tapes had arrived home, including the one in which Carl had said, 'I don't know what I will do when I get home, but I do know that my work here is finished.' That took on a new meaning for me now.

My parents met me at Washington Dulles Airport on Saturday, September 14. How good it was to see them, and looking so well. We drove to the home of Esther Kraybill's parents in Virginia, where we spent one night and attended their church on Sunday morning. They were like sponges soaking up all information about the Kraybill family. We drove to EMC to meet Co Thanh and Anh Quang who were delighted to see someone who had 'just come from their home.' They wanted to be updated on everything that had recently happened in Nhatrang with the Tin Lanh church and the clinic. We spent another night at Esther's parents' home.

On the Monday, we drove to Akron, Pennsylvania to meet with Paul Longacre and Paul Leatherman at the MCC office for debriefing. Dad and Mom were so pleased to meet the people related to my assignment. Then we drove to Elizabethtown to pick up my parcels at Dr. Kraybill's parents' home. They, too, wanted to hear firsthand about their son's family and security at the present time. I thanked them for kindly keeping my parcels for me.

Since Dad had relatives in Pennsylvania, we spent one night with them. In the evening, I had to be in Philadelphia to give a presentation on the work in Nhatrang because the doctors at St. John's Lutheran Church had sent many parcels with medical supplies for the clinic.

Wednesday was a full day's drive home. I was emotionally worn out before getting home and wasn't prepared for the changes in my absence.

My three sisters, Brenda, Donna, and Susan, had grown so much and Rob was still living at home. Clare and Linda gave me a niece during my time away. What a beautiful child! Mom and Dad were just so glad to have me safely back home.

Invitations for speaking engagements were already waiting for confirmation from me. Culture shock! Newspapers couldn't give me all the information I wanted about Vietnam. Soon the letters were going the other direction. I really missed Vietnam but was equally happy to meet friends here. Their lives and interests were different than mine. Where did I belong?

Since people were keenly interested in Vietnam, my work, and what MCC was doing there, I had more invitations to show my slides and talk than time permitted. My nursing classmates had a reunion on September 21, where I spoke for one and a half hours.

In November, I began working on the eighth-floor female postoperative ward at KWH. It was a balancing act to work full time with many evening speaking engagements.

I received a long letter from Katy in Nhatrang saying that VNCS had had a three-day conference in Saigon in which she was able to participate. It was decided that should anyone want to return to Vietnam for a second term, they would be required to have specialized training in their field. Katy knew that I was considering returning because I had not really adjusted to life back home and missed Vietnam. I also knew that Tharon was still working in the outpatient clinic because they did not have my replacement yet.

By mid-December I requested to have my holiday time and regular days off together over the New Year. I planned to drive to Pennsylvania to spend some time with Doc, who was also struggling with adjustment. Meanwhile, Paul Longacre was visiting my church over Christmas because his sister was married to my pastor. Because I was working over Christmas, I was unable to meet him, but my parents did. They told him that they thought I would be going back to Vietnam. Paul confirmed that at the VNCS conference held in Saigon a month previously, it was agreed that anyone returning to Vietnam would need to have specialized training in their field.

On the night of December 30, before I was scheduled to drive down to Pennsylvania to meet Doc, I decided to cancel my trip, feeling that I would be going back to Vietnam. I went to bed convinced a phone call would come from the MCC Akron office the next morning asking me to return to Nhatrang for a second term. The phone call came!

Would I consider returning to Vietnam for a second term? If so, could I leave in two weeks? Part of the package would be that, within my first year back, I would have to have more training in my field. My immediate response was that, yes, I would go back, but I wanted to resign in good standing at KWH and needed to give them at least three weeks' notice.

The next day, I handed in my resignation to KWH and started the process of preparing to return. This time, I knew exactly what to pack. It was an exhilarating feeling: I couldn't wait to see everyone again in Vietnam. When the KWH staff found out that I was returning to Vietnam, they were not surprised. Frankly, the last four months in Canada had me feeling exhausted. It was a balancing act between culture shock, work, and having forty speaking engagements. The adjustment was more difficult than when I went to Vietnam. Even though people were keenly interested in Vietnam and what MCC and my role had been, I felt I didn't belong. I had left my heart in Vietnam.

MCC Akron quickly made travel plans for me.

CHAPTER 3

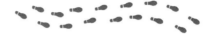

My Second Term in Vietnam

On Friday, January 24, 1969, I left again for Vietnam. It was emotionally draining to say goodbye once more to family and friends in Canada. Crossing the international date line, I arrived in Saigon on Saturday, January 25, where I was met with familiar faces saying, "We knew you would come back!"

That evening all my energy and emotion of the last several months left me exhausted, and I was so sick with vomiting that the staff said I would not be able to fly to Nhatrang the next morning. I was determined to go, and I did. When I arrived at the airport in Nhatrang on Air Vietnam, much to my surprise, no one was there to meet me. Knowing that sometimes the unit members attended chapel at the American base, I decided to hitch a ride to the military base. Sure enough, our van was in the parking lot, so I put my luggage in the back of the vehicle and proceeded to walk toward the chapel. As unit members were walking in my direction, they didn't even recognize me. They were stunned, as they were unaware that I was returning for a second term.

Eating the noon meal together, I discovered they had been praying for someone to take Tharon's place in the outpatient clinic starting the next day because she was to begin teaching in the nursing school. What an answer to prayer! I was amazed that the news that I was returning had not yet reached the unit.

Monday, January 27, 1969, I was back working with Katy in the out-patient clinic. There had been significant changes in the Western and Vietnamese staff.

In a letter home, I wrote:

Recently Nhatrang was attacked, but we didn't have anything out our way: we heard lots about other areas. Wednesday was graduation for our first nursing class: tomorrow they write their final exam and an admission exam will also be given.

The Kraybills are leaving for vacation, and Ruth leaves this weekend too. Unfortunately, Das cannot go on vacation, because his visa has not arrived.

Sunday morning, I got up early, so Das and I took Ruth to the airport. It sure was hard to see her leave, but she will be back in six months. In the afternoon, Katy and I took the Kraybills to the airport for their two-week vacation. In the evening, the majority of the unit went to a Korean restaurant in Dave Whybrew's honour—in the US Air Force, Dave had been a staunch supporter and volunteer for our work. I had once played a trick on him: when Doc had prescribed meds for him, I added an additional pill that makes your urine turn blue. He became very alarmed about the blue colour and consulted with Doc who soon figured out what had happened. Dave never forgot this, and I guess felt he had to get even with me before leaving . . . so Dave and Das put three toads in my bed. I caught the guys in my bedroom, but didn't see anything amiss. The next morning Das asked me if I had several friends sleep with me last night. Then he told me what they had done, and I didn't even know it! It became a laughing matter that I had slept with three toads that they assumed were flat now!

Katy and I worked in the clinic alone today, with Dr. Piburn filling in between surgeries. In the afternoon I made rounds in the TB hospital alone.

I still chuckle in the TB clinic because there are many patients returning for their appointments to discover that I am back. It's the same with the outpatient clinic. Patients get excited, jabbering and looking in the windows to be sure it's me. Ong Kien just tells them that it's Co Marcy's younger sister!

When Emma and I left, followed by Doc, it was decided that we would write a letter to be circulated between all of us and the unit. Today, it arrived from Doc who had taken an assignment to Biafra. He wrote that he was glad that I could return to Nhatrang because this is probably where I belong, although he is sorry that they didn't draft me for Biafra. Sounds like he is really missing Nhatrang. He wrote that he did surgery for thirty-six hours with enough time for a banana and a glass of water: no sutures were available, so sewing thread was used.

Dr. Beetz, Medical Director of Mission Overseas, came to discuss two to three month's education plans for me in my first year back in Vietnam. The most likely place is India, for practical training in public health. He recommended the Vellore School of Nursing. I need to correspond with the dean of nursing regarding three months of study after one month of language study before Dr. Kraybill leaves. My job is the same, plus organizing the warehouse and setting up a filing system until I leave for India.

I'm embarrassed by the small number of letters I've written since returning. The workload has been so heavy. Sometimes I wonder whether I would like to work in another place in Vietnam, but Chi Cuc expressed concern that I stay here as a liaison between old and new staff.

Today when riding the motorbike into town, a young Vietnamese guy pulled up beside me and in a questioning tone of voice said, "Co Marcy? I thought you had gone home. Why don't you come to my house?" so I had to explain that I had gone home and returned. People are still discovering that I am back. On Tuesday, I go to Saigon for further language study for one to two months.

We had a deep discussion one evening with a well-informed and learned theologian and politician. He thought that the US should pull out of Vietnam because they were not appreciated, that the Vietnamese were being driven to communism rather than away from it. He had had interviews with politicians on both sides in Paris, Cambodia, Laos, and in Vietnam. He felt that the NLF were on the level and seeking peace. He also said that people in Washington admitted that it was an error to enter Vietnam. There were many negotiations going on that the general public were not aware of. Some that even the Republic of Vietnam didn't realize.

In the Republic of Vietnam there was a movement in the central area, and, if they gained enough power of support, there could have possibly been another coup. They wanted a coalition government. I wasn't really sure what the general public knew back home. When he talked with North Vietnamese and the NLF in Paris, they all agreed that voluntary agencies could remain in Vietnam if the South Vietnamese people voted for them to stay. They agreed, realizing how rundown the country was. Several VNCSers who had returned from an out of country vacation said that Vietnam was in sad shape in comparison to its neighbouring countries. There had recently been many isolated terrorist activities throughout Saigon with activity stepping up. There were different possible reasons, such as Ho Chi Minh's birthday on May 19, and pressure regarding the peace talks in Paris.

A week previously, I had an interview with the personnel director and still knew no more than before. There was a possibility that I may be assigned to another project after two to three months in India at the end of the year. There was still no replacement for Dr. Kraybill, although apparently, Akron had a possibility.

Our language group was informed that we would no longer be VNCS after January 1970 due to differences in philosophy: MCC would be independent from CWS and LWR.

When I finished my language studies in Saigon, I went back to Nhatrang. One Saturday afternoon, the unit rented a boat on the other side of Nhatrang, ate a picnic lunch on an island, cruised around for a while and, in the evening, we ate out on the rocks. Ted and Gloria, two VNCSers, were visiting from Saigon: Ted played the guitar well, and we sang folk songs together. It was great!

After taking Ted and Gloria to the airport, Dr. Harold and Esther Kraybill, Das, Chi Cuc, Liz, and I went to a beach house for a Vietnamese meal. Much to our surprise, there was a Vietnamese military entertainment group there—band, singers, and all. Chi Cuc and I enjoyed it so much that we stayed on and had Das, with two of Dr. Piburn's children, pick us up later.

I went back to work in the clinic. Katy was now in Saigon for two weeks of language study.

In mid-June, Dr. Piburn and his family were on vacation, so Dr. Kraybill and I ran the clinic, which was running about 200 patients per day. It sounded like American troops were starting to pull out in numbers of 25,000. It seemed to be a known fact that the American Air Force would be leaving Nhatrang in September, turning it all over to the Vietnamese. The American Army would be staying.

The Kraybills left for good July 30. It was hard to see them go. Bob Miller, our director, had recently visited, and he confirmed that I had to go to India at the end of September to audit a postgraduate course in public health nursing for three months.

According to our July clinic report, Dr. Kraybill, Co Huong, and I had set a record for screening patients: we saw 5,100 patients, of whom 1,000 had TB. One Thursday, we saw 300 patients!

In early September, I wrote to update my parents:

> I've been making changes to suit Dr. Piburn's needs and am teaching two nationals to do some screening in the clinic. There is a new nurse in Saigon who will be replacing me

while I am in India, but we'll only have two weeks overlap, which is scanty. She will need an interpreter because I have been functioning without one. I'm in the process of breaking in Mrs. Piburn, who will be in charge of the TB hospital. Rumour has it that I will be starting a new project on returning.

I went to visit Ba Cu, who informed me that Lt. Lan, her son, is back in Nhatrang and wants to see me, but to be very careful because he wants a Western wife so he can leave Vietnam. I laughed.

Bill Herod, a former VNCSer, says he is returning to Vietnam in mid-September. He says, "With most friends I have to spend a great deal of time and effort explaining 'why'—somehow I think that you, Ruth, and a few others will understand."

It is September already, and it will soon be a year since I arrived home in Conestogo. We are expecting a Dr. Stuckey to arrive the middle of this month.

I received a note from Saigon that the remainder of my things had arrived in Kevin's barrel—all of my Tampax included. Mars, the Filipino working in the Saigon office, who opened Kevin's barrel and saw all the contents, came out exclaiming, "This can't all be Kevin's!" Joe, the Paxman assigned to our unit in Nhatrang, went to Saigon to pick it up. I'll soon know what clothing I have and can buy what's necessary en route to India. My ticket takes me to Singapore, where I'll have a week's vacation before flying to Madras: then, by train to Vellore.

I've just been informed that the post certificate course that I would be taking in community health and family planning is ten months, with the second semester from the end of September through December. Then I have two weeks' vacation to take before returning to Vietnam. Katy plans on meeting me in Bangkok in January.

Two nurses have arrived in Nhatrang: Sue, my replacement, and Martha, who will replace Tharon in the nursing school.

This is my last letter from Nhatrang. Das dropped me off at the Wycliffe Bible Translator's home because they have a piano, which I enjoyed playing until noon. After lunch, I invited several Vietnamese friends and a TB patient, Em Cuc, to go for a car ride with me to Ninh Hoa, about thirty km north of Nhatrang. The road has been paved, and it is now a lovely drive, through a mountain pass, banana groves, and fishing villages along the seaside. The most enjoyable part of the trip was seeing and hearing the others' reactions to the beautiful scenery.

We returned home in time to go to our Chinese Vietnamese friend Anh George's place for a delicious seven course Chinese send-off meal before I headed to India for my three-month program in community health at the School of Nursing at Christian Medical College and Hospital in Vellore, South India.

Public Health Study in India

I left Saigon on September 20 for India. After a ninety-minute flight to Singapore, I was in a completely different world. New compact cars everywhere—a clean city. There was no litter due to heavy fines. It was a fascinating city representing Chinese, Malay, Indian, and British nationalities, primarily.

After a three and a half hours flight to Madras, I was met by an Indian gentleman who put me up at a hotel overnight. The next day I had a three-hour bus ride to Vellore. The first thing that hit me was all the cows—everywhere! The bus was continually slamming on its brakes and honking its horn just in time to dodge them. The nurses there informed me that it wasn't uncommon for a bus to land in the ditch in order to avoid hitting a cow.

The hospital compound was huge. There were more doctors than nurses—it had to be the only hospital with that problem. The next day, I was to get a tour of the hospital, starting with the outpatient department. I was to have every Saturday afternoon and Sunday off. There were two Canadian University Service Overseas (CUSO) nurses, and I was rooming with one. My bed was on her porch on the fifth floor of the nurses' residence—it had chicken wire netting enclosing it so I was exposed to everything! Wake-up call came at five a.m. from the loudspeaker of a mosque a block away.

To acknowledge Canadian Thanksgiving, I decided to write home to my parents.

Happy Thanksgiving! There are three of us Canadians, so we are going out to celebrate this evening. To exit the hospital compound, though, we need to walk past about twenty beggars with leprosy, maimed and disfigured. It is impossible to give to just one, so we keep on walking. Painful. I can hardly bear to look at them.

One has to see India to believe it. A country of people, children— who are adorable with their big brown eyes, jet black hair, and flashing smiles—and poverty. The majority of homes that we visit are of the workers or untouchables, which means a thatched home made out of mud, one blackened cooking pot, and one change of clothing, if they're fortunate.

Last week we had rain for two days and many people were flooded out of their homes. One home we visited had six children, the youngest nine days old. It was one room with a big hole in the roof: the dirt floor was one big mud hole. It was so sad. The average income is about $8 US a month.

Malnutrition is a major problem in India. The government is pushing a family planning program to sterilize people because, by 1985, India's population is to double. She can't even feed all her people now.

Wood is so scarce that they use dung patties made of cow manure! Last week, several of us were riding bicycles in the countryside when we saw a woman with a basket on her head, walking on the road behind a herd of cows. She was picking up the fresh manure by hand. The manure is then made into patties and put on the outside wall of the house or on the ground to bake in the sun. This is only one example of how resourceful these people are.

I ride a bicycle six km every day to the leprosarium. I cannot possibly capture the sights and sounds on paper. The villages I pass through are primarily mud thatched homes. No such thing as privacy: it is survival. The caste system doesn't make it possible for the untouchable children to go to school. Faces tell you they are hungry. Life is so unfair. I see how workers are not treated with respect at the hospital. Maybe if you grew up in this culture it wouldn't impact you the same way.

Our meals, in the canteen beside the hospital, leave much to be desired. Very few vegetables and no fruit. I cannot complain because there are many people here who would do anything to eat what I have.

There are so many people who live outside: no home, hard to tell where they sleep. I can understand why Ken Shantz made the comments he did about it. These people don't have a chance. One of the biggest medical and govern-ment programs is family planning: sterilizing people. Young girls get married at the age of thirteen to fifteen in the vil-lages and look old at the age of twenty-five. I am so glad I wasn't born in India.

One day I accompanied the hospital bus with a team of doctors and nurses giving immunizations in several villages. I was impressed with the public health program that day, until I discovered that only children of families who could afford to pay a small fee received the immunizations. The poverty is so overwhelming.

A third-generation medical missionary in India, Dr. Ida Scudder, started the Christian Medical College and Hospital in Vellore in 1918. She dedicated her life to working with patients with Hansen's Disease, commonly known as leprosy, and the hospital has become one of Asia's foremost teaching facilities. There have been several books written about Dr. Ida Scudder: one is Dr. Ida: The Story of Dr. Ida Scudder of Vellore and Ten Fingers for God.

I am feeling a bit unwell with a fever, headache, and sore throat. As long as I don't pick up anything worse in India, I'm alright. You wouldn't believe the filth. Buses drive down the road like they are on a track the hell drivers use, dodging goats, cows, dogs, and bicycles. No one looks to see what's coming or where they are going! One of these days I'll get up enough courage to take a photo.

On November 6, I wrote:

Greetings from the little village of Kawanur, about twenty miles from Vellore. Yesterday, several of us were driven out by the hospital van for varied stays, mine being the shortest, from Wednesday through Sunday. It's quite an experience being stuck out here as the only Westerner with an Indian diet, few vegetables and no fruit, but lots of rice and chili. Water is only served with the noon meal, so the burning sensation from the chilies continues for a while. The schedule is breakfast at six forty-five a.m., with chapati, a whole wheat pancake with a scant amount of spicy chutney; tea at ten or ten-thirty; lunch at one p.m., with rice, a small portion of vegetables, and a little chutney; rest until three; the evening meal at seven, which consists of the same as at lunch with a little meat. Oh, for some delicious fresh fruit!

When I go into the villages with the hospital staff, I am asked if I come from "America", the rich country. The second question is, why I don't wear gold? It's an Indian custom to invest your money in gold, bangles, necklaces, earrings, more rings, and toe rings. All I had on that day was a small pair of gold studs in my ears and my KWH School of Nursing ring. I wanted to say that I don't have that much, but they would never believe me. They think everyone coming from "America" has to be rich, especially if you go to India.

Last week I was out making home visits with the nurses. This week I'm hoping to see a home delivery. We've had two here at the centre, but so far, none in the homes. Today there was a Well Baby Clinic in a village three km from here. We walked and came back by bulla cart, which makes our Mennonite horse and buggies back home look plush with their springs. It's a real education being here. I'll never criticize the Vietnamese again for being slow because the Indians are slower, if that is possible.

I will always remember my experience in the village, making home visits for expectant mothers. The mud thatched homes, with no doors, open to the elements. Each had a small mud area built up with space for a cow dung patty to cook their rice in a little black pot. One emaciated expectant mother did not have any extra clothing for herself, let alone for her baby that was due. We discovered on our next visit that she had her baby later that same day, but we were not called. It was a girl, so it had been left in a ditch to die: had her baby been a boy, she would have kept it, even though the family did not have enough to feed themselves.

One day, Laura, my roommate, and I hiked with two Australian friends, and then shared a meal of cabbage, carrots, potatoes, and ham sent from Australia. It was delicious! We took a "line" bus back to our hostel. Everyone made eyes at us when we dared return at nine-thirty p.m. Apparently, in India, no respectable young girl was out after dark!

Carl's mother wrote a lovely letter that contained some news about Doc. He would be returning home early from Biafra for a rest. I received two more letters from TB patients wanting me to return to Nhatrang.

My experience in India was proving very humbling which was evident in my letter home.

I am once again thankful for health and friends: someone to talk to on paper who understands what I am trying to say, even if it's not written well, or someone who can read between the lines and get the message. We don't know how fortunate we are. We are so wealthy in our way, especially when you see how little these people have. Imagine growing up and never being able to afford a well-balanced diet.

I'm dying to hear some good music again. The Hindi temples have their music playing over the loudspeaker starting at five a.m! Only eight more days left in Vellore, then on to Calcutta to meet Vernon Reimer, MCC Director for India, a fellow Canadian.

Dawn, the CUSO gal is going to give me the names and addresses of several CUSO friends in Bangkok. Katy is definitely coming to Bangkok from December 27 - January 3, 1970.

I have learned much while in India. Putting educational benefits aside, it gave me a good chance to evaluate the Vietnamese situation objectively, mentally, and physically. I feel much better equipped to return and do my job justice.

The My Lai massacre in Vietnam seems to be making global headlines now even though it actually happened on March 16, 1968. Why didn't they do something about it earlier? It was one of the most horrific incidents of violence committed by American soldiers against unarmed civilians. Close to 500 women, children, and old men were brutally killed. It needs to be addressed. I sometimes wonder how effective a Western person can be in a foreign country. It really takes a national to reach a national.

Laura and I get into some good discussions. The other day in class, we were discussing pit privies (outhouses) and types. One was a seat with a pail underneath that requires emptying every day. Well, Canada isn't such a far cry from India—maybe only fifteen years ahead. How well I remember the smokehouse and outhouse. Then, in winter, down in the cellar, to a seat/pail, beside the coal bin. I had been petrified one night when a skunk met me at the foot of the stairs. Laura howled when I told her. She shared how she came from down East from a family that was so poor that her father never had to pay income tax.

On Friday, December 19, Laura went with me to Madras by train. We splurged and went out for Chinese food in the evening and saw the movie, Bullet. The next day I flew to Calcutta. I only had the MCC office address and telephone number. Of course, the office was closed. Fortunately, an Indian gentleman who spoke some English, and had been on the same flight, took it upon himself to be responsible for me and questioned some people living near the office. Finally, one peasant man said that he didn't know the name of the street but could direct us to the Reimers' home. I got there only to discover that they weren't there. They finally arrived, and they were a delightful couple. We went to the Methodist church Sunday morning, where I met the Metzler family who had served at First Mennonite Church in Kitchener, Ontario. What surprised me was that Everett Metzler, Director of the East Region of India Peace Corps, even knew who I was!

I discovered in Calcutta that my visa for Vietnam would not be issued here, so I decided to go on standby for Thailand late Monday afternoon and succeeded in getting a reservation.

Early Monday morning, the Reimers, their children, several other Indians, and I piled into their VW van and drove forty miles out of Calcutta to distribute 600 Christmas bundles in a village. Too bad the people who made up the bundles couldn't see the faces of those receiving their precious gifts. I joined a medical team giving immunization shots for cholera. In the afternoon, I flew to Bangkok, Thailand.

India made a profound impression on me. The massive poverty, especially the untouchable class that had no hope for the future, was painful to accept. I could not bring myself to take one photo during my time there. Life was too unfair.

I went to the Vietnamese Embassy in Bangkok and got my visa. I stayed at the Bangkok Christian Guesthouse, where one CUSO volunteer, Bob, happened to walk in for Christmas dinner, and then invited me to the "Ghetto" for a party with other CUSO volunteers. We ended up going out for another Christmas dinner!

I wrote about this Christmas celebration and my travels with Katy in Thailand, in my letter home to mom and dad.

Just after Christmas, I went with 'the gang' to a coffee house, where two CUSO volunteers were playing their guitars and singing. You will never guess who I met there. Fern Hilliard, who attended Conestogo Elementary School with me! She came in July for a two-year term with CUSO and was teaching English at a school four hours north of Bangkok. She invited Katy and I for a visit. Katy arrives tomorrow, so I'll see what she says. Then, on Sunday, another volunteer from Kitchener has invited us to go for a boat ride on Bangkok's many canals. He and another CUSO gal invested in a boat. Sounds like fun. I am not really stranded like I thought I'd be.

It is a new year, 1970, and a new decade! Oh, all the changes that took place in the Sixties. One cannot help but wonder how much further man can go. Reaching another planet seems impossible.

Due to a visa issue, Katy was unable to arrive until December 29. We decided to take a bus trip to Chiang Mai, a twelve-hour bus ride from Bangkok. We sure didn't get much sleep, but it was fun because the bus was full of young people. The town of Chiang Mai is known for its woodwork, pottery, and silver work. One morning, we toured a Meo tribes' village. It was fascinating and the people were very much like some of our Thai tribes' people in Vietnam. The old men were smoking their long bamboo "pot" pipes (with water in). We toured the King's Palace and a large Buddhist temple. There were beautiful waterfalls with rocks and trees surrounding all these places that were 17,000 feet up a mountain side. What beautiful sites! The last stop was the university campus.

Later in the afternoon we just wandered around, did a little shopping, and decided it would be fun to rent motorbikes the next day. We rode out about ten km into the countryside where they made silk on hand looms. Unfortunately, on our way back, Katy's motorbike broke down and we had no idea what to do. We were in the middle of nowhere. Unexpectedly, police patrolling the area in their jeep stopped to help us. They kindly fixed the motorbike and we hightailed it back to town before anything else could happen and decided it was best to stay near the town.

Early the next morning, we took a bus back to Bangkok. The secret of taking these day long overland excursions is not to drink because there are no johns in sight!

Katy and I went to see Hello Dolly, which was really terrific. Sunday morning, we went to a Southern Baptist church, which left a little sour taste in my mouth. The pastor's wife was vocal in her thoughts regarding having only American Southern Baptist doctors running their hospital so they can continue to have a warm friendly feeling. Wow! Then in the Sunday School class there was prayer for 'our boys' in Vietnam but not a word for the Vietnamese, North or South.

Return to Vietnam

Katy and I flew from Bangkok to Saigon on January 5, 1970.

Soon after, Bob Miller, VNCS Director, informed me that they wanted me to do some traveling within Vietnam to survey some places for possible projects. The first place was in the Mekong Delta. Bob Miller said that Bill Herod, who had recently returned for a second term, was doing a survey in the Delta for VNCS, that was getting pressure from Stateside to open projects there. He wanted me to accompany Bill to check out a request from a Tin Lanh pastor for VNCS to assign a nurse or doctor.

On January 7, Bill and I drove down to My Tho near the coast, a good hour's drive from Saigon. The delta was in such contrast to the Vietnam I knew. It was flat! Rice paddy after rice paddy, thatched roofs and mud houses that were well kept up.

We registered at a hotel, which proved rather interesting because everyone considered us to be married and insisted on calling us Mr. and Mrs. ARVN troops patrolled on the third floor outside our bedroom doors all night. Bill had a beard and could pass for being much older than he was. We told some of the soldiers that we were Germans, that Bill was forty and had been in Vietnam twenty years already, and they believed us. I'm sure they were watching to see if we would end up sleeping in the same bed. Our rooms were next to each other.

All went well until Bill got up early and went to the market to buy some bananas. He had informed the desk clerk at the hotel not to bring breakfast up to his room until he returned. There must have been some misunderstanding because the 'nosey' man from the night before brought our breakfasts. Bill was gone so he came to my bedroom window (no glass, just decorative iron grill), pulled back the drapes, stuck his face in the window, and hollered, 'Where is he?' I was still sleeping under the mosquito net. It was such a shock! Bill thought it was funny!

There was much reconstruction at that time because much of My Tho city had been destroyed during the Tet offensive in 1968. We first went to meet the pastor who had requested that VNCS support his project. Unfortunately, he was at a conference. Then, Thay Luong, a friend of mine from Nhatrang, who was a student pastor there, kindly showed us around the area.

The next day we drove to Cai Be, ninety-minute drive southwest of My Tho. Asian Christian Service (ACS) had a tremendous team there—an Indian doctor, two Australian nurses, two Indonesian nurses, and a Thai pharmacist. They said that VNCS had been seriously negotiating with them, but I felt that the project did not need a full time Western nurse because it was functioning well.

When Bill and I returned to Saigon we reported to the VNCS office and met the director of ACS to hear his opinion. It didn't look like I would be working there. VNCS administration would be having a meeting regarding the My Tho clinic, after which Dean Hancock, VNCS Personnel Director, would inform me of their decision.

I flew to Pleiku via Nhatrang to pick up some of my things. It was great to get back and see everyone again. Sue was managing the clinic and had made a few changes. It was good to have a new face and ideas. India had given me time to think things over, and I was quite content to go elsewhere and start a new project: but at the same time, was really hoping to be reassigned to Nhatrang.

While in Pleiku, I covered for two nurses while they were on vacation. The Saigon administration also decided that, during my time there, I was to go to Dak To, north of Kontum, and evaluate the possibility of developing a public health program there.

Pleiku was cold! In January, it was only 66 degrees in the house, and I froze. Nhatrang never got that cold. Pleiku is in the Central Highlands, close to the borders of Laos and Cambodia.

The hospital had twenty beds and most of the patients were from Montagnard, Jarai, and Bahnar tribes.

The four months in India had given me a chance to get rested and look at the Vietnam situation objectively. I had to go all the way to India to realize how exhausted I was, mentally and physically. All of the adjustments of the last year had been a little too much and had affected me more than I was aware of. I felt like a new person, and I had come back to Vietnam appreciating the Vietnamese.

After Pleiku, I was to return to Saigon, report, then go north to Quang Ngai to do a survey of the refugee camps: while there, I was to try to get to Tra Bong. Those were three possible assignments, along with Di Linh south of Dalat. I was not permanently assigned anywhere at that point. I was anxious to dig my teeth in and do something.

In my letter to my family on February 6 I wrote about spending Tet in Nhatrang.

I tried to get to Nhatrang for the first day of Tet on February 6, but instead I made it on the seventh. It was wonderful visiting and being invited to homes of friends for two days. It's the usual custom to visit each family at Tet and wish them good health and prosperity for the coming year. It's also their custom to serve tea, candied fruit, rice and bean cake, watermelon seeds, etc.

Sunday morning, Tom, Paxman assigned to Nhatrang, and I went to early Mass at the new Catholic Church, then to the Tin Lanh Protestant Church in town. The pastor, whom I knew very well, invited us both for dinner that evening. When we returned home briefly at noon, Katy said that we had two invitations for dinner that evening, but she had turned the one down. I said, but I'm going to Pastor Kiem's for dinner. We didn't know what to do because Chi Thinh had gone to market early in the morning and was busy preparing her food already. Katy and I went to her house to say we couldn't come (she, her sister and brother-in-law work at the hospital). Then Chi Thinh said, if we can borrow your car, we'll take all our food to Pastor Kiem's place and invite ourselves for dinner too (her one sister was married to his son). We ended up having dinner together at his home. It was so good to meet everyone.

Tuesday morning, I returned to Pleiku. Joe, one of the Paxmen, took me to the airport via the fish market. I sat in the back of the C123 with the soldiers and this big fat fish, approximately two feet long, head and tail included, fresh from the sea to give to Chi Thinh's sister, who lived across the road from the Pleiku Hospital.

From Pleiku, I flew by helicopter to Kontum and spent the night there en route to Dak To, which is north of Pleiku, near the Cambodia/Lao border. Bill Rose and Ron Ackerman were working there in community development.

I had no sooner arrived, when they conscripted me into the Dak To VNCS Physical Fitness Program to see whether

I'd qualify for their unit. It included digging irrigation ditches, hoeing a peanut patch, etc. All their work is with tribal people known as Montagnards. Ron is concentrating on agriculture in one village: their gardening land is outside the village compound. To get to their village you have to cross a swinging bridge, which was in pathetic condition until they recently rebuilt it. It's now made with barbed wire going out at a 45° angle on either side, with bamboo spaced every foot length and flimsy planks on top of that. Nothing to hang onto! The guys said that I passed the test in agriculture, but I got about one third of the way across the swinging bridge and just couldn't go any further. This swinging bridge was fifteen to twenty feet high and about sixty feet long. There was a Land Rover full of people watching from behind and some elderly villagers laughing on the other side, so I knew I had to go all the way. When the bridge stopped swinging, Bill hollered, "Well, Marcy, what do you propose to do?" He came and helped me. Oh, the pain!

We had no sooner crossed when a villager drove across it on his motorbike, which made me feel like a heel! Bill came out with the brilliant statement, "Marcy, looks like these people will have to come to you if they want help." Truer words have never been spoken.

Montagnards are known for their rice wine. The villagers continually come to their gardens drunk after dinner— many never make it back in the afternoon.

Work here will be a real challenge. It will mean learning another language.

I'm heading back to Pleiku to organize the warehouse for one day: then Wednesday and Thursday I will go with the C & M A nurses who work with leprosy patients in Jarai and Bahnar tribal villages in the district.

In a letter to my parents, I wrote:

> *Thank you, Mom and Dad for your support. Somehow, I don't feel worthy of it. I wonder if coming to Vietnam was the coward's way out. One can run away from all the tensions existing at home and quietly exist here with the prestige and publicity that goes with working overseas, especially in Vietnam. Truly, anyone working in the ghettos and slums back home has a much more difficult task: there's no prestige with it. It's equally, if not more difficult to communicate and be effective with those people and they are every bit as needy as anyone in Vietnam. One can be as great a service to mankind at home as abroad.*

After applying for a new passport in Saigon, I flew to Quang Ngai.

Once there, it meant harvesting rice in some places, in others, plowing or planting with other vegetables. The rainy season was over and all was lush green. There were swaying bamboo trees like we didn't see in Nhatrang. Beautiful countryside. Although I did not have a keen appreciation for making surveys and writing reports, it was a real opportunity to get to different areas and learn about the various minority groups, like the Jarai tribes in Pleiku and Sedang in Dak To: in Quang Ngai, the Vietnamese were also very unlike the Vietnamese in Nhatrang.

There were eighty-five officially recognized refugee camps in the province. Most of them had been created five or six years earlier, and a few had only formed within the last six months. Some of the living conditions were absolutely deplorable: inadequate nutrition, not enough of any food. But truly, these refugee camps were better off than much of India's population, where there was chronic starvation and severe malnutrition. Our Western countries were at one end of the spectrum and India and Biafra at the other.

It must have been very hard for these people to flee for their lives, leaving their homes and personal possessions, many of their homes destroyed. There was so much destruction from the war. Rubble from Tet 1968 remained untouched. Many homes we went into had bullet holes patched in the walls and ceilings. We saw much less of this devastation in Nhatrang.

Bob Miller (another Bob Miller) and I gave out several monthly scholarships for students who could not afford to go to school in a village less than four km from where the My Lai massacre occurred.

One afternoon our unit drove up a small mountain, several kilometres outside of Quang Ngai city. At the top, I had the feeling I was on top of the world looking out to the sea only eight to ten km away: behind us, the mountains that had literally been deserted. People had fled to the area along Highway Number 1, with the coastal region still reasonably insecure.

I returned to Nhatrang to attend the graduation ceremony for ten students from the nursing program. The Saigon administration was well represented. We also had a farewell party for Das who was returning to India on completing his term.

I spent much of my time at this point completing my reports on what I saw at Pleiku, Dak To, and Quang Ngai.

On March 25, I was officially assigned by the Saigon office to start public health work in Quang Ngai. We knew it would be difficult because we did not have permission from the provincial medical chief to start medical work there.

I arrived in Quang Ngai in April. It was a dusty, dirty 'crumbly' town, even by Vietnamese standards. There were some rich people, but, by far, many were poor peasants. You got the feeling that you were living in town no matter which street you drove down because they were lined with houses, but, actually, we were right on the very edge, then rice patties for half a mile, then a river.

The unit was very happy to see me return, and I was grateful to be wanted and needed. Geisala, one of the German volunteers, a home economist whom I met while making my survey, was on my plane en route to Quang Ngai. She told me they had recently had over $1,500 US worth of material and equipment stolen from the building where they held their sewing classes. They knew where the thieves were storing the stolen equipment: apparently their night watchman and interpreter were involved. They fired all their staff and told the students no more classes. Even though the Germans reported this to the police department, nothing happened. They suspected that the police got their share of the loot too.

I wanted to introduce the unit members of Quang Ngai to my parents in this letter home.

Our unit consists of: Bob, formerly a Methodist minister, married to Co Anh, a home economist from Saigon with a four-month-old baby, called An Dao, which means cherry; Co Van, a home economist and my roommate; Glen, an American social worker, and our unit leader, who is setting up a nursery school in one of the resettlement camps; Doug, also American, an economics graduate, and me.

Sunday was Easter and Father requested a Vietnamese helicopter to go to Ba To in the highlands with the Montagnards— it's about a thirty minute helicopter ride. He invited us to go along because it is not safe to go by road. Bob, Co Anh, Co Van, and I went and celebrated an Easter service in their cathedral. We were met by a Jeep on arrival, in a valley with a river and mountains on both sides. We drove through a Special Forces Camp, then the river—no bridge—so we drove right through, up the other side, through the village, stopping every few hundred yards, telling people to come to worship. Then we beat the gongs to let everyone know. It was a beautiful place. Two hours after we had had our service, it was deserted because the NLF came in every night. All the people go to the district head-quarters to sleep. It must be terrible to live with that fear.

Two nights ago, we had quite a bit of action—lots of mortars, rockets, and small arms fire. The hamlet chief for our area, who lives less than a block away, was assassinated. I was sleeping until I heard the whistling sound of incom-ing artillery, then a boom, and I saw a big flash outside. I jumped under the bed— nothing happened. The remainder of the rockets were outgoing. Finally, at four-thirty a.m. or so, it stopped.

When we got up in the morning, we discovered a rocket had landed in the middle of the path between the building I was sleeping in with Co Van and the neighbours. It was embedded in the path, and our lives were spared because it never exploded. Thank you, God for your protection.

The bombing continued all day. I have never heard the likes of it before. We surely live sheltered lives at Nhatrang. All of Quang Ngai was insecure at night. Thankfully, our reputation was well established: I was told that the situation has been much worse than now.

Last Friday, I went with Bob to give out several of his scholarships in the area that is known for making sugar cane. They had two water buffalo in a yoke walking in a circle. In the middle were two women feeding the stocks of sugar cane into three clogs. As the wheels went around, they squeezed out the juice that ran through a small pipe leading to a big barrel or keg. They had an underground oven made of mud and the sugar cane syrup was boiling in woven bamboo baskets that had been pitched. Then they would scoop it into the next basket until it reached the right consistency. Finally, it was scooped with an ancient metal helmet and notched onto the end of a long pole. It was fascinating.

Today, Glen and I went to see Dr. Khai, Provincial Medical Chief, to discuss whether he would agree to VNCS having a public health program. Although he is agreeable, there is so much red tape to navigate before it can be cleared.

Bill Snyder, from Akron, wants to meet with all MCCers on his visit to Vietnam, so that will mean another quick trip to Saigon.

Last night was an unusual evening. We ate Western food! Inflation is so high that sugar, flour, and shortening are next to impossible to get. Fortunately, we had some number ten size cans (one gallon size) of army goods given to the unit, including some salmon, so I made salmon patties and we had a white cake mix that just needed to have water added, *and we also had a tin of blueberries, so I added some to the mix instead of the water, and, for topping, I thickened the remaining blueberries with flour and added a little sugar and butter for a glazed topping. It was such a lovely treat!*

We learned that two weeks ago when Ron and Bill at Dak To were driving home, they were shot at: four flat tires and several bullet holes through the windshield. Fortunately, Ron ducked just in time. The car motor wasn't damaged so the guys kept on driving on four flat tires until they got home. It's the first time that VNCS has been targeted.

The weather is getting hotter. In the evenings, the air barely moves. I teach English five evenings a week: one class three times a week is at the Tin Lanh Church, and I also do private tutoring twice a week. They have difficulty saying 'c,' so 'cities' comes out 'shitties' every time; 'ph' comes out 'f'. It's a pleasant and enjoyable change, which also gives me a chance to learn more Vietnamese.

Last weekend, we had a pleasant surprise. Brennon, a VNCSer, and Jackie, a Wycliffe Bible Translator, arrived from Saigon. Jackie is assigned to the Cua tribespeople in Tra Bong, who live in the mountains, sixty km northwest of here. Due to security and added group responsibilities, she and Eva, who are the only two assigned to the language, had been unable to concentrate on translation. She came to make several tapes and visit friends there. Now, Brennon has been assigned there. Tra Bong is a beautiful valley surrounded by mountains and rice patties: a river flows through town with a lovely fresh smell to the air—frequently the scent of cinnamon—and Tra Bong is known throughout the world as producing the world's best cinnamon. Due to NLF taxes, they have not been able to export for several years, but are now awaiting approval again. It has the shortest airstrip in Vietnam: one thousand one hundred feet! We went by helicopter. Caribou planes (Canadian planes designed to land on a one-thousand-foot runway) can land there but no large military aircraft.

The tribal women there were fascinating with their beads, as many as forty to sixty strands of bright coloured beads around their necks: some even had hip beads. The children were so friendly, all eyes and smiles. Vehicles were scarce. As we drove down the street in an open Jeep, we kept collecting kids like an avalanche rolling down a hillside. They sat on the hood, fenders, etc.: every conceivable place. We had to tell them we couldn't drive them. What a completely different world just a ten-minute helicopter ride away.

We spent close to an hour in a Cua long house, which was built on stilts four feet off the ground, was made of bamboo with thatched roofing, and was large enough for five families.

In early May 1970, I began working full time at the Canadian TB centre run by the Canadian government. On my first visit, accompanying the doctor on his rounds, one patient recognized me from Nhatrang! The Canadians informed me that our mail had not been coming due to a postal strike in Canada. At the TB centre, I was working on a file system, to identify delinquent patients who failed to keep their appointments. With gaps in their prescribed treatment, stopping and starting with their medications, they ran the risk of becoming resistant to therapy. In addition to jeopardizing their own health, their families could also become infected. Continuous treatment was necessary until they had a negative sputum test and/or X-rays showed positive recovery. I spent most days scanning charts.

It was only a ten-minute bicycle ride from our unit house to the Canadian TB centre. The Canadian doctor bought a bicycle that I was able to use.

Katy wrote me to say she only had a few months left in her term, and she wanted to come for a visit. Last weekend, Co Van and I drove to Tam Ky, seventy km north, to visit our unit there: Dennis and Maurice. It was a good experience to sleep on bamboo beds with a reed mat. They lived in real Vietnamese style.

I was glad that I was living in Vietnam instead of Cambodia. The news was reporting that Vietnamese were being massacred inside Cambodia. Apparently, fifty to one hundred Vietnamese were being allowed to return to Vietnam each day, but they were interrogated at length and treated brutally as prisoners of war, before being allowed back.

Brennon, who was assigned to Tra Bong, was our former VNCS correspondent in Saigon. While he was still in Saigon, he decided to ride a scooter to 'parrot's beak' in Cambodia with Mike Morrow, a freelance writer. They arrived in the afternoon, and the American military allowed them to cross the border but said not to go more than twenty km inland. Brennon told me that they saw so much destruction, caches of rice and many people held hostage being interrogated. This was the result of Norodom Sihanouk, ruler of Cambodia, allowing the NLF to build their strongholds on Cambodian soil. Then, a week later, Mike asked Brennon to go again, which he was unable to do. Mike and two other reporters decided to go together in a Jeep. Sadly, they were last seen being led off by the NLF, thirty-two km inside Cambodia.

The atrocities committed in the war were appalling. When I was in Quang Ngai, I agreed to accompany an American Quaker doctor on his weekly visit to a large political prison because his wife was pregnant and couldn't go. There were 1,200 prisoners! One room was so full, with about 650 women with children, that they could not all lie down to sleep at the same time. The torture they must have endured!

My letter to my parents on June 15, 1970 was on a lighter note.

> Your Christmas parcel just arrived. Thank you! Popcorn: what we have all been craving! Brennon went out to the kitchen, and the next thing I heard was, "Marcy! Marcy!" He couldn't believe that it really popped.
>
> Guess what my latest project is? Raising rabbits! I brought four bunnies with me on my last trip from Saigon. Unfortunately, I had to sleep in a hotel in Danang for one night. The maids discovered there were bunnies running around in room 503! Before long, the desk clerk and maintenance staff were up on the fifth floor. I hope it didn't ruin

my reputation there because I might have to stay there again sometime.

I received a message from Saigon following my brief conversation with Bob Miller, two weeks ago when he was leaving Quang Ngai: He asked how I would feel if I was asked to temporarily fill in at Pleiku for four to five months. Now, I was clearly asked to do so.

I decided to write to Saigon regarding their decision because there was no point in getting halfway through the posters and lessons I'd been preparing to be taught at the district level for health care workers here in Quang Ngai, if I was going to Pleiku. The answer arrived yesterday: Pleiku definitely needs me now. Will I please move there? They await my answer.

I feel like a hypocrite because I told the Canadian team I would work with them for one year. The request from Saigon did not say that I have to go, but my conscience does not allow me to stay here knowing that they need me in Pleiku. VNCS projects should take priority before loaning personnel to other projects. I have discussed it with the unit here that wants me to stay, but Glen agrees with me and feels he likely would make the same decision.

Half my term will be history by August. What have I accomplished this time? It has meant hopping around since returning from India, adjusting to new situations and people. I felt like I was getting my teeth in Quang Ngai . . . then off again. I regret having to share my decision with the Canadian team later today. Whatever my job for my second term is, I'm sure there is a plan.

At the end of June, a few days before I was set to leave Quang Ngai, there was a party at Doctor Jutras' (from the Canadian TB centre) house. It was a farewell for three staff and a welcome for two replacements and myself. But as it turned out, it was my farewell too.

It was hard to leave Quang Ngai already because I had made contacts and felt I was able to establish a rapport with many of the workers. My weakness or strength was that I tended to become too involved and found it hard to cut ties.

The District Superintendent of Nhatrang Region came to see me to ask if I'd allow him to request of Bob Miller in Saigon that I not be transferred to Nhatrang until November or December, but I doubted that that wish would be granted.

I left Quang Ngai on July 2 for Hue, on business for the Canadian team, then flew to Dong Ha for a weekend break before starting my new assignment in Pleiku. Dong Ha is the most northern town in South Vietnam, next to the demilitarized zone (DMZ) or the 17th parallel. At the time, there was one huge refugee camp of over 20,000 refugees living in appalling conditions. Not enough food. There was a very definite need for public health. Three VNCSers, Wayne, Gunnar, and Kevin were busy setting up a school for mechanics for Vietnamese and Montagnards. Early one Saturday morning, two Buddhist monks came to the house to relate a recent happening. It had happened in one of the well-to-do areas of Quang Tri Province. Villagers had gone out to their rice paddies and fields at approximately eight a.m., and North Vietnamese troops had come into their village demanding rice and money. As soon as the American military became aware of this, they strafed the area and completely flattened fifteen villages.

The three VNCSers had been working closely with the Buddhist sect, who had an excellent social service project in the area, using it as a model for the province, helping people to help themselves. The boys also agreed it was one of the most beautiful areas in the I Corps. The narrow lanes had been arched with bamboo and the homes were well structured. Now the homes had been flattened, large jugs used for storing rice were broken with charred rice everywhere, stalks of bamboo in shreds, frayed from the bombs. We did not want to go to see the bombed area, but the monks insisted that if we gave aid, we must see where it goes. There were 250 families, homeless and hungry.

The two monks had come to the house to request any assistance we could give. We did not have food, clothing, or medicine, but Kevin said we could go to the American Marine dump where good pieces of wood could be salvaged. When we got there, the only lumber to be seen were empty ammunition boxes from various sizes of rockets. The boxes were still intact, including the casings. The whole scenario seemed paradoxical. The Americans bomb one day, and then, we, supposedly acting as a reconciling force, could only provide rocket boxes! Later, we were able to scrounge some flour, bulgur, cooking oil, and some US surplus commodities.

In a nutshell, the North Vietnamese Army did no harm to the villages, but the Americans bombed and completely destroyed fifteen villages: seventeen civilians were killed, four North Vietnamese killed, and 250 families left with nothing. The horror of war!

I had to return to Danang via a military flight. To get manifested, I had to say what organization I was with. When I answered with, "Vietnam Christian Service," I knew I would either get a negative response or appreciation for being helpful. The nineteen- or twenty-year-old young man responded immediately, "I've been reading the Old Book (Bible) lately. I never used to read it back home. I used to make fun of Christianity, but I've seen what this war has done to many guys and war's not the answer." In further conversation, he mentioned that most of the guys in his unit smoked pot, many deliberately killed Vietnamese civilians while out on operation, and that they were still looking for the answer.

Transfer to Pleiku Hospital

On July 6, 1970, I arrived in Pleiku. I had hitched a ride from the American Air Base into town, where I hired a Lambretta to the hospital. The team was surprised to see me because they didn't know I was coming.

Dr. Kleinbach, her husband, Russ, and their child were scheduled to leave for the US in two weeks. We shared the unit house with Akiie (Aki) Ninomiya, a twenty-three-year-old from Tokyo, Japan, who was the unit coordinator. He looked after the unit and hospital finances, the generator, broken down vehicles, supplies, etc. His reason for serving was due to the Japanese involvement during WWII and they were responsible for taking many Vietnamese lives.

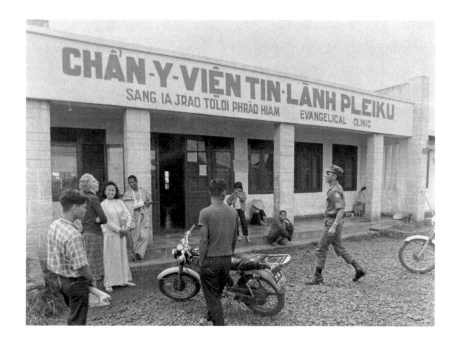

Pleiku Evangelical Clinic.

We were expecting Dr. Joanne Smith T., from Saigon, to fill in until Dr. Margaret Fast, from Manitoba, would arrive on July 29. Zelma, a black nurse from the US, was assigned to the hospital. We shared evening and night duty. I asked her one day if she wasn't afraid to be on call at night. Without skipping a beat, she answered, "If I keep my eyes closed, they will never find me!"

I was primarily working in the outpatient clinic: surgery and organizing the warehouse. Other VNCS members included Sally, our public health nurse, and Reverend and Mrs. Workman, who worked in agriculture. They all lived two blocks down the hill in a duplex.

One day, when our unit members were gone to say farewell to Dr. Kleinbach, Russ and family at the airport, our house was broken into. They came in through my bedroom window, prying off the shutter, breaking a board, and pulling a steel bar out. My stolen possessions included a small transistor radio, my camera, $30 US, $10 in Vietnamese piasters, and $2 Canadian. Besides that, they stole three other radios, a small tape recorder, two cameras and about $200 in Japanese currency. We knew it was the Army of the Republic of Vietnam (ARVN) by the foot tracks. Apparently, this had happened several months ago too. Fortunately, they didn't take any of my clothes.

I knew what to expect at the hospital because I had filled in for the nurses in February, but it was still a real learning curve. Because Vietnamese discriminated against the tribal people, referring to them as 'moi' which means 'savages', the outpatient clinic treated Vietnamese in the morning and tribal people in the afternoon. This meant that I needed an interpreter for the afternoon, which generally worked well.

Montagnards lead a nomadic life, living in outlying villages and walking to the clinic. They relied on bartering in town for their needs. They were basically self-sufficient, raising their own chickens, pigs, vegetables, and rice. They had a school in their villages teaching up to fourth grade. I soon learned that they were hard-working honest people with a great sense of humour. I wished I could have communicated in their Jarai and Bahnar languages.

When Montagnards came to the clinic, they needed to register to open a file. One would think that would be easy, but as nomads they generally did not know their age, full name, or address. It was a challenge even for our Bahnar receptionist, who spoke both languages.

When it came to dispensing medicine, one had to say to take a pill when the sun came up, or when it was shining directly above, or when it set. I was really impressed with a patient who said that he noticed ants came where he had just urinated. He was diabetic! I soon discovered that they too, like the Vietnamese, wanted to die at home if recovery was unlikely so that their spirit would not feel lost and roam.

Our unit house was situated on top of a hill overlooking the hospital and the town of Pleiku. Directly across the road was an ARVN artillery division that fired every evening, with the cannons vibrating our whole house and rattling the windows. Above us was a military radio station that was a target, as was the ARVN artillery base across from us. Even if you were sleeping soundly, you learned very quickly to distinguish between the sounds of incoming and outgoing artillery. Aki worked very hard with his assistant to make a large bunker outside our back door. In the end, Dr. Margaret Fast, Aki and I, decided that we would never have the courage to run outside to the bunker if attacked. Aki ended up lining a closet in his bedroom with sand bags, big enough to accommodate the three of us if necessary.

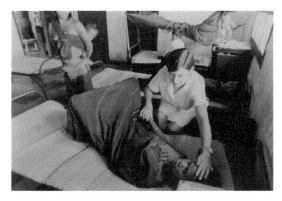

Marcy with Montagnard patient.

Work was very heavy. I had organized and cleaned up the hospital and clinic, then the warehouse. It was tiring going through several years of unfinished work and adjusting to new people and new situations.

Even though Pleiku was not a tourist spot, we did have many international visitors who were interested in learning about the different ethnic groups in the Central Highlands. I wrote about the guests in this letter home.

In early September we had a rash of VNCS guests from Saigon, including Hiro, a Japanese working with 'shoe shine boys,' homeless boys in Saigon. Doug was down from Dak To over the weekend. We had a fun night with Margaret trying to do the limbo. She hadn't done it for some time. After we all had our turns. Aki taught us some judo—just in case, he said. Breakfast conversation frequently revealed that our guests spent part of the night under their beds instead of in them. The loud artillery all night could be nerve racking. Doug shared that security was a major concern in Dak To since several road mines and rocket attacks have been happening as election nears. Gradually, the perimeter was tightening, with complete villages moving closer to town.

Katy came here via Quang Ngai and brought my parcel. What fun unpacking it. We all went wild over the fresh strawberry jam and started a 'fish story' about strawberry

jam by telling Aki that it only took half a Canadian straw-
berry to fill the jar. He said I must tell my mother to send
ten strawberries!

Margaret and I just came back from the town market.
I bought a long black skirt like the Montagnards wear that
can be worn with a blouse or sweater.

We have been invited to the US Air Base for a 'wet' go
away party, but we feel it's best not to identify too closely
with the military because our security rests on our reputa-
tion. Most of the US Air Force will leave Pleiku by the end
of December. Sally came back from Saigon saying there is
a German nurse in language study who will be assigned to
Pleiku. Katy just left for Canada.

If the MYF is interested in a project, would they like to
raise funds for a pressure cooker, which we need to sterilize
our supplies for cataract surgery? We could probably buy
one in Singapore when someone goes through. Brenda,
would you entertain the idea of coming to Vietnam for a
short stint as a volunteer?

Tonight, September 15, the children at the orphanage down
the hill are getting ready for the Mid-Autumn Festival. They
had their little torches lit and a whole line of them composed a
dragon, wearing a huge dragon head. They paraded down the
street beating their drums to an old Vietnamese song. Aki and
I went for a walk down the road to follow them. Tomorrow
is really the festival day, but it's apparently the custom for
the dragon to go out and ask for money. You are supposed to
pass money through the dragon's mouth. I never knew this
because at Nhatrang, the children were never allowed outside
the orphanage property. We were rather embarrassed because
neither one of us had any money with us. The kids couldn't
figure out who we were.

The greater part of a week's vacation was spent at
Nhatrang. It was wonderful to get back and see famil-
iar faces, talk with friends, and see how the hospital has

changed. Yong, a Bahnar Montagnard who has been with the Pleiku Hospital from the beginning, flew with me to Nhatrang. As I have mentioned previously, there is much prejudice between the Montagnards and Vietnamese. It did Yong a lot of good to meet some of the competent Vietnamese staff at Nhatrang. I think he used me as a scapegoat for his feelings toward the Vietnamese, so I'm glad he saw how much the Vietnamese meant to me.

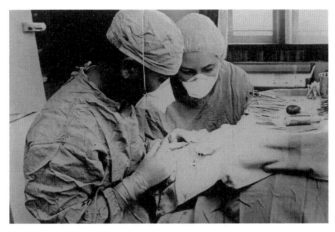

Yong doing cataract surgery with Marcy assisting.

I did have an ulterior motive for taking Yong to Nhatrang. He was Bahnar with only grade four education, but he spoke seven languages! He was a very committed Christian and was hired at Pleiku Hospital as an interpreter for Dr. Luez, who studied cataract surgery with Dr. Gehman in Nhatrang. When Dr. Leuz returned to Pleiku to do cataract surgery, he had Yong assist him: then, recognizing Yong's potential, he arranged for Yong to study and assist with cataract surgery with an American Dr. at 71st Evacuation Hospital in Pleiku. When Dr. Luez left, Yong's ability was recognized by Vietnamese doctors in town, who started to refer their patients to him. I had worked in the operating room in Canada and felt capable of teaching Yanh, a bright Bahnar girl, to assist Yong. They made an excellent team and never had a complication during my time in Pleiku. My dream for Yong was to become an "Y si", the Vietnamese equivalent to a nurse practitioner, which did come to pass.

I continued my correspondence:

Aki came to join Yong and I in Nhatrang on Friday, where we visited the Ponagar temple tower at Thap Ba, an ancient Khmer temple complex built between the eighth and eleventh centuries by the Champa beside the first bridge. Because its history was written in Chinese characters, Aki could read it and told me more about it in twenty minutes than I ever knew during my term there. He had also studied much about Southeast Asian architecture because his uncle was an anthropologist. We also visited the big Buddha, went snorkeling, and saw beautiful tropical fish. Aki also brought a radio and camera that Dr. Smith T. had bought for me as a gift because mine had been stolen in Pleiku.

The next morning, Aki, Yong, and I left Nhatrang by bus for Qui Nhon, where we stayed with Anh Tin's parents: Anh Tin was a former staff member at Nhatrang. After arriving around noon time, we walked into town with Yong carrying my camera, which he had wound tightly around one hand. Suddenly, two young boys came by on a motorbike and tried to get the camera from Yong, which he had to let go or they would have dragged him down the street. He was really upset, and I was a little too. Yong decided to go home, and Aki and I went to the market. On the way home, the same two boys on the motorbike swiped my Montagnard shoulder bag that had 5,000 piasters, my ID card, good earrings, the cross jewelry from my sister, our laboratory drug order, and our bus tickets for Pleiku the next day. Earlie,r they had tried to pickpocket Aki's back pocket, so I kept his money in my shoulder bag, but, fortunately, he had just taken it out or we would not have had any money to get back to Anh Tin's parents' home. It had all happened so fast. We had to return before three p.m. because we were told that the NLF came into town around four and they are not allowed to have foreigners in their home. We did not carry on a conversation and were confined to a room until morning.

Regarding a possible trip for Brenda, I will write to Paul Longacre in Akron and question VNCS Director, Bob Miller, whether it could be considered a voluntary service assignment.

In October, Dr. Margaret made a quick trip to Saigon regarding medical business because the Vietnamese government was making it so difficult to access needed drugs.

One Tuesday morning about three a.m., I heard a car drive up the lane: then a pounding on the door. It half frightened me to death because earlier in the evening we had had a drunken Montagnard come to our house knocking on the windows. But this turned out to be an ambulance from 71st Evacuation Hospital, the American military hospital where we took patients for consultations. They said that Gloria, our VNCS worker in Kontum, had been shot at twelve-thirty, and she had been evacuated by helicopter to Pleiku. She was asking for Zelma to come and see her as soon as possible so Margaret and Aki drove down the street to get Zelma at her house, then drove out to the hospital. They knew it was not safe to travel at this time but they went anyway, knowing the circumstances.

Gloria had been critically shot high in the spine: they were giving her blood. Zelma accompanied her by helicopter to a larger American military hospital in Qui Nhon, under the care of a neurosurgeon. At seven a.m. they did spinal surgery, but her spinal cord had been severed, and she was paralyzed from the neck down. By mid-morning, her mediastinum was widening so they did major chest surgery. They were unable to locate the bullet, but she was obviously bleeding from a major blood vessel. She had a tracheotomy and was on the bird respirator, which was keeping her alive; but she was in no condition to be evacuated to the United States. Zelma stayed with her because they had a special relationship. Apparently, Gloria was alert and aware of what was happening.

This was a very difficult time for us in Pleiku to lose another VNCS staff person. I wrote home about how we were struggling.

Sadly, Gloria passed away at the Qui Nhon military hospital on October 22. Zelma has now gone to Saigon in hopes of accompanying the body back to Kansas. Because it will take seven to ten days for clearance, she will likely be gone about three weeks. I hope to take some vacation when she returns. Vietnam has been getting to me recently. I am getting short with people for no reason at all: just weary I guess.

I was fascinated to learn that my sister, Brenda, had seen a movie on North Vietnam. I suspected that it was propaganda, but I agreed that the Americans should pull out. They were just prolonging the war. Too many lives were being lost: people imprisoned without trial month after month, year after year. Atrocities will always happen when there's war, but it was so much worse there because the war was so dragged out. Historically, POWs have usually been released in several years, but in Vietnam the war went on for twenty plus years.

It really bothered me to go with the Quaker doctor to the political prison in Quang Ngai—mothers and children imprisoned only because they happened to be in a free fire zone when they weren't supposed to be. Planes flying over villages, giving them twenty-four hours' notice to leave their homes, and if they didn't, the consequences were either to be killed or arrested. Unfortunately, many villagers had been in that position and many of the women in the prison had been arrested. They had been accused of supporting the NLF and were arrested when, in fact, they just did not want to abandon their ancestor's spirits on their soil.

At this time, I was getting into a serious relationship with Aki, another unit member assigned to the same project in Pleiku. In a letter to my sister Brenda, I explained how delicate the situation was:

I am glad that you are still thinking about coming over because I think it would do a lot of good for more young people to see how the underprivileged live. It would change their outlook on life. There are several possible scenarios that are undecided at this time that would determine the best time to come—likely after you finish Grade 12.

Confidentially, I am seriously considering marrying Aki. Please keep this confidential within the immediate family— if it gets back to our administration in Saigon indirectly, I might find myself going back to Quang Ngai! I don't know how my family would feel about me marrying an Oriental. Aki is really very Western in many ways and even in much of his thinking. Marrying him would likely mean spending most of my life in Southeast Asia. He has studied law and wants to be a social worker, which means an additional two years of university. After that he would like to join the staff at Japan Church World Service.

When Bob Miller comes tomorrow, I'll inquire as to how you could fit in the VNCS program.

Nights in Pleiku in November can be cool. I am enjoying the heat of the fireplace burning up all kinds of trash. Much has happened since my last letter. With Sally leaving next weekend, her replacement has arrived. Ursula is a German nurse who has spent ten months in Danang with a Catholic religious order and has a three-year commitment with VNCS.

I had plans for a two-week vacation in Singapore with Martin Rock, VNCS's Secretary, until Ursula brought my mail from Saigon. There was an invitation to Das's wedding in Calcutta, India, on December 5. Because the date matches my vacation time, Martin and I decided to surprise Das, if we can get our visas on time.

Dr. Margaret has not returned from her meeting in Nhatrang about ordering drugs. Soon we will not be able to order them through the Vietnamese government. Our twenty-bed hospital is overflowing, and we see about 100-125 patients per day in the outpatient clinic.

As planned, I went to Das's wedding in Calcutta with Martin Rock. Das had been our lab technician in Nhatrang. It was a lovely wedding, and it was great to see Das again. After shopping and sightseeing in Calcutta,

Martin and I flew to Singapore and spent a week there. I had forgotten how relaxed it can be in a normal situation—no war, people were happy. Singapore was so clean and orderly, traffic followed the rules: everything was green, fresh with flowers, and people spoke English. We took a boat trip to an island and had a picnic lunch there. We spent two afternoons at the Botanical Gardens reading and feeding the monkeys, saw *The Sound of Music* and *Romeo and Juliet*, and went ten pin bowling.

I returned in time for the hectic Christmas season. There were so many church programs, including our hospital's. Christmas morning, we decided to go with Yong (our medical assistant) to his Bahnar village. The VW was loaded down and as we drove out the lane, Aki said, "What if we have a flat tire?" We would be far away from villages, and our jack and tools had recently been stolen. We pulled into the gas station and, lo and behold, we had a flat tire. We eventually found someone who had a wrench that fit, but we had lost precious time and we got to the village very late. The service was outside a little wooden church with just a few benches near the fence. We were in our dry season with gusts of red dust continually. Although we understood nothing of the service, it was very interesting. They had a little skit with Mary, Joseph, the king, wisemen, and shepherds. It really amused me when the king appeared dressed in a pink housecoat, obviously from a missionary barrel.

A parcel from home arrived just before Christmas with lots of goodies. We all enjoyed the cherry filled chocolates and chocolate bars.

Aki left for Japan on December 27. As the eldest son, it was important for him to be there for the burial of his father's ashes at a Buddhist temple to commemorate the one-year anniversary of his death. He also wanted to talk to his mother about me and get her reaction.

I planned to write Paul Longacre a letter to get his thoughts on Brenda's possible visit. The big question was, was it worth spending the money for a two-month visit? Another thing to think about was security. Things were tightening up in our area, Kontum, fifty km north, and Dak To, northwest of Kontum. Our two VNCSers told us the perimeter was closing in: Tet was getting closer and action was expected sometime just before or after the holiday. Pleiku was near the Laotian/Cambodian border and there were North Vietnamese infiltrating the area. They were expecting them to try to have a military victory in the highlands to push their advantage in the Paris Peace talks. With the Americans leaving the area, we could feel it.

My letter to Paul Longacre, dated January 3, 1971:

> *Dear Paul, I trust you are sitting when you receive this letter. After two years of waiting, the shock may be too great! It is once again the time of year here in Vietnam when Tet is less than a month away. Candied sweets are appearing in the market: bright plastic flowers are available at every little stand and the prices are all rising. Because it is traditional to wear new clothes for Tet, Margaret and I, your representatives at Pleiku, took the opportunity to buy your 'Tet' suit at the market, all five yards of it. 'Mung Xuan Moi' (Happy New Year) to our 'Guam Doc My' (American Director). If you need instructions on how to put it on, we will send it in a plain brown wrapper marked 'Personal' (the gift was a Montagnard loincloth).*
>
> *It hardly seems possible that I've been here for six months. The work at Quang Ngai was interesting and a challenge. I found the people there much cooler: more anti-Western than anywhere else I have been in Vietnam. My being somewhat accustomed to the country and the advantage of speaking some Vietnamese certainly were in my favour.*
>
> *In May 1970, Doug Cook came to Quang Ngai, wondering whether I'd consider filling in at Pleiku until November. After considerable thought, it only seemed reasonable that our VNCS projects take priority before going on loan to another organization. I guess my conscience pricked me toward going to Pleiku because it is more MCC than VNCS administered. It always appeared to have terrific potential, but never got on its feet after the Tet Offensive in '68.*
>
> *The name MCC seems to mean more stability to the nationals and missionaries. Public relations are good with the national church, missionaries, the provincial hospital and the team there. The 71st Evacuation Hospital closed its doors to nationals at the end of November, which has*

eliminated considerable running around for Aki. It had provided an excellent source for medical consultations for Margaret, who found it difficult to be the only doctor. At the same time, it was difficult for Aki, who has definite feelings about identifying so closely with the American forces, the same question that has always been posed. We opt to associate only as much as is necessary for medical work.

The Jarai young people from the church near the hospital painted the inside of our hospital as a project. They did a terrific job. You would probably see a tremendous change in the whole compound. The warehouse is in order and the house still has plumbing problems. Don't they all in Vietnam? The hospital is full, plus the guest house: the average census has been running around thirty-two. In the outpatient clinic we see 120 to 140 persons per day, the majority still being Vietnamese, although more Montagnards are coming. What a challenge to see it pick up during my six months here.

Yong has been doing eye surgery. He's very good and fast. He was in the process of studying at 71st Evacuation Hospital when I arrived in July. Since November he has been doing cataracts on his own with a doctor supervising. We're presently investigating the possibility of him taking a nurse practitioner course at the University in Saigon.

We've got an outstanding number of good workers and staff. They are conscientious, and if they're asked to do something, you know it will be done. Goodness, it sounds like I'm getting biased too. Montagnard prejudice against Vietnamese.

Aki is doing an excellent job. Considering he's a city guy, it's amazing he's so mechanically minded. Dr. Margaret and I still have to push the VW van in the morning before going to the clinic to get it started. If it wouldn't be for Wayne Kiem's old salvaged Jeep, we'd be up a creek. By all appearances, security is much the same, although some people say things are tightening up. Time will tell.

Three weeks ago, I returned from a vacation to Calcutta and Singapore with Martin Rock. We went to Das's wedding because he had no family to support him. He was surprised and pleased to have two familiar faces from Vietnam. After a week in Singapore, it felt good to get back to Pleiku and its red dust.

I have an eighteen-year-old sister, Brenda, who is keenly interested in coming to Vietnam next summer for approximately two months. She will have just completed Grade 12. I made the suggestion to her and my family that she come, after having observed what the C & M A did this past summer. They had five young girls, some of them nurses: one, who came for two months at her own expense, with the mission providing room and board, was considering nursing. Two of the girls who were assigned to Pleiku were surprised by what mission work entailed and felt that they had gained much from this experience.

Would MCC consider such a project worthwhile? The girls last summer worked with persons with leprosy with their handicrafts and sorting clothing in a warehouse. I would be interested in your reaction.

Happy New Year to you! Greetings to Doris and family.

Awaiting your reply,
Marcy Weber

Paul's response dated January 12, 1971.

I appreciated reading about your very positive comments about the way the hospital program is developing. Also, the good way that you have been able to maintain relationships with Pastor Sang and the establishment there.

Your comments on Aki's contribution and activities are interesting. Keep working on him. We need more

Mennonites in Japan. I am pleased to hear that your team has developed a good team spirit.

Your comments about the quality of staff is also very favourable. This good quality of national staff will move the Pleiku medical project ahead many strides.

Thank you for the gift. I took it home to try and put it on so I could model it sometime. Doris grabbed it when I brought it into the house and said it would make a perfect wall hanging. That's where it is now. The colours just match our living room. I'll try to get it back during Tet for one wearing.

I received a letter from Doris and Das after their marriage. They expressed real appreciation for your coming to their wedding.

Concerning the possibility of your sister Brenda visiting you: I received a letter from Doug Snyder in the MCC office, Kitchener on this too. Your family has talked to Doug about it. You and your family will need to evaluate the cost of this two-month trip over the value it will be for your sister. Through your wide experiences, the Weber family has been broadened to the need for and opportunities of overseas service. Will a two-month visit add enough to compensate for the expense? This is a question you and your family will need to answer.

I am confident that between the Chan-Y-Vien Tin Lanh and Tin Lanh leprosarium you will be able to find meaningful work for Brenda during her short stay. I gave a copy of my letter to Doug Snyder, and to Bob Miller, and I'm also copying him on this letter. I would like him to react to this visit. You probably have discussed it with him already.

Doug asked about the cost. I told him that we could not provide anything toward the travel costs. We could provide the cost of lodging while in Pleiku and possibly board. I suggested you and Bob work out the final details.

I understand that no final decision has been made on
whether Brenda will come to visit you. You have discussed
the possibility with your family and are evaluating the pros
and cons of it. We appreciate being requested for counsel at
this early stage.
    God's blessings to you and Margaret for the New Year.

Paul Longacre,
Director for Asia

Yong continued performing cataract surgeries. Yanh assisted, and I circulated, making sure that they had everything they needed. It was encouraging to see the work expand and the standards raised. Everyone who visited
remarked how clean it was, which was truly a compliment at that time of
year in the dry season when there were clouds of red dust most of the time.

To give you an idea of my life outside work, let me tell you about where
I was living. One night, I sat at home alone in the kitchen because it was
the only place with electricity in the house. It was the eeriest feeling to
stay in that large dark house with all kinds of noises, a strong wind and
artillery being fired from next door. There were so many windows in the
house and they were not tight. The night before, the regulator broke for
the electric voltage and the Vietnamese couldn't fix it, so Mr. Workman
hooked up the water pump and one lamp to the generator. It was quite a
mess. We had 110 volts in the house and 220 in the hospital. I would be
glad when Aki returned and could look after the generator. I had been
looking after the unit and hospital finances while he was gone, as well as
the maintenance - buying barrels of diesel fuel for the generator, butagas
for cooking and kerosene. Invariably, every time I went to buy them, they
were out of butagas or the truck from Saigon has not arrived yet or there
was no electricity to pump the fuel. Two more days and Aki would be back.

On January 19, I wrote:

The hospital has slowed down considerably. Now that Aki
is back it takes a load off me. No more finances or running
around for fuel. Fortunately, we had one running vehicle to

pick him up at the airport. The generator died two nights after he returned.

Tet is February 12, so the clinic is slowing down. We've had so many injured civilians come since Montagnard villages are being mortared. Recently, I really had to question the value of Western people being in Vietnam. Perhaps if we all left this war would finish sooner. Security is becoming a concern. Proof that it's not just rumours is that large refugee camps are being created with 3,000-4,000 persons per camp. People have nothing and it has been so cold.

Ursula, our German public health nurse, discovered a camp when en route to another village. She has since gone out to help several times. Eighty persons died in two days from cholera. So tragic! Originally, this village was located only ten kilometres away from our hospital. We have been protected until now and pray for continued protection.

On March 20, 1971, I wrote:

Many Montagnard villages are being moved by ARVN troops via helicopter and dropped on pieces of land that have no grass or trees, just barren hills. No protection from the elements. Pleiku is one of the camps with 5,000 refugees. They've been there for almost four weeks without any commodities provided by the government, like rice, meat, housing: no decent water supply—no sanitation! Finally, they were given some corrugated tin, due to the cold weather, but, in reality, it made them more visible and a target for shelling. At one point, forty people died in two days due to dysentery, malnutrition, dehydration, etc. Ursula has been going out to the camps, but we are not medically equipped to handle this situation: not enough staff or medicines. Zelma isn't back yet from vacation, and Ursula has been bringing in ten to twelve patients a day. Previously, we had twenty-nine beds in the hospital, but, when Zelma returned, we had sixty inpatients. Intravenous was hanging from nails on the walls with two to three patients in a bed. It was chaos!

I made a quick trip to Saigon and met several agencies with Bob Miller, such as Asian Christian Service, World Vision, and USAID, to scrounge medicines and personnel. Miraculously, ACS had closed their unit in the Mekong Delta and we received a significant amount of their drugs. MCC agreed to send more medical supplies, meat, and refugee relief, such as blankets and clothing, too because we had depleted our stock in the warehouse. Within two days three shipments arrived at Pleiku airport. Thank God.

We desperately need IVs in the hospital. Miracle of miracles! The 71st Evacuation Hospital made an error in ordering their medical supplies, so they gave us a Land Rover full of them.

Aki is in Saigon getting treatment for a whiplash injury he sustained in December when an American GI gave his Jeep a push to get it started. Unknown to Aki, the American was high on drugs and gave a major jolt, resulting in a whiplash injury that wasn't apparent initially. It has been aggravated by his job here in Pleiku, which requires him to do everything that he is not supposed to, such as turning his neck to drive, heavy lifting, no tension, etc. Hopefully, the physiotherapy treatment in Saigon will be helpful and he can return next weekend. He is due back on April 1.

VNCS and USAID Public Health Department have filed a report protesting the abuse and neglect of the Montagnards by the Vietnamese. The Vietnamese government originally promised commodities and medical services that never materialized. The government plans to add about 5,000 more people to this camp and create three to four more similar camps. According to other sources, this is also happening in several other highland provinces.

The VNCS and USAID file was discovered by the Vietnamese military because it also made headlines in Time *magazine. We had a high-ranking Vietnamese military official visit us, inquiring if we had reported the refugee camp situation. Aki said no, but he threatened us, saying we would be in danger if we did not keep quiet. Later, we discovered that a temporary camp had been set up with all the commodities to show reporters that the previous report was unfounded!*

Security and the war are very fluctuant now. We have several new refugee camps in the area with extremely poor environmental conditions—no food. They are eating weeds, there's scanty dirty water, no security: people are so sick that anywhere from four to ten people die each day during the few hours Ursula can be in the camp.

We have sorted clothing and blankets for the camps. There have been mines planted on the roads going to the camps: I say roads, but, really, just a few tracks across open fields. Vehicles have been blown up by landmines. Knowing this, we placed sandbags on the floor of our vehicle as protection. One morning Ursula, Bill Herod, and Mr. Workman went to the C & M A missionaries' home to borrow their megaphone to use at the camp, which made them about ten minutes later than scheduled. A military Jeep hit the land mine that was meant for our vehicle.

Aki noticed a bullet hole in Ursula's vehicle. We knew that the time had come that we had to debrief Saigon office on our present situation. They made the decision that we can no longer go to the refugee camps. This is so painful because we know these people are not having their medical needs met. Are we to treat patients in the hospital, and then after recovery, take them back to die? It is genocide, but our hands are tied.

Holy Week in Pleiku

Our experience during Holy Week is still vivid in my memory.

On Saturday, April 3, the day before Palm Sunday, Dr. Margaret went to Saigon for one month of Vietnamese language study and Dr. Allen Stuckey, his wife, Jeannie, and their son, Jonathan, arrived from Nhatrang to cover during Dr. Margaret's study.

Our outpatient clinic was very busy on Good Friday morning for the Vietnamese. Because military personnel generally went to their own clinics, it was unusual to see a Vietnamese military officer come with his young daughter to be seen. He was very insistent she be seen immediately, and he circumvented the system by walking into the doctor's office when he was examining another patient. Dr. Stuckey kindly informed him to please wait his turn because his daughter did not appear seriously ill. When the officer realized that the doctor would not change his mind, he left in a huff.

The Stuckeys, our guests, Ron Ackerman from Dak To and Bill Herod from Saigon, were sitting around the unit's dinner table around eight p.m., chatting, when a Vietnamese military officer entered the house through the unlocked door through the kitchen. Aki and I were in his room and at first unaware that anyone had entered the house, until Aki and I heard a voice shouting "Oi."

Aki exited his room and saw a Vietnamese military officer. Aki asked what was going on and was promptly told by Bill to sit down and put his hands on the table like everyone else, which he did. Apparently, the officer, who spoke good English, had been trying to convince Dr. Stuckey to go to his home for a meal to say thank you. Dr. Stuckey had been politely refusing his request until Aki had appeared. The officer, becoming a bit nervous, pulled out his revolver, released the pin, walked over behind Dr. Stuckey, and pushed the gun into his neck saying he had to go with him. Sensing something was very wrong, Dr. Stuckey still didn't want to go, until Bill told him that he should do so.

As that was happening, I appeared to see a young Vietnamese soldier, standing with a gun, facing the table. As I stood in front of him, I asked, "Ong muon gi day?" (What do you want here?) He replied, "Khong biet." (I don't know) I said, "Khong biet?" (You don't know?)

As Dr. Stuckey was led out by the officer, I told the soldier covering me that he didn't have permission to do this, which was a crazy thing to say. I tried to follow, but the gun pointed at me was real, so I stopped. The officer escorting Dr. Stuckey out the door hollered, "Do not leave this house because soldiers are guarding outside."

We then heard a Jeep start and a gunshot as it drove away. In a state of shock, we locked our kitchen door and turned off the lights. I was designated to tell Jeannie that her husband had been taken at gunpoint. We decided that someone had to report this to our unit leader, Mr. Workman, who lived two blocks away. After looking out our windows for any movement or activity for at least fifteen minutes, Bill and Ron volunteered to go to report to Mr. Workman. They walked out of the house with their hands behind their heads, then quickly drove to the Workman's, who insisted that this needed to be reported at Military Assistance Command Vietnam (MACV), near the airport. About an hour later, Bill and Ron returned to our house as we continued to wait in darkness behind our locked doors.

Suddenly, a motorbike drove right up to our back door. We heard, "It's Dr. Stuckey. Let me in," in perfect English. We were unsure if it really was him, but it was! He had been beaten, had wounds on his face, a bloodstained shirt, and no eyeglasses. He said that he hoped no one had reported what had happened or our lives were in danger.

We told him we had reported it, so Bill and Aki quickly drove to Workman's to report that Dr. Stuckey had returned, and then went on to MACV to request that this incident not be reported further because we had been threatened. Needless to say, nobody slept that night: we were all on alert.

The next morning, Dr. Stuckey asked Aki to take him to a cemetery, a good block down the hill, to look for his eyeglasses and wrist watch.

I was designated to phone Saigon to report this incident to Bob Miller. Because we did not have a telephone, we needed to use a phone at MACV. When I tried to make the call in English, the Vietnamese operator would not connect me, so I decided to hang up and try speaking in Vietnamese. She connected me right away. Bob was stunned with the news and agreed to come to Pleiku as soon as possible.

Bob Miller appeared in Pleiku on the Monday and interviewed each one of us about the incident. It was agreed, on Aki's recommendation, that

Dr. Stuckey return to Nhatrang as soon as possible for everyone's safety. We were told not to report or talk about the incident with anyone. So, within days, Dr. Joanne Smith T. arrived to cover until Dr. Margaret would return.

In 1973, we had a VNCS reunion in the US. Everyone was billeted in different homes, and Dr. Allen Stuckey said that Aki and I must stay at his parents' home to hear his and his family's side of the story related to this incident.

Allen said that when he had been taken at gunpoint, he was driven to a Buddhist cemetery with his hands tied behind his back, forced onto his knees, and the four soldiers who had been in the Jeep were ordered to beat him, which they were hesitant to do until forced. Allen was questioned by the officer if he knew why he was being beaten. He didn't, until the officer told him. The reason was that Dr. Stuckey had refused to see his daughter immediately in the clinic that morning. The officer finally agreed to let him go if he promised not to tell anyone about what happened. Then the officer and four soldiers drove off in their Jeep. Allen said that he had a vision of Jesus and how he had been beaten. This was the evening of Good Friday. Believing that he was not alone, he started walking toward the entrance gate of the cemetery, when he had a vision that his mother knew something had happened to him. He was met by people living across the road who wanted to cleanse his wounds. He refused, but he asked for a ride to Chan-y-Vien Tin Lanh (our hospital), but, due to a misunderstanding, he was driven on motorbike to the Jarai church down the road first, then kindly driven to our unit house.

On Easter Sunday, when Allen had worshipped at the Jarai church, he had a strange feeling in his throat while reciting the Lord's Prayer. He discovered later that he had received the gift of speaking in tongues on Easter morning.

Apparently, at the same time that Allen was being beaten in the cemetery in Vietnam, his father was going up the steps in the barn in Kansas at six-thirty a.m. on Good Friday to feed the chickens, when he heard a voice saying, "Allen needs your prayers." He stopped and looked around, but he didn't see any one, so he continued going up the steps when he heard a voice say, "Right now." Frightened, he knelt by a bale of straw and prayed for Allen. He felt something had happened to his son and waited for news from Vietnam, but nothing came. On Allen's first Christmas home, he related the whole experience to his family. Then his aunt shared how she had been vacuuming at home when she felt that she had to pray for Allen at the same time that he was being beaten.

Later, we pieced the puzzle together. The Vietnamese colonel that did this had studied for two years in the States, had been treated disrespectfully, and was angry that he could not have his daughter seen immediately in the clinic. The thing was, Dr. Stuckey was just being fair, not rude. We also discovered that he lived at the base across the road from us!

In a conversation with Dr. Stuckey in 2020, he still vividly remembered what I had said to the soldier covering me, telling him that he didn't have permission to do this.

The incident has had a lasting impact on Dr. Stuckey: little was known about Post Traumatic Stress Disorder (PTSD) at that time. He said that when he wants to talk to God, he goes into a room alone and speaks in tongues, which gives him a feeling of peace. He regrets that he cannot share about this gift with his home congregation, feeling they would not understand. I might react in the same way as his congregation if I had not known Allen personally. I now believe in the gift of speaking in tongues.

The day after Easter, an Indonesian nurse and a Vietnamese nurse arrived with their personnel director. They were staff of ACS, our sister organization, that had discontinued many of its projects in the Mekong Delta and was at that point primarily providing finances for other existing programs. They were coming as a result of my frantic visit to Saigon to recruit staff and medicine for a refugee camp.

Then in mid-May, I received good news from home and replied immediately.

> *Yesterday, I was shocked and delighted to receive a thick letter from home containing the news that Brenda has decided to come to Vietnam this summer. Wonderful news! I was already making plans for a vacation to Bangkok in June, which I will change to dovetail with plans of her visit. This will mean applying for a passport, then a visa—a two-month one saying she is a volunteer would be best, and*

immunizations for smallpox, typhoid and paratyphoid, cholera, and plague—we are treating contaminated cases in the hospital at present, mostly people coming in from refugee camps. I am getting excited already. In regards to travel plans, Menno Travel Service, Ephrata, Pennsylvania, will help. Brenda does not have to be afraid to travel alone because I have contacts.

So much has happened since my last letter. First, Aki is being transferred to Saigon indefinitely because of his whiplash injury. Secondly, Dr. Margaret developed hepatitis while in language study. She is continuing to study and doing quite well. Thirdly, we now have an Indian doctor, Dr. Pradan, a reinforcement from ACS, as well as Mars, a Filipino to replace Aki, which makes me the only Western person in the unit. With all these changes, it has been difficult and tiring. I also have the added responsibility of being the unit leader. On Friday, I will fly to Saigon to take an orphaned Montagnard boy to a psychiatric residential setting, to talk over problems in Pleiku with Dr. Margaret and the administration and to attend a Memorial Service for Ted, a VNCSer.

Ted was a social worker assigned to Di Linh, who had started an agricultural project with the Koho tribespeople. The success of the project caught the attention of the local Vietnamese. Two weeks after Ted was married, their house was unexpectedly entered when the village was attacked, and he was shot. The two girls and Ted's wife hid in a closet so they were not discovered. Fortunately for Terry, another VNCSer, he was not at home that evening, so his life was also spared. It hit me that of the trio, I was the only one left alive. Both Ted and Gloria made the ultimate sacrifice being in Vietnam.

Rainy season is coming soon, thankfully, because we are almost out of water at the hospital. One reason is the Montagnards unscrew the taps, which depletes the water supply in the water tank. They have never seen water come out of a tap before and are frightened of the 'spirit' coming out of the pipe. Other times, we find tin cans placed in the hole of the squat toilet to prevent the spirit from coming out. One of Aki's jobs was to pour a little water into the well to prime it to pump water into the water tank for the hospital and our home.

Since Aki has been sent to Saigon for treatment for his whiplash injury, and it seems to be getting worse, he will likely be sent back to Japan. As for me, I've never felt more rundown, really in a state of mental and physical exhaustion. It must be obvious to the VNCS administration because they have asked me to leave Pleiku for a few weeks. Our whole unit has changed, which makes it very difficult for the national staff to adjust. I'm at the point where I can't sleep: eating is strictly mechanical with frequent nausea and vomiting. Knowing my present state, I plan on requesting an earlier termination date. I'll be in Saigon on Friday and can talk things over then.

By May 23, I had been in Saigon for one week, on the advice of Bob Miller, for some rest and recuperation. The previous week, I had finally mustered up the courage to inform Bob of my relationship with Aki. He was shocked and, of course, asked many questions—he sort of claimed me as his daughter. He read my written request to terminate at the beginning of November. On reviewing my history with MCC, he felt it would be no problem. Aki would be returning to Japan for further treatment. He was still having pain and would likely terminate with VNCS because he needed long term therapy. The time frame for everything was undecided.

Aki and I met with Mr. Miyazaki, YMCA Director in Vietnam, and his wife, personal friends of Aki's who had done marriage counselling for several international marriages. After talking with each of us individually, they stressed that a timetable was necessary: that Aki and I needed to make some decisions before talking with Bob again. We decided that Aki would finish his term with VNCS: he and Mr. and Mrs. Miyazaki thought it would be great if we got married in August so that Brenda could be there representing my family. But I didn't know if my conscience would allow me to leave MCC on such short notice because they needed time to recruit my replacement.

The time had come to talk with Bob Miller, the VNCS director. I wrote to Brenda about future plans in several letters in May and June.

Tomorrow Aki and I will talk with Bob again and suggest the possibility of me terminating in August. I want to know how my family feels about me marrying Aki. In the future, he wants to pursue studies in theology and social work, most likely in Waterloo. He received letters from Wilfrid Laurier University and Waterloo Lutheran Seminary today.

Aki and I have invited Bob and Jean Miller for a Japanese dinner on May 28 to see how Bob will respond to the possibility of me terminating in August.

Regarding your travel plans Brenda, Bob mentioned that it would be prudent if MCC and my family had an agreement if anything happens, confirming that MCC will not be responsible. We received a telegram that your visa has been issued.

***

I returned to Pleiku today to find a letter with your itinerary, Brenda. I am so glad that you will stay one day with Emma in Vancouver before continuing on to Hong Kong.

Things are moving faster and in a different direction than I ever would have suspected, even a month ago. When Bob was here for a board meeting, two days ago, I asked if I could leave in August. He just about fell over. He said that I deserve to leave, but his only concern is the nursing staff situation at the hospital. Sonia, the Indonesian nurse, would stay until the end of December.

My original plan was to take vacation with you in mid-August, but MCC policy does not allow a vacation when terminating, so that is not an option. If I want to travel with you, it would seem logical to take vacation when coming, otherwise we run into the matter of exit and re-entry visas for Vietnam. To eliminate this issue, I am recommending that you follow your flight schedule to Hong Kong, and Aki will meet you at the airport because he is en route back to Japan. He can help you change your ticket and flight number, apply for a Thai visa and find lodging. I will meet you in Bangkok. We can travel in Thailand for about ten days and stay with my nursing classmate, Donna Patterson, before flying to Saigon. Then I will leave Vietnam with you, travel to Tokyo via Hong Kong. You can enjoy a few days with Aki in Hong Kong, much more interesting than if you are with a Westerner because he can read Chinese—but he can't speak it.

I am officially engaged! I will send out announcements after Aki has copies of our photo developed in Hong Kong. Brenda, now that a wedding is in the picture, bring a good dress and a pair of shoes.

***

I just received a letter from Aki today saying that he will meet you in Hong Kong and make arrangements for you there to travel to Bangkok, Thailand. In the event that there would be a foul up (very remote), Aki will be staying at the Chinese YMCA—there are four in Hong Kong. His full name is Akiie Ninomiya. If you quickly send me your airline, flight number, and date of arrival, I'll pass it on.

I have written to Paul Longacre with a copy to Bob Miller, requesting early termination at the end of August. He will do his best to arrange for me to leave then.

I feel much more like myself now after getting out of Pleiku for two weeks. With the rainy season starting, the clinic has slowed down, and we're working a regular schedule. Things will probably stay at this pace for a couple of months. As long as I can work at this pace, I'll last. The refugee situation is so sad. It is genocide and is heavy on my heart! Zelma leaves for good at the beginning of July, so there'll be more work for me in the hospital, plus extras to get done before leaving. See you in Bangkok!

On Saturday, June 12, Aki arrived in Pleiku for his farewell and soon after, he left for Saigon. It gave us an opportunity to discuss last minute things before he departed for good.

Regarding our wedding, Aki was going to request to have it at the chapel of the International Christian University (ICU) in Tokyo because he knew the chaplain and dean well. We were planning a small wedding of twenty-five to thirty guests because he had a small family and mine would only have Brenda present, with a tea party to follow. We would have a reception in Canada at a later date.

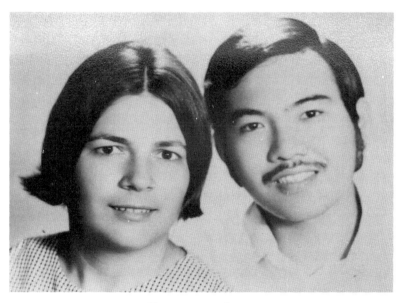

Engagement photo.

A letter that Aki wrote to my family, dated June 15, 1971.

Dear Mr. and Mrs. Weber and family,

I'm very happy to hear that Brenda is coming to Asia and thank you for your hospitality.

I am the happiest boy in the world because I can marry with the nicest girl in the world, Marcy!

International marriages can have many problems but our purpose of life is devotion for our neighbours in the world under God's mission.

I will do my best for Marcy's happiness as much as possible.

We will have our wedding on the fourth of September in Tokyo. I'm sorry that you can't attend, but I'm glad that Brenda can be there.

Now I haven't any fortune, but I have a strong heart, courage, will, and love for God and Marcy.

Please bless our marriage life.

Sincerely yours,
Akiie Ninomiya

Brenda's Visit

On July 11, 1971, Brenda and I arrived in Pleiku from Saigon, much to our relief. We had been booked on Air Vietnam, and the flight was cancelled, so we had rebooked for the next day. We finally boarded the airplane and were ready for take-off when they announced that we needed to disembark; we left two hours later. Poor Mars, who waited at the airport in Pleiku for us!

We had ten days in Bangkok, staying with Donna Patterson, my nursing classmate, and her family. We used public transportation to get around the city to see the Grand Palace, the Temple of Dawn, the famous floating market in the canals in Bangkok, etc. One Saturday, we went to the largest weekend market in Southeast Asia when Brenda needed a toilet. We found a public pit privy set up at the market, and Brenda joined the queue. Her turn finally came. She went in, turned around, and came out saying, "There is only a hole in the ground." I said, "That's it." So, she had to join the queue again. One became so accustomed to things that you forgot what was new to someone coming for the first time.

One day, Donna drove us to the bridge over the River Kwai near the Thai and Burmese border to see and hear its history, as well as an international cemetery en route. There is a movie called *Bridge over the River Kwai* if you want to know more of its history. Brenda and I tried to balance our sightseeing and rest because we were both tired.

Donna introduced me to a seamstress who made my wedding dress for $20 US from lovely ivory coloured Thai silk: I was also able to have a pair of white shoes made to go with it. Until then, my footwear had only included thongs or sandals! I bought a veil later in Japan.

I was waiting for confirmation of the wedding date for September fourth because Brenda's school began September sixth.

Aki and my future plans regarding going to Canada remained undecided, it was looking more likely that it would be spring 1972, pending Aki getting a scholarship and being accepted at Waterloo Lutheran Seminary in Waterloo.

Brenda was too tired to write home about her visit to date so I acted as her scribe and wrote to our parents to let them know that she was still alive.

It's been over a month already since Brenda left Canada. Last weekend she flew with Mars, the Filipino replacing Aki, to Nhatrang to meet the unit members and see the hospital where I worked for four years. She fits right in here, and she seems to be enjoying it.

Yesterday, Dr. Margaret, Brenda, and I went to market, then visited Chi Cuc, a good Thai friend. Brenda had met her sisters when visiting Nhatrang. We then went to the hospital to pick up Dr. Margaret, only to find four women—two were young girls—brought in from Plei Blang Ba refugee camp four km away. Apparently ten or so women were walking down a path to get bamboo sprouts when they hit a landmine. *Two were killed instantly, one died shortly after arriving at our hospital. What a horrible heart wrenching scene. Innocent people are dying all the time, to no avail: all they want is to be able to live, have a place to call home, enough to eat, and peace, but they are deprived of it all!*

This morning we drove out to Yong's Bahnar village. We discovered that new Christians are being persecuted in the village. These dear people have a bleak future with genocide being practiced on the ethnic minorities.

Thank you so much for the money sent with Brenda from the St. Jacobs' Sunday School to purchase a pressure cooker for the hospital. We are most grateful for the support from back home.

Brenda has asked me to write that she went to a leprosarium on Saturday with the C & M A missionaries and their two summer volunteers, then to the Bahnar tribal village today and yesterday: it was the first time for her to see a person die. She also mentioned the crackdown the American military was having on drugs here in Pleiku. All the soldiers are being quarantined on the base for one week to identify the hard users with a new temporary ward opened to accommodate the large number.

All of a sudden, I find myself getting near the end of my term, leaving me with mixed emotions. I really love these people and am not mentally prepared to leave so soon. At the same time, I realize that it's time to go. The hospital is moderately busy now, which gives me time to get everything in order and keep up with the pace.

Aki writes that his neck is getting better with treatment. I keep wondering if he remembers everything in preparation for the wedding. Never dreamt that things would turn out this way. It looks like Anne Falk may be coming to Pleiku for six months while she waits for her visa for Indonesia.

Because Aki has legal family matters to oversee as the eldest son, due to his father's passing, we will not be able

*to go to Canada this year. This is my opportunity to get to
know his family and Japan: anyway, he would not start
university in Canada until September 1972. At this time, it's
not possible to be definite about future plans.*

It was so difficult to know that my time in Vietnam was running out. Staff kept asking when Aki and I would be returning—after the wedding or next year? They couldn't believe it when I said most likely never.

At that point, there were only two and a half weeks left before we left Vietnam for Tokyo. I thought it would be easier leaving Pleiku than Nhatrang, mainly because I didn't have as many Vietnamese friends: many Montagnards, of course, but they were all connected to the hospital. Yong was going to Saigon with us for a four-year nurse practitioner course.

I wanted to go the Jarai church once more before leaving, so Brenda and I went one Sunday, sitting through a service where we did not understand anything.

We were unable to book Brenda's return flight because Canadian Pacific did not have an office in Saigon, so it had to be done in Hong Kong.

The future looked bleak for Vietnam when listening to the South Vietnamese Army and civilians talk and with the presidential election that was happening at the beginning of October.

A letter arrived from Aki saying that everything was in order for the wedding and that all he needed was me.

A letter to my parents dated August 17, 1971:

*Brenda will likely leave Tokyo the evening of September
4 after the wedding, but I will confirm this in Hong Kong
and send a telegram. Just plan on a trip to the airport on
September fifth.*

*On Monday, August 23, the hospital staff had a farewell
party for me at the unit house above the hospital. What
an emotional time. They had spent a month's salary to buy
Coke, steamed rice cakes, and fruit for everyone. They know
how to have a fun time, but it was too painful for me. Yong
presented me with a hand woven Montagnard skirt and top*

from the staff, made by his wife. She had spent a month weaving them, making the top extra big so as to fit me, but it was still too small! What a lesson in giving! People who have so little give so generously. It was sacrificial giving! To graciously accept their sincere gratitude for my short time working with them in Pleiku was truly overwhelming and humbling. I was moved to tears. I was thankful that Brenda could share in this event.

Wednesday, August 25, Mars drove Yong, Brenda, and I to the airport to spend one day in Nhatrang saying goodbye to dear friends, and then the next day, we flew to Saigon for goodbyes there too.

CHAPTER 4

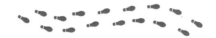

Goodbye Vietnam: New Challenge

On Friday, July 27, Bill Herod drove Brenda and I to the airport in Saigon, bound for Hong Kong. Bill helped us with our luggage and the check in at the counter. I was processed, but when they checked Brenda's passport, there was no exit visa! The VNCS office had failed to get one for her! The airlines would not let her on the flight. Fortunately, Bill was still there and said he would make sure that Brenda would be booked the next day for Hong Kong. I could not believe what was happening, but I trusted Bill. I still do not know to this day how Bill got an exit visa on a Friday afternoon when government offices were closed, but I do know that Brenda arrived in Hong Kong the next day! What a relief, because we were scheduled to fly to Tokyo the following day. At the airport we were able to make Brenda's booking on Canadian Pacific and had Everett Metzler, a missionary based in Hong Kong, send a telegram to my parents.

After Brenda checked into the YMCA with me, she passed on a message from the VNCS office. Brenda did not need a visa as a tourist to Japan, but I needed to have one because I intended to stay in Japan for a longer period of time. Brenda recalls me crying all night thinking that I would not be allowed into Japan for my upcoming wedding.

Sunday, August 29, Brenda and I discovered at the airport that my visa was indeed not an issue to enter Japan, but that I could apply for one after entering the country. Aki was a welcome sight at the Tokyo airport. What a relief to arrive safely after all the emotional events leaving Vietnam.

We took a taxi to his home in Sangubashi, Tokyo, where we stayed with Okasan, my mother-in-law, and Akira, my brother-in-law. We were welcomed by Okasan, but communication was difficult because her English vocabulary included "good morning," "good afternoon," and "thank you." It was a good orientation to live in a truly Japanese house, sitting on the floor with tatami mats, learning the proper way to sit and sleeping on futon on tatami mats, reed woven mats.

I needed to buy a veil and Okasan said that tradition dictated that I must carry a pair of white gloves: they did not have to be worn, but I had to carry them, so for the wedding ceremony I dutifully carried a pair of white gloves that were too small for my hands.

Tradition also included having two couples as matchmakers, whom we needed to visit before the wedding. The next day, we visited Reverend Takamine, Acting Executive Director of Church World Service Japan, his wife, and Mr. Ogawa, Executive Director of Agape Vocational Centre, and his wife. Tradition dictated that Okasan had to accompany us to their homes going through the formality of requesting them as matchmakers. Of course, I did not understand a word that was exchanged. On departure, I asked Aki what Okasan had said. Much to my shock, she had apologized "for her stupid son!" One of many firsts in my steep learning curve on Japanese tradition!

The same evening, we met with Reverend Toshi Arai and his wife, who were officiating our wedding. Rev. Arai and Aki had arranged a lovely ceremony for September fourth at the International Christian University (ICU) Seabury Chapel for approximately twenty-five guests. I was relieved. But although Aki's last letter to me said everything was taken care of and all he needed was me, when I inquired about the reception, lo and behold, nothing had been organized! This was five days before the wedding!

Mrs. Arai, an extremely organized pastor's wife, came to the rescue. She agreed to make my bouquet of flowers, order a cake, and buy the needed items to make a simple snack of sandwiches, cake, and tea following the wedding ceremony. Arrangements were made for my sister, Brenda, and Cookie, Aki's best man, to make the sandwiches the night before the wedding.

Aki had made a resolution to quit smoking, which was difficult because Okasan and his brother were both heavy smokers and we lived together. Aki had his last cigarette the night before we married and has not smoked since.

The bilingual wedding ceremony was simple but new to Aki's non-Christian friends, many of whom came uninvited. His cousin, Kiyohiro, came from Okazaki. Guests representing me included Brenda, Anne Falk, a colleague from Vietnam, Margaret Workman, whose parents worked with us in Pleiku, and Mr. and Mrs. Carl Beck, Mennonite missionaries in Tokyo. Another guest was a professional photographer, Mr. Taku Ogawa, who had visited us in Pleiku with his colleague, Mr. Wakabayashi, who had been killed in a helicopter accident in Pleiku and had written an article about Aki in the *Catholic Journal Magazine*. Mr. Ogawa offered to be the photographer for our wedding.

The reception was held in a triangular shaped room, which eliminated the traditional headache of assigned seats according to status. Because Okasan was not involved in the arrangements for the ceremony or reception, she was very nervous. In the end, she and everyone enjoyed the informal setting with the brief traditional speeches: Brenda, Anne, and I sang one song (I do not remember what it was).

After the reception, Akira, Aki's brother, accompanied Brenda to the airport for her return flight to Canada so she could attend school the day after her arrival.

Our honeymoon was determined by the wedding gifts of cash received. We spent the first night at a hotel near Aki's parents' home. I heard Aki make a phone call to his brother: he had forgotten our train tickets for the next day at home as well as his pajamas, and asked if he could bring them the next morning.

We travelled by train to Nagano, where we stayed at a national youth hostel to see Mount Fuji. My memory of this place was the public bath, new to me, one for women, another for men, plus a family bath. Unfamiliar and feeling uncomfortable with the custom, we used the family bath. We never did see Mount Fuji due to poor weather. After riding bicycles around Lake Shirakawa, known for its beautiful birch trees, we took a train to Okazaki to Kiyohiro's home to meet relatives. He had been so impressed by our wedding that, on returning home, he had his parents make an arranged marriage for him to Tomiye San. They were married three months later!

After the honeymoon, I was expected to fill the role of the eldest son's wife in the home, which meant being responsible to run the household, learning where to shop daily for food, keeping the house clean, especially the ofuro (bath), etc. Okasan took me grocery shopping within walking distance. Each shop had a specialty, such as fish, tofu, meat, fresh vegetables: one was expected to shop daily. Okasan showed me how to cook some simple Japanese dishes, including the basic miso soup (fermented soybean paste). One was expected to serve many little dishes with each meal, many that were new to me.

Then, one day, a sixty-six-year-old relative arrived. Okasan told me to make the evening meal, which traditionally was my job. The relative had no teeth and high blood pressure so my menu was limited to shopping for fish and vegetables. My dinner consisted of rice, grilled fish, and miso soup with a spread of different dishes from the refrigerator. Shopping for food without language was a challenge! Okasan didn't want to lose face having a daughter-in-law who couldn't serve a meal to a guest, so she found an excuse to come to the kitchen to see if I was ok. The meal had to be served in the living room on the low square table called a kotatsu, with everyone sitting on zabuton (cushions) around it. One had to get on one's knees and bow to serve, then politely exit. It was an art I soon learned. The meal ended by serving green tea.

I soon learned that the Japanese are very concerned about their appearance, especially with regards to clean clothing and bathing. Having a bath every evening was the ultimate pleasure. You bathed yourself clean outside the tub, rinsed yourself using a basin to dip hot water from the hot bath, which was heated with gas, then immersed yourself up to your shoulders or neck in the hot tub. Their preferred temperature was always hotter than body temperature, which I couldn't tolerate. Family members enjoyed sitting in the hot tub called an ofuro until they were like red lobsters, then hopped into bed. With the onset of cold weather, I did learn to appreciate the hot ofuro because there was no central heating in the house. After the bath, one generally went to bed so the hot body would warm the futon. The kotatsu table top could be removed to throw a heavy blanketlike cover over the table, replace the top, and plug in the electric heating unit attached on the underside. It kept your feet warm. One tended to wear the same amount of clothing in the house as outside due to no central heating.

I recall the neighbour across the street, who arrived at our doorstep with a large box of potatoes as a wedding gift saying, "I know Canadians like potato chips, so I thought you would enjoy these potatoes."

Every month, one elderly lady came to settle accounts with Okasan. After being in Japan for about a month, I understood a fair bit of Japanese, but I spoke much less. When the lady arrived, I knew that I had to serve her tea, so I asked her in Japanese if she wanted tea. Because she declined, I prepared to exit with the tray and tea cups. Okasan immediately said to her, "If you want tea, you better say yes or she will take it away."

The lady's immediate response was, "Yes, yes." Very embarrassed, I served her tea. Obviously, I had unknowingly made a major mistake previously. Apparently, one must ask three times, and the guest will respond affirmatively after the third inquiry. I never made that mistake again.

Aki and I needed to support ourselves financially. He was working at the Japan Church World Service office, but I needed to seek employment. We agreed to meet Mr. Miyazaki, head of the YMCA, who had given us marriage counselling in Vietnam and was now living in Tokyo. He offered a one-year contract for me to teach English at the Takatanobaba YMCA part time. The students, primarily young adults, were delightful and eager to learn, especially one gal, Sachiko, who said that she hoped to go to Canada one day. The students gave me helpful cultural information as they practiced their English. One day I asked them where I could buy large size shoes because I only had sandals and cold weather was coming.

The students agreed that the best place would be the Washington Shoe Shop in Shinjuku. So, one Saturday, Aki and I went. No shoes my size but they could have a pair made. One of the staff traced my foot on a piece of paper, then disappeared and soon returned, asking to trace one more time. Then we waited. The gentleman came out a third time, very embarrassed, asking if he could please check one more time because he had never seen a foot this size before! Buying shoes in Canada was also problematic, so this was no surprise.

Six weeks later, I had a pair of loafers that fit perfectly and they wondered if I wanted another pair made. I now had shoes, but no winter clothing. Thrift shops were non-existent in Japan, so Aki and I shopped to supplement some of Okasan's clothing given to me, including a winter coat.

I recall teaching one day on the fourth floor when I suddenly felt very dizzy and had to hang on to the desk to keep my balance. Looking at everyone's faces, I realized that it was an earthquake. After about twenty seconds it subsided. The students knew that one does not try to run down steps during an earthquake, so we stayed in the classroom.

Earthquakes were new to me. One night while sleeping, Aki and I were thrown back and forth, which frightened me. His response was that as long as we were moving sideways, the earthquake was not directly below us. Fair comfort that was!

Nightmares from Vietnam continued to haunt me off and on, but I was able to relax more than previously.

In late September, I was contacted by a missionary working as personnel secretary for several mission boards in Tokyo. He was frantically looking for an English-speaking nurse to work the night shift for a patient who required special care. Would I please consider working for an American who was hospitalized at St. Luke's Hospital in Tokyo? The patient was serving with the World Council of Churches in Geneva and was on an Asian tour when he began to feel ill in the Philippines, but he had decided to continue travelling on to Japan. On arrival, he was taken by ambulance to the hospital, too weak to move on his own, and had a cardiac arrest soon after admission. Could I please start working immediately? I needed to discuss this with Aki because I had just signed a contract with the YMCA.

Aki and I agreed that I would work the night shift at St. Luke's Hospital, thinking it would not be long term. I taught English class in the morning, went home to sleep until late afternoon, then, after eating the evening meal, Aki would faithfully accompany me to St. Luke's every evening in time for my eight p.m. to eight a.m. shift.

The patient was a forty-year-old man named Jerry, who was later diagnosed with Guillain-Barre Syndrome. He had rapidly developed paralysis of his limbs, had difficulty breathing, couldn't speak, and was unable to swallow. When I came on duty, he had a tracheotomy with an iron lung on standby outside his room. He had had two cardiac arrests already, and he was so weak that he was unable to even blink or close his eyes. His eyes were closed, but he could hear my voice. His wife was notified and she made arrangements for their wheelchair bound daughter in Geneva so she could be in Tokyo with her husband.

This was definitely different nursing than I had done in the last several years and went on for weeks, then months, with minimal improvement. Finally, I was able to communicate with Jerry by his very faint squeezing of my hand. When I sensed that he wanted to communicate, we would go through the letters of the alphabet, and he would squeeze my hand when it was the correct letter. He managed to say that he wanted to write a book about forty nights with Marcy! He had a sense of humour! By early April, he was drinking clear fluids: by the end of May he was booked on a flight back to Geneva. He had four seats to lie down and, on arrival, was transported by ambulance to a hospital there.

You might wonder how I got along living together with my mother-in-law. Well, I had very little time awake at home for months. When I was, Aki was generally there too. My first New Year in Japan was a memorable experience. You spent three days cooking osechi (New Year's dishes) so that you didn't need to cook for the first three days of the new year. You also cleaned the house with the last cleaning done around eleven p.m. before the new year, which included sweeping in front of the house as well! The whole family was glued to the TV on New Year's Eve for the special program and to hear the ringing of the bells at temples around the country to bring in the new year. We also ate soba noodles after eleven-thirty p.m. to connect the old year to the new.

Aki and I discussed future plans and always came to the same conclusion. Because Aki wanted to study theology and social work in Canada, it seemed best to go there in the summer of 1972, with studies beginning in September if he was accepted. (When Aki had applied to Waterloo Lutheran Seminary and the Graduate School of Social Work at Wilfrid Laurier University, he had not realized it was the only place in Canada that offered the combined degree.)

We anticipated spending much of our life in Asia, so it seemed logical to study in Waterloo to be near my family while we were in Canada.

Move to Canada

We left Tokyo, Japan on June 12, 1972 for a fun trip home. We flew to San Francisco and purchased $99 three-week Greyhound bus passes. It was shocking to see the size of people and culture shock from the portions of food served in restaurants. After touring the Redwood National State Park, we took a bus to Portland, Oregon, where we stayed and reconnected with my friend Jessie from Pleiku, who was now married. After three days, we took a bus to Vancouver. The welcome extended by Canadian Immigration at the border was wonderful! Emma, with whom I had worked in Nhatrang, met us at the bus terminal. What fun we had reminiscing and seeing the sights in the Vancouver area. On our bus to Banff, we were stunned to hear seven different languages spoken as we walked to the back of the bus. Canada definitely was a multicultural society!

In Banff, we stayed at a hotel near the train station. Unfortunately, I had a bottle of nuoc mam (fish sauce) in my suitcase that decided to perfume our clothing. What an odour on opening my suitcase! We then took a bus to a village where you can walk to Chateau Lake Louise. While walking uphill, we noticed the traffic stopped in both directions: one passenger pointed to us and we looked—a big black bear had come up out of a deep ditch and was quite close to us. One car offered to give us a ride, which we gratefully accepted! Lake Louise was absolutely breathtaking. We enjoyed a canoe ride toward the glacier, the picturesque flower beds, and a meal in the cafeteria. We returned to Banff for the night and did some sightseeing locally the next day, including the sulphur springs.

The Greyhound then took us to Edmonton. The noise from the hotel next to the station made it impossible to sleep, so we decided that we would go directly to Saskatchewan to stay with my Aunt Barbara, Uncle Howard, and cousins, Elaine and Raymond. It was wonderful to finally see their home because our family had never been able to travel out West together.

They showed us the area and introduced us to their relatives. What a flat countryside with hardly any trees.

After several days we were headed to Winnipeg, where we stayed with Katy, a colleague from Nhatrang, and her husband Jake. Katy was still struggling with adjustment to Canada after Vietnam.

Tired of travelling, we decided to travel straight through from Winnipeg to Kitchener. It was the longest bus ride! My three sisters were at the bus terminal in Kitchener to meet us.

What a reunion! Mom and Dad were delighted to welcome us to live with them until we could find a place of our own.

We were thrilled to learn that Aki had been accepted at Waterloo Lutheran Seminary. The Graduate School of Social Work acceptance pended on his first year in Seminary. Kitchener-Waterloo Hospital employed me to work in the O.R. starting in September. We lived at home with my parents while we excitedly started to piece our life together in Waterloo.

Meanwhile, my parents had planned a wonderful wedding reception for us at the St. Jacobs Community Hall for 125 guests, which included my pastor, Glen Brubacher of St. Jacobs Mennonite Church, and Paul Frey, soloist, with the Mennonite Youth Fellowship serving the catered meal. It was wonderful to meet family, relatives, friends, and former nursing class-mates, even though I felt like a fish out of water.

Fortunately, we soon found an upstairs apartment in an old house on Park Street, Waterloo that looked good to us, but Mom declared that we could not possibly live there. After Vietnam, to us it looked fine. It was located halfway between the seminary and the hospital, so we could both walk to our destinations.

We started going to auction sales to furnish the second and third floor apartment. My uncle Orville generously gave us a new bedroom suite as a wedding gift. My parents bought us a Chinese set of dishes. We eagerly looked forward to entertaining. Our routine was for Aki to walk to his classes at the seminary and me to KWH to work in the O.R.

Aki's seminary orientation of three days included a picnic meal, whereby leftover food was just dumped in the garbage, which upset him: Vietnam was still a reality. Later, when preparing his first sermon in methodology class, he was told to be careful, that a good sermon does not make a congregation feel guilty.

Aki found the classes difficult and frustrating because, initially, he understood so little. After three weeks, he wanted to give up. Other seminarians talked a lot in class, and he felt that he was going to be a failure because he had difficulty joining in the discussion. Much to his surprise, at the end of the year, he was top of the class, which meant he was accepted into the Graduate School of Social Work in the combined degree program, M.Div. and MSW.

I came home one morning after being on call in the O.R., having worked all night, stunned to find Aki still in bed. He was sure that class was cancelled due to a snowfall of five centimetres! Welcome to Canada!

With no money to buy a car or TV, I bought a crokinole board for Christmas. Life was routine and simple. We walked to Waterloo square to do our laundry and grocery shopping. We joined First United Church due to its proximity, and because the worship was comparable to the United Church of Christ in Japan.

Through an introduction to a Japanese faculty member, we made additional Japanese acquaintances. Dr. Mike Shimpo, a sociology professor at St. Jerome's College, and his wife belonged to a house church, and they wondered if we would be interested in becoming members.

It was this group that welcomed us and became a family: Walter and Ruth Klassen, faculty at Conrad Grebel College, Arnie and Lou Dyck, faculty at U of W, Fred and Lorrie Snyder, Arnie and Linda Snyder, as well as Marg and Norm Warren. We met every Sunday evening, rotating homes, eating soup and sandwiches as we shared and had a Bible study.

In September 1974, when we moved into the University of Waterloo's married students' apartments, my Aunt Agnes who was employed at Children's' Aid Society (CAS) telephoned. She was moving to another division there and wondered whether I would consider applying for her position in Infant Care. This job involved having a car and working with foster homes with the children under care. I decided to apply and was hired. I said goodbye to my colleagues in the O.R. and was soon orientated to work that was another new experience. Three of us in the Infant Care Division were nurses because many infants and young children had medical issues, whereas the older children needed social workers.

I thrived on the challenge, but I struggled with several older children who had multiple problems—in addition to complicated medical issues—that the social workers were quick to pass on to the nurses. Conditions that some young children experienced were incomprehensible to me. As time passed, my caseload increased to forty infants and young children, making it difficult to provide maximum quality service. I had several contested cases that required me to appear in court. My name proved problematic for the judge who invariably called me Mrs. Pneumonia!

At this time, the first Vietnamese refugees, nine young men, arrived in Kitchener after spending four months in the States. We became involved with helping them get settled. One day, we discovered one of them walking around in public in his pajamas, which was fine in Vietnam but not here in Canada. These young men were very creative and made lamps out of tin cans, etc. They were so appreciative of being here that they invited the local government workers as well as ourselves for a meal in their apartment. They rolled a sheet of plastic down the living room floor and we all sat on the floor to eat our simple meal that they had worked hard to prepare.

Meanwhile, I became pregnant and was under the care of Dr. Young, who had been my mother's doctor, had delivered me, and now was to deliver our baby! Aki and I took lamaze classes so he could be present for the birth of our first child. We were blessed with a daughter, Melody, in June 1975.

September meant I was back to work and Aki was in classes again. We then struggled with consistent child care for Melody: Egyptian and Chinese ladies living in the same building provided child care. Occasionally, Aki got permission to take her to class because his classes were small.

Dr. Delton Glebe became Aki's mentor in pastoral counselling, especially death and dying. In Aki's last year at Seminary, he studied Paul Tillich for Systematic Theology under Dr. Dick Crossman. This study became the backbone for his situational theology.

Aki's combined degree program required four field placements. The first one was at the House of Friendship in Kitchener, a Mennonite NGO working with homeless men. The second one was to work at an inner-city project, Wesley Centre in Hamilton, operated by the United Church of Canada. His experience of taking five delinquent teenage boys along with two assistants camping at Algonquin Park for a week would pale in comparison to any fiction book as well as make a book in itself! It was a turning point in the lives of the boys, as it was an eye opener experience for Aki and his assistants. Another placement was at the Children's Aid Society (CAS) in Kitchener, where I was currently working. The final placement was at the Interfaith Pastoral Counselling Centre, also in Kitchener.

During this time, Aki became a candidate for ordination with the United Church of Canada (UCC), Waterloo Presbytery, Hamilton Conference. In his interview, he was grilled on his faith history, which was Buddhist, Catholic, United Church of Christ in Japan, now seeking to be ordained by the United Church of Canada having studied at a Lutheran Seminary. When asked what excited him most about the church, I cringed on hearing his immediate response, which was, "Not Sunday morning!"

He definitely was forthright in his responses! He passed the interview so the next step was to be assigned to a three-year commitment. Much to our surprise, Aki was assigned to the Okanagan Presbytery, in British Columbia, to a seven-point charge with Japanese Canadian Churches based in Kelowna. Ordination by the Hamilton Conference was the climax in May 1976. I said farewell to colleagues at CAS and the dear children under my care, started packing, bought a reliable car, and said goodbye to family and friends again.

Life was in the fast lane. Aki graduated with the combined degree, MDiv. and MSW in April, and I with my PHT, Putting Hubby Through: he was ordained in May, and in June we were bound for Kelowna, BC. It was an emotional goodbye to family, our house church family, and friends.

Assigned to the Okanagan Valley

Melody was one year old when we started driving to British Columbia. We stopped in Winnipeg to see Katy and Jake again, relatives in Saskatchewan, and then the final leg to Kelowna. I wanted to cry after crossing the Rockies: it was like saying goodbye to Canada and to my profession. I was now a pastor's wife, no longer a professional in my field. Even though I wanted to be a mother full-time and enjoyed homemaking, it still hurt.

The manse where we would be living was located behind the Kelowna Japanese United Church on Highway 97, the only road through the Okanagan Valley. People were happy to see us, and we met the retired pastor who continued to attend the Japanese language service.

We soon learned that there were two Sunday morning services in Kelowna: the Japanese service at nine a.m. and the English one at eleven. Twice a month, a Japanese service was held in Vernon, thirty-five km north, at the Vernon United Church at two p.m. and twice a month in Summerland, thirty km south, at their United Church at two p.m. Sundays were a challenge because the Issei, first generation Japanese Canadians, were generally appearing at our back door as early as eight-thirty a.m. I did not attend the first service, in order to get organized to teach Sunday School to some children at eleven a.m. and prepare lunch, because, immediately after the second service and chat time, it was quickly close the church, eat lunch, and hit the road for the next service.

Aki insisted on doing family visitation after the third service, which meant that we got home around six p.m. I sincerely appreciated the home visits and the stories, but, at the same time, Sunday meant survival. It was especially challenging having a one-year-old with all the services. On Wednesdays, Aki alternated Bible study with Issei in Westbank and Winfield.

When there was a fifth Sunday in the month, which happened several times a year, Aki had services in the Kootenay mountains with Issei who had been interned there during WWII. He stayed with church members in Midway, Greenwood, and New Denver and was usually gone for five days. Aki listened to their tragic life stories from which they had never fully recovered. In New Denver, the church building had housed two families that had been interned there.

The Japanese Canadian families living in Kelowna were the only families who had not been interned in WWII because they were living more than 100 miles inland from the coast. All others had been resettled. I listened to so many stories that made me cry even though they were told without bitterness: a very sad missing chapter in Canadian history books that left me with great respect for these dear people.

At the time that Aki was assigned to Kelowna, the previous pastor had told us that the church would close in six months. Ironically, we experienced a growth in the English-speaking congregation and had solid support from the Issei. We enjoyed the people, and Aki did much home visitation. After two years, we discovered that Aki's work load had extended to include evenings. We needed to schedule an evening for ourselves, so we decided to join a beginner's class in square dancing once a week, which proved hilarious.

An annual church event valued by the community was our church's fundraiser, the chow mein bazaar. All able church members spent three full days feverishly working to meet the demand for their famous chow mein! That was how Aki met Mr. Tanaka, an active Buddhist leader who offered Japanese dance classes, and who was a key player in the newly formed Multicultural Society. The judge overseeing applications for Canadian citizenship asked the Multicultural Society to organize new citizenship classes for new immigrants. Aki became the coordinator, teaching Canadian history, politics, culture, and geography. When immigrants said their Oath of Citizenship, Aki was designated by the judge to congratulate them. After the second time, the judge became infuriated when he discovered that Aki, who was representing Canada, was not a Canadian citizen himself!

Aki was now at a crossroad regarding his citizenship. We agreed that it would be best if he would become a Canadian citizen so that all our family members would have the same. The memory of seeing Vietnamese families divided because of different citizenships at the end of the war was the deciding factor for us. Aki immediately received Canadian citizenship. When Timothy was born in June 1978, we all had the same citizenship.

We were blessed to have a seventy-six-year-old retired Japanese pastor, Reverend Ito, who came from Japan as an evangelist for the Issei, stay in our home for a week. He was such a spiritual person whose presence filled the room. I vividly recall going over to the church one afternoon to sit in for part of the service. I noticed a church member sitting at the end of a pew several rows ahead of me, who was slowly leaning towards the centre aisle. I walked up and didn't get a pulse, so I immediately asked

Aki to call for an ambulance while I stayed with the member and laid him flat on the pew to start CPR. Rev. Ito appeared and put his hands on the member and prayed, reciting John 11: 25: "I am the resurrection and the life. Whoever believes in me will live, even though he dies." The ambulance arrived, which Aki followed to Emergency at Kelowna General Hospital. The patient was hospitalized because he had another cardiac arrest after arrival. Knowing the patient was under medical care, Aki returned to the church where Rev. Ito was still preaching!

When the patient's wife returned home in the evening, she discovered their home had been entered. The only missing item was her husband's prized coin collection, which he looked at every day. Panicking, she called Aki, wondering how she could break the news to her husband. Aki volunteered to tell him at the hospital the next day. The patient's amazing response was, "Praise the Lord. He took my coins but gave me new life." His wife was stunned but relieved. The patient then asked Aki what he had been wearing on his chest when he was in the ambulance with him. The fact was, Aki had not been in the ambulance with him. The patient drew the symbols that he had seen, which were the symbols for Alpha and Omega, the beginning and the end that were on one of Aki's stoles. This incident made a spiritual impact on the Issei members as well as ourselves.

This incident soon spread to the other Issei congregations. Aki's custom was to visit all sick Japanese Canadians in the hospital, regardless of their religious affiliation. One Buddhist lady in the Kelowna Hospital was very ill, in an oxygen tent with no clear diagnosis. He held her hand as he prayed with her. He later learned that she had felt a warm sensation in her hand when he had prayed and that this warmth spread through her whole body during the night. The next morning, she was healed and discharged with no specific diagnosis.

Another time after a church service in Vernon, a member asked Aki to please visit a Buddhist patient in the hospital who was in an oxygen tent with IVs, having difficulty breathing and unconscious. The doctor had told the family that he likely had just a few days to live. Aki held his hand and prayed with him before returning home. The next morning at seven a.m., the phone rang from the church member who had asked Aki to pray for her friend, saying, "Taihen Da! Taihen Da!" (Shock, shock!). Apparently, the patient was sitting up in bed, eating breakfast and feeling fine. He said that he had been trying to catch "a scarecrow" in his sleep and had finally managed to catch it. Aki asked his church member to take a photo of Jesus on the cross to show the patient, suspecting that might be what he had seen. Yes, it was! He had caught Jesus during his sleep! He was discharged later that day feeling well. This miraculous healing changed his life. His whole family, including his adult grandchildren, were later baptized and became Christians. His hope was to meet his daughter in Japan whom he had not seen since she had been forcibly sent to Japan after WWII. We learned later that he was able to spend four months with his daughter in Japan before he returned to Canada and passed away peacefully.

Another miracle in Vernon happened when Aki baptized a ninety-year-old Japanese Canadian grandmother who had no teeth: several years later we learned that she got nine new teeth after baptism!

The presence and power of the Holy Spirit was amazing! One elderly lady in Kamloops, who was bent over for so many years, had been unable to sleep on her back. Aki had a prayer with her before returning to Kelowna in the evening. The next morning, we received a phone call from her—she had woken up with a straight back! Miracles happened in Westbank, Summerland, and Midway too. We praised God for His work and miracles performed in His ministry in our midst.

We were informed that a Vietnamese refugee family with seven children had arrived in Kelowna, so we befriended them and acted as a resource. They were delighted to know we spoke Vietnamese. Several months later, a member from the Vernon congregation told us that a young Vietnamese couple was living there, so we invited them for a visit in our home. In conversation, we discovered that he had graduated from Saigon University. I asked him if by any chance he knew of a Montagnard man named Yong who took the nurse practitioner program at Saigon University. He said, "Yes, he was my roommate, and he was able to return to Pleiku on the last plane before the government fell in 1975!" We finally knew that Yong had graduated and returned safely to his family.

In January 1979, Aki received an invitation from Reverend Buma, Executive Secretary of Japan Church World Service in Tokyo, who had recommended that Aki go to Vietnam in 1970. He was asking Aki to come as associate director of Agape, a residential sheltered workshop for 100 persons with disabilities in Kanagawa Prefecture near Tokyo. Aki's immediate response was he was not interested in working with persons with disabilities. A month later, the second letter arrived and Aki gave the same response. When the third letter arrived, Aki went outside, praying, "God, you know that I do not want to go to Japan, so please send me a sign. I will follow your guidance." When he opened his eyes, he saw several sparrows and had peace of mind knowing that if God looked after the birds, he would look after him.

Aki's commitment to the citizenship classes, offered through the Multicultural Society, had reached the ears of Premier Bill Bennett in Vancouver who invited Aki to participate in the Provincial Multicultural Society's Conference at the Vancouver Hotel. Aki received a phone call from the premier's secretary, apologizing for failing to send an invitation earlier. The program had already been printed, and it indicated that Aki would lead the premier's procession for an evening program, wearing his clerical gown. Miraculously, Aki could fit in a brief trip to Vancouver for his involvement.

When Aki was walking in the hallway of the hotel toward his room, he met two Asians in wheelchairs. He asked them in English where they came from. Because they didn't understand, and judging from their appearance, he asked them in Japanese. They said they were from a centre outside Tokyo. When he asked them what centre, they told him Agape. This was the centre where Reverend Buma wanted him to come to work! Aki discovered that three of the twenty persons with disabilities in this tour group came from Agape: he had met two of the three.

Aki quickly phoned me, saying, "Marcy, we are going to Japan. This is the sign from God that I asked for." On returning to Kelowna, he immediately resigned as pastor, which stunned the church elders. There were several factors that culminated in Aki's decision to resign.

Early in 1979, we had applied to the Division of World Outreach of the United Church of Canada because Aki was feeling the need for a new challenge. Our application stated that the only country in which we did not want to work in Asia was Japan because Japan was a developed country compared to Nepal, where there was an opening. Our application was acknowledged, but there had been no further communication. So, when Aki was certain that he had received a sign from God, his resignation was timely because his pastoral charge needed a bilingual pastor. He knew of a bilingual seminarian to be ordained in May, who would be assigned elsewhere if he did not resign now. The other UCC pastors in Kelowna told Aki that he was downright irresponsible resigning because he had not yet been accepted by the Division of World Outreach (DWO of UCC).

In April, DWO UCC had arranged for comprehensive assessments of persons applying for overseas work. In May, we were informed that we were accepted with our assignment undecided. Rev. Buma had done his homework and requested that Aki be assigned to Agape. The Japanese congregations were stunned that our departure was becoming a reality. They had appreciated our ministry and community involvement. The newly ordained bilingual pastor was assigned to replace Aki, and we had exactly three weeks to pack up and move to Toronto for orientation. Again, God had worked in mysterious ways.

It was hard to say goodbye to everyone with everything happening so fast. In June, I took a linguistics course at the University of Toronto, while Aki studied vocational rehabilitation for persons with disabilities at Goodwill Industries headquarters in Toronto. The director invited him to participate in the International Goodwill Industries Conference in Ohio, USA, where he met the Reverend Dr. Harold Wilke, a social activist who was born without arms and believed in disability rights as a movement. Many years later, Dr. Wilke was a guest in our home in Japan.

In July, our family attended the Missionary Orientation Conference at Cedar Glen, Ontario, which included persons serving with other mission boards. One couple, Stan and Marty Murray, serving with an American Baptist Mission Board, also assigned to Japan, became special friends. Stan, years later, visited us in Bangkok, Thailand. It was a stimulating, challenging and empowering experience to share with international persons of other faiths. We learned about liberation theology from a Catholic priest.

Playing in the last game of volleyball on the last day of orientation, Aki tore the cruciate ligament in his left leg, which required major surgery at Toronto General Hospital. I was at a loss how to cope with Aki's needs in the hospital in Toronto, and our children, Melody and Timothy, ages four and one respectively, in Conestogo at my parents' home. After a week, Aki was discharged with a cast from groin to toe at about an eighty-degree angle. My parents graciously and willingly agreed to accommodate our family of four until we could leave for Japan—which was definitely not going to happen as originally planned.

This was a difficult and frustrating time for all of us. Aki spent time in bed with the uncomfortable cast. After three weeks, it was replaced for an additional three weeks. We celebrated when the cast was finally removed, which left him with a leg that was at an eighty-degree angle, but at least he could get around much easier with crutches. He was given vigorous exercises to do 100 times a day that would hopefully leave him with a straight leg. Aki was determined to have a speedy recovery but soon learned that it was unusual for persons who had this surgery to have a straight leg again. Many times, we have marvelled at God's arrangement for such a complete orientation to work with persons with disabilities, which included Aki having to use a wheelchair and crutches. This delay also gave our family the opportunity to re-establish relationships and for our children to spend time with grandparents and relatives.

CHAPTER 5

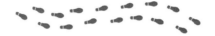

Mission to Japan

Finally, on November 4, 1979, our family was able to leave for Japan with one crutch, three months later than originally scheduled. On arrival, we went directly to Agape where we would be living in a compact family unit for staff in a prefabricated building with minimal furnishings. Aki was on duty the next morning already, and I was left to do shopping locally with two preschoolers and no knowledge of the language. This unreal experience is still a vivid memory.

Agape had 100 residential persons with disabilities: seventy used wheelchairs and thirty commuted daily. One of Melody's comments several days after arriving was, "So many people in Japan are in wheelchairs." Clients soon became our extended family, especially for our children who thrived on the wheelchair-bicycle-tricycle races and ball games.

Aki was busy as head of the managerial department and enjoyed the challenge of organizing the first Asian Vocational Rehabilitation Conference in April 1980 as a result of his connection with Goodwill Industries in Toronto. Nine countries participated, along with experts from the International Labour Organization of the UN. An outcome of the conference was the birth of the Asia-Pacific Council of Vocational

Rehabilitation for Disabled Persons. Aki also organized an annual Asian exchange program.

Around that time, Rev. Buma attended the Rehabilitation International World Congress held in Winnipeg, Canada, where more than 200 persons with disabilities representing many countries participated. They wanted to raise their voices and make changes to the program that had been organized by medical and rehabilitation professionals. Because the organizers refused to do so, the persons with disabilities decided to meet simultaneously. Wanting to have a voice of their own, Mennonite Central Committee (MCC) made it possible by offering space and funding with Henry Enns assigned as general secretary to establish a self-advocate organization of persons with a disability, which later became known as Disabled Peoples International (DPI).

We got to know the residents at Agape well because we lived in the same compound. One resident, Gen San, was a Korean who had lived on Cheju Island, Korea, until he had been forcefully taken by the Japanese military before WWII to work in a military factory in Kawasaki, Japan. After the war, feeling depressed, with no money or family, he attempted suicide by throwing himself in front of an oncoming train. He survived but lost a leg. For this reason, he felt that he could not return to Korea because it would bring dishonour to his family as a person with a disability. After rehabilitation, Gen San was employed to work in Agape's vocational workshop. Because he could not commute to work, he lived in the same longhouse that we did (there were four units for the single staff, and we were in the family unit at one end with the Japanese bath for all of us at the other end). Gen San could eat his meals at Agape's cafeteria from Monday to Friday, but Saturday and Sunday he was on his own, which meant he thrived on sake and dried squid. We decided to regularly deliver some cooked meals to him. At the age of sixty, arrangements were made for him to move to a nursing care home where he was happy but still lonely. He had never talked much. We visited him twice a year on our trips to Tokyo to Okasan's home and offered to take him to Cheju Island, but he said that he had lost contact with his family.

In June, Kazuko, an accountant in the office, who used a wheelchair, and her fiancée, using crutches, had a beautiful wedding. Many of their friends with disabilities formed a band and played two songs that the bridegroom had composed. Overwhelmed with emotion, I had two thoughts: one, who is a person with a disability? Many persons have healthy functioning bodies but lack the happiness and strength of character so often found in persons with a disability. It was so obvious how much each person playing a musical instrument and singing was totally lost in the music in pure enjoyment. What a blessing they were!

The second thought I had was Corinthians 12: 12-31: "Christ is like a single body, which has many parts; it is still one body, even though it is made up of different parts . . ."

I continued the challenge of language study part time. Aki overheard my telephone conversation one evening when I put an accent on the wrong syllable, changing the meaning from husband to prisoner. I wonder how long he had been my prisoner!? Melody was also my teacher, as she learned quickly from her friends at preschool. It was interesting that the mothers from the lower income families extended friendship to me, whereas those living in good housing did not even greet me.

Unofficially, I was the nurse on call for clients who became ill in the off hours at the workshop because our unit was beside the residential building for all the clients. I'll always remember one client who was unable to eat, so I made some strawberry Jell-o and bought some fresh strawberries for him. He later shared how touched he felt by this unexpected act of kindness. As a wheelchair user, his family had deserted him, and he was all alone.

Besides the work at Agape as the rehab director, Aki spoke at many churches and participated in many social welfare conferences and study groups. It was our hope that the church would open its doors to persons with disabilities because they have many gifts and much to teach us to deepen our faith.

A highlight was Agape's Christmas service and party. Entertainment was enjoyed by all with the musically talented clients voluntarily participating. Our family's contribution was "Little Drummer Boy" with Aki playing the mandolin, me singing, and Melody and Timothy beating plastic cooking bowls with chopsticks until Tim put the bowl on his head!

The United Nations declared 1981, the International Year of Disabled Persons (IYDP) that opened with the motto "Full Participation and Equality." It was a difficult year for our family that resulted in many unexpected changes. Aki's stand for justice cost him his position at Agape in April, and we had to leave. He wanted to return to Canada but I refused, saying, "We had a clear sign to come to Japan for a reason."

We were temporarily assigned to a vacant missionary house in Tokyo, waiting for God's guidance. Aki had been promised a chaplaincy position at a Christian hospital that just needed to be rubber stamped at their board meeting. Aki felt confident that this was right; I didn't think it was but did not want to oppose him. Surely, we were not called to Japan for chaplaincy work! In the evening, two weeks later, the phone rang with the message that the chaplaincy position was not approved, primarily because Aki's qualifications threatened another chaplain. Aki hit rock bottom. I felt elated but couldn't verbally express it. What a relief, because it just hadn't felt right.

Then, early the next morning, the phone rang again. It was a former director of Agape, who had left for the same reason we did, looking for Aki to work for two central offices in Tokyo: the Japan Council of the IYDP, International Year of Disabled Persons by the United Nations, representing 108 organizations for persons with disabilities and rehabilitation institutes, and the International Abilympics (an international skill contest for disabled persons) Office by the Ministry of Health, Labour and Social Welfare.

One of their exciting projects was the Japan Study Program for Asian Leaders in Rehabilitation, with Aki acting as chief coordinator, where we made lifelong friends, most notably our Thai friend, Suthida Srimulchai, a social worker at the School for the Blind in Bangkok, Thailand. This friendship with her family continues to this day. Aki was also assigned as the central office coordinator for the International Abilympics (Ability + Olympics) contest which was the first global skill contest for persons with a physical disability to promote employment of persons with disabilities. He screened the applications for the 841 participants from fifty-six countries, which included paraplegics, amputees, persons with cerebral palsy, and persons with visual and auditory disabilities.

One severely disabled contestant, Emmanbokuku from Mauritius, came to participate in the watch repair competition. Aki believed persons with a severe disability also needed representation in the event, which is why he invited him. Besides being a paraplegic, Emmanbokuku only had the use of his right hand. Aki went to meet him on arrival at the airport only to discover his electric motorized wheelchair had to be dismantled to fit into the luggage area of the bus. But the real challenge was for Aki to get Emmanbokuku's 200-pound dead weight into the bus! With pushes from behind, he finally succeeded.

En route to his accommodation, a bright full moon was shining between two high rise buildings. Emmanbokuku was in awe that the Japanese could even create an artificial moon. Aki assured him that it was the real moon. Everything was a first for him—flying, riding a bus, and travelling overseas. The next hurdle was an accessible washroom in his room. A portable toilet solved the problem. Emmanbokuku told Aki that his wife was seven months pregnant and if he had a son, he would name him Aki after him. Years later, Aki visited Mauritius: Emmanbokuku had just passed away but he met Aki, Emmanbokuku's eight-year-old son.

To participate in the watch repair competition, Emmanbokuku had to lie down in bed and use his chin and right hand to do the repair. He was amazing! Aki considered his participation as most valuable to show how even persons with a severe disability can be productive with the needed support.

There were seventeen skill contests as well as an exhibition site to include skills not represented in the skills contest. At the same time, a three-day international Abilympics seminar was held, which greatly contributed to promoting employment of persons with disabilities.

Meanwhile, I had been busy helping in the translation of Japanese articles about persons with disabilities and being a resource person for the Japan Red Cross Language Volunteers for the International Abilympics. This involved weekly sessions for five months with twelve university students.

At the same time as the Abilympics, our third child was due, and Aki wanted to be present for the delivery. Fortunately, much to the relief of all the staff, Matthew arrived three weeks late.

Most IYDP programs and projects finished, but the true IYDP had just begun. Aki decided that he wanted to continue working with persons with disabilities, which felt right. We began editing an English report of a national long-term plan of action for the IYDP.

Aki then volunteered to attend the first World Congress of Disabled Peoples International (DPI) in Singapore, in December 1981, where more than 400 delegates from sixty countries met. They established their constitution, dividing themselves into five regions, with the Asia-Pacific as one of them. Their motto was "A Voice of our Own." Aki attended as a volunteer with the forty-five-member Japanese group of persons with disabilities. Senator Edita Yashiro, a wheelchair user, was elected as Chairperson of the Asia-Pacific Region and Aki became the Regional Secretary and liaison to the global community. Each region was required to organize a regional conference within two years. As a result, I ended up editing English correspondence until someone was hired to do so. This proved to be an education for me and many names began to have faces!

The Singapore conference was a turning point in Aki's thinking: he knew that persons with disabilities were capable of making decisions and living independently in the community. It was their human right to do so and be empowered, not controlled by professionals such as medical, vocational, educational, and social workers. Rather, they were to be the service providers. Persons with disabilities had the right to make decisions regarding their own lives: to be supported, not controlled. In the Bible, Jesus did not control persons with disabilities, rather he empowered them, sending persons who were healed back to their home or community. Aki decided that he wanted to work with persons with disabilities at the grassroot level.

During the conference, Aki received a phone call from Hamada Sensei, whom he had never met, representing Kobe Seirei Social Services Community (KSSSC) in Kobe, Japan. Mr. Hamada had been given Aki's name from Japan Christian Social Work League because they were seeking a professional social worker to work with persons with disabilities and wanted him to come for an interview. Aki, feeling positive about this, immediately phoned me from Singapore, wanting me to also be present for the interview. Arrangements were made for Aki to fly to Osaka directly from Singapore: The children and I would meet him in Kobe. Because

Matthew was only six weeks old and with two more young children, I enlisted the help of Sachiko, one of my English students in 1971, to accompany me and the children on the Shinkansen (bullet train) to Kobe.

As a result of our visit, we agreed to move to Kobe at the end of March 1982. God answers prayer! We looked forward to sharing this challenge with the Christian community in Kobe. God had put us in situations of tremendous challenge. Although we had felt inadequate at times, God had seen fit to use us as instruments in His work, and we knew He would continue to do so.

New Life in Kobe

Aki began working with Kobe Seirei Social Services Community (KSSSC), a Christian organization that began through the vision of a small Japanese church in Kobe. Nishi Kobe Church felt that faith meant action to help those in need, so they identified persons with disabilities as most needy. After fundraising for several years, and campaigning in the streets, they finally had enough money to buy a piece of land in Wadayama, in Western Hyogo Prefecture, about 100 km north of Kobe. Several church families quit their jobs in Kobe and moved to Wadayama to construct a residential sheltered workshop, Keisei-en, for fifty persons with disabilities, of which twenty were blind. At the time of our assignment, they had built a nursing care home, Shinsei-en, for fifty persons with severe disabilities next door to Keisei-en.

KSSSC was now in the process of opening more centres in Kobe on land given by the city: Aisei-en, a nursing home for fifty persons with severe disabilities, and Seisei-en, a vocational training workshop for fifty persons who were intellectually challenged.

Much of Aki's energy had gone into introducing a social casework system in each institution. In Japan, the basic social welfare situation for persons with disabilities was still primarily institutionalization, which was the cause of isolation and lack of socialization. Aki taught a holistic approach: community inclusive development leads persons with disabilities to be part of the community and participate in social activities. He also introduced a personal service concept instead of institutional service, which meant that all services should be based on individual needs, not the institution. Spiritual and personal fulfillment were becoming the basis of our social work approach, rather than materialistic services.

This was a new concept. All parents wanted was to have their young adults accepted in an institution for life. Aki was promoting assessment and appropriate job placement for those with potential. Some parents protested and withdrew their children. Within a year, four clients were successful in getting job placements in society: six were on field placement at three different companies. Aki was putting three rings in a box: the client's training, the family support system, and the employer's understanding and acceptance of persons with disabilities. The pride and joy of each person who got employment made all the hard work worth it! This resulted in our organization becoming a threat to government institutions that accepted the highest functioning persons with disabilities who graduated from special education schools and were not working toward mainstreaming.

Sundays were full days. In the morning, our family attended Nishi-Kobe Church because their church had started KSSSC. After a simple lunch at church, our family drove to Aisei-en for an afternoon worship service with the clients and their families, followed by tea time for fellowship. Clients enjoyed interacting with our children. As chaplain, Aki would conduct worship services two to three times weekly, Sunday afternoon at Aisei-en and Wednesday at Seisei-en, the vocational workshop for fifty intellectually challenged persons.

Aki published a small booklet, *Pastoral Guidance; Living with Disabled Persons* promoted by the Hyogo Conference of the United Church of Christ in Japan as a resource handbook for ministers: how to understand and communicate with persons with disabilities, make churches accessible, and include all resources available in the community. They continued to be reluctant to complete the booklet due to finances. In the end, it was such a success with a surplus of $1,000! Aki is now promoting the next book, *Pastoral Guidance 2; Living with Old Age.*

In March and April, Aki went to Thailand to help them prepare for the first DPI Asia-Pacific Congress. He worked hard to convince associations of persons with disabilities, such as the Association of Physically Disabled

Persons, the Association of the Blind, the Association of the Deaf and the Parents' Association of Intellectually Challenged Persons, to join together to form one national group to become the organizing committee for the congress to be held in November 1983.

Our family was finally settled after moving to Kobe at the end of March 1982. Our house was perched part way up Mount Rokko, between the inland sea and the mountains. There was a steep cliff behind the house that only boars could navigate. My primary roles were homemaking, meeting the family's needs, providing accommodation for our international guests—some with disabilities—and supporting Aki's work behind the scenes.

Melody enrolled in Grade 1 at Canadian Academy, a five-minute walk up the mountainside from our home: Tim, who had special needs, enrolled in preschool at the same school. Matthew kept me company at home.

I introduced a *Quiet Book* to the Parents' Association at Seisei-en, a handmade cloth book originally made by intellectually challenged persons in Victoria, British Columbia. The parents met at the centre every week for peer counselling and to make their own version of fifteen pages as a fundraiser to build a halfway house. The orders came in faster than they could produce the books for 10,000 yen per book. What a celebration when they had raised 1,000,000 yen and orders were still coming in!

In January 1983, at a Christian women's conference on peacemaking, I shared some of my experiences in Vietnam as a "Voice of Reconciliation" and had the opportunity to co-chair the 1984 conference with the theme "Now Choose Life."

In March, Ed Long, an American lawyer, severely disabled with muscular dystrophy and confined to a wheelchair with limited use of his hands, stayed in our home for one week. We had him speak about his life experiences with clients, staff, and family at various centres for persons with disabilities, churches, and at Canadian Academy where Melody and Tim attended because he was a pioneer in the independent living movement in Boston, USA.

At the Easter Sunday worship service, Aki baptized Mr. Yamasaki, a client at Aisei-en and the Clients Association President. He was the first person with a disability whom Aki baptized. He had been employed until an accident left him a paraplegic: he lost his job and his wife left with his daughter. He was lonely, bitter, and angry. He really missed his daughter. Aki met him after he was transferred to Aisei-en, and we included him in several family outings. When we were on home assignment, he became very ill. Finally, his married daughter was located and she visited him, along with her daughter, his granddaughter. Yamasaki San passed soon after.

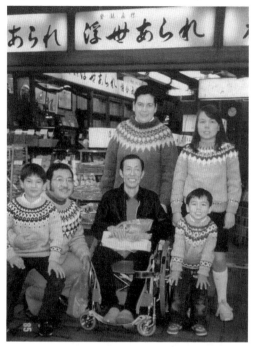

Mr. Yamazaki (centre) with our family: left to right, Tim, Aki, Marcy, Melody, Matthew.

Many North Americans who visited took the opportunity to join the worship service with the intellectually challenged persons. Aki introduced the guests by means of a world map on the wall. He had taught the clients where Japan and Canada were located and used them as reference points for other countries. Many Americans found it rather humorous that the clients could find Canada but not the United States.

You will recall Aki's prayer prior to our assignment to Japan, "Lord, I don't want to go to Japan, but if it really is Your will, please give me a sign." The sign had come in the form of Mr. Hasegawa, in a wheelchair, a resident client at Agape Workshop who was part of the tour group Aki had met in Vancouver. He said that his life changed since meeting us. He left Agape, lived independently, married, had a son Naoto, and supported his family by taking private contracts for typing in his own home. When they first married, they had decided to invest in an electric typewriter with 3,000 characters. Because of Mr. Hasegawa's perseverance and determination to become an accomplished typist, he had the honour and dignity of supporting his family through the use of his right hand.

His family's visit with us in Kobe for five days was memorable. It was the first time they had travelled on the Shinkansen bullet train to Western Japan. We were amused by Naoto, then age two, who took advantage of the fact that neither of his parents could run after him when a reprimand was needed. We were also amazed at his profound perception and sensitivity toward them, helping them as best he could, acting as their hands and feet. A heart-warming five days!

Around this time, Mr. Varghese Abraham from Kerala, South India, came to Japan for four months as the first exchangee of the Japan Christian Social Work League (JCSWL) and stayed in our home while training at Seisei-en. Mr. Abraham was the superintendent of the Nava Jyothi School for Mentally Disadvantaged Children, sponsored by the Mar Thoma Syrian Church. He had graduated from seminary but worked as a social worker with intellectually challenged children. While he was in our home, our children would rehearse the song, "Father Abraham had seven sons . . ." Although it was a new song for Mr. Abraham, he knew it well before leaving Kobe! His presence opened the eyes of the Japanese to the needs in Asia.

Before we left for home assignment in Canada, a significant event occurred: the government granted KSSSC independent status from the Hamamatsu Seirei group. The neighbouring community who had opposed the building of our centres two and a half years earlier was invited to the ceremony. They were beginning to understand and accept our work: some of them became volunteers at our centres. One weekend, approximately 100 of the neighbours came to construct a special garden for wheelchair-bound clients to do gardening. In return, KSSSC offered a large field on the property to the community children for soccer and baseball. Church ministers in the community were now beginning to cooperate with us too. Because we were scheduled to return to Canada for home assignment for a year in July, the local ministers agreed to continue the chaplaincy work on Aki's behalf.

In early July, we were an excited family en route to Canada, arriving in Vancouver, where we rented a car to drive to the Okanagan Valley to visit families of our previous ministry. We were surprised by the wide-open spaces, the few cars on the road, and people driving on the wrong side of the road! Tim was shocked to see that Canada had McDonalds too. The children couldn't believe the number of French fries in a serving. I couldn't believe how carelessly the food was served, such as coleslaw falling off the side of the plate. It was culture shock after living in a culture that required perfection in everything.

Aki had culture shock when he attended the general council meeting of the United Church of Canada in Morden, Manitoba. The focus was on whether a homosexually oriented person could be ordained. This topic was never an issue in Asia.

We moved into the home of a church family in Waterloo that was on a year's sabbatical leave, which matched our needs. Melody, in Grade 4, came home from school one day in tears, asking who she was. At this time, boat people from Vietnam had settled down in the area with several students in her school, and children had called her Chinese. We assured her that she was a blend of Caucasian and Japanese, but she was not Chinese. Tim enrolled in Grade 1 at the same school, benefitting from special services, but he did not qualify for an assessment because he had not been in the system the previous year. Matthew attended a preschool at a local church.

September heralded a new era. Deputation began, which meant speaking about our ministry at Hamilton and Toronto conferences. We shared our initial unwillingness to go to Japan, frustrations and despairs, the joy of seeing the fruit of our labours, and how hope and happiness changed the lives of those who had been empowered and accepted Christ into their hearts. Slides made it real.

In addition to deputation, Aki attended the DPI meetings in Jamaica and Australia along with Senator Yashiro, DPI AP Region Chairperson. DPI had extended its mandate to include the human rights of persons with disabilities because it had non-governmental consultative status with the Human Rights Sub-Commission of the United Nations. DPI took action regarding the plight of mentally ill persons in Japan by taking the issue to the U.N., who then officially approached the Japanese government. Through this experience, we learned how to improve the human rights of persons with disabilities.

At the second Asia-Pacific Regional Convention of DPI in Adelaide, Australia, a mandate on the Human Rights of Disabled Persons was adopted and a Human Rights Committee for the AP Region was set up. Funding came from Canadian International Development Agency. However, because many delegates with disabilities expressed concern for their welfare due to possible repercussions from their governments, it was imperative to carefully study and develop this area. In the AP region, many persons with disabilities did not have the right to education, employment, medical treatment, transportation, housing, and marriage: many faced discrimination by society and their government, legally and illegally. There was a long way to go, but the first step had been taken, so our work and ministry continued.

Our children enjoyed getting to know their grandparents and relatives this school year. They especially liked Grandpa Weber's turkey farm, chasing turkeys in the corn field, etc. Playing in the snow was also a new fun experience.

Aki had left Canada toward the end of February 1985 to visit the U.K., India, and Bangladesh for his research on integration of persons with disabilities into the community. England was advanced in community living but attitudinal discrimination continued to be an issue. He found more natural acceptance in rural communities in India and Bangladesh. Aki was hoping to develop an agricultural community-based inclusive system in Asia through DPI and U.N. agencies. He was impressed with Bangladesh's cow and chicken banks, micro finance projects run by the Blind Association whereby a family had to return a newborn calf and some chicks to the bank to keep the project expanding and promote sustainability.

Aki held a leadership training seminar for persons with disabilities in Bangladesh that focused on the integration of the rural community with persons with disabilities with community-based initiatives. His memory of Bangladesh was of an extremely poor country where there was no food on shelves in the market.

KSSSC continued to develop and opened another vocational training centre for intellectually challenged adults. Aki continued to train and supervise new staff and organize daily morning devotions and weekly worship services. After one year, six clients were able to get job placements.

He continued his chaplaincy work at Aisei-en and supervision at Seisei-en. We were sowing seeds of the Christian spirit in the community.

In April 1985, Aki became a part-time lecturer at Kwansei Gakuin University (KGU), teaching social work about persons with disabilities in the Department of Sociology and Pastoral Counselling at the Master's level in the Seminary. There was much to be done in the area of Christian social work, but there were few workers. Technologically, Japan was well developed, but the human rights of persons with disabilities were deeply neglected. We wanted to pursue Jesus' work in Japan and Asia.

Immediately after completing the school year in June 1985, the children and I returned to Japan where they discovered that both Japan and Canada were their home. They were surrounded by their familiar things and friends again. Matthew, who enrolled in a Japanese preschool, was soon chattering in Japanese. I was green with envy as I struggled with my lessons.

You will recall that Aki had met Rev. Dr. Harold Wilke, born without arms, at a Goodwill convention in the US before we went to Japan. He had developed the use of his feet as hands to write, drive, eat, and dress himself. He was scheduled to stay in our home during his time in Kobe. The children asked endless questions before he arrived, but then sat speechless much of the time he was with us, especially when he ate with his feet on the table with a fork between his toes. Although they had considerable exposure to persons with various disabilities, they had never seen anyone use their feet to eat and telephone, etc.

Our Indian neighbour, wanting to be a volunteer, approached me to see if she could do so at Seisei-en. She enjoyed the experience so much that three more of her Indian friends joined her.

The greatest challenge was to get local ministers to understand that working with persons with disabilities in the community was mission work. KSSSC now had seven centres for persons with disabilities, one community centre, one coffee shop and a day care centre. The coffee shop, opened in a regular shopping plaza, employed three intellectually challenged adults who had graduated from Seisei-en full-time. The organization's policy was that if clients had had five years of training but were too low functioning to be mainstreamed, they would open a day care for about ten persons, which would open the opportunity for ten new clients in the training program. I had been hounding Aki since 1981 about opening a bakery and employing intellectually challenged persons. That had been my daily prayer and continued to be my vision.

A day care centre was made possible by using the 1,000,000 yen raised by the Parents' Association with the sale of the *Quiet Book*. They were so proud of their ability to contribute toward this new addition. God had been blessing our work. At the time, we were providing services for more than 400 clients. KSSSC invited Christian social workers from Korea, India, and Malaysia, who worked with persons with disabilities for an exchange program.

I found myself busy supporting Aki and the family, with three children who were very happy to be back in Japan. Our concern was whether Timothy's academic needs could be met in middle school. The positive side was he was motivated and never gave up, even with extra help!

I continued to take language study part-time. Studying kanji characters was fascinating: one learns so much about culture through language. I learned enough to become aware of how little I knew! It was a good feeling to no longer be illiterate, although there was still so much to learn!

Much of my time was spent in the home, having many international guests who provided stimulating and excellent learning experiences for me. I enlisted the help of the children at times so they could learn to cook. This paid off for Tim at the Japanese Sunday School event for Thanksgiving. Each grade was to take a vegetable to the church to contribute to a pot of stew. The church provided the rice and meat. Each child had to prepare his or her own vegetable. Tim had peeled his in no time, much to the chagrin of his classmates (I guess helping mother in the kitchen does have its advantages). Another classmate was not so fortunate and ended up having a suture job on his right index finger.

The highlight of 1987 was Dr. Jean Vanier's visit to Japan for a Christian retreat with the Catholic Church, who invited our staff to participate. They were moved by his sharing of his life with persons with disabilities.

Christmas in Kobe

Christmas was as busy in Japan as in Canada. Matthew and Timothy were preparing for a concert at school. Melody was practicing her trombone for the junior band's concert. Each centre also had their own Christmas program that they practiced for weeks in advance. Their performances always surpassed the commercial ones. I will never forget one of Seisei-en's pageants. I recognized the client playing the role of Joseph, which I must share.

Joseph was finally able to commute by bus to Seisei-en independently, which was a major achievement. This had been working well, until April, when high school students started their new school year: their excited chatter on the bus when meeting their friends again had totally disoriented Joseph. He got off at the wrong bus stop and started walking. When he did not appear at Seisei-en as scheduled, everyone became concerned. Aki joined the search with staff and family: police were mobilized, but Joseph eluded everyone until the next morning. Feeling hungry, he entered a convenience store five km away and stole an ice cream bar. The owner checked his carryon bag and discovered Seisei-en's phone number, which was how he was finally found, much to everyone's relief. Apparently, he had walked all night and, of course, was happy to be back home and played the role of Joseph well! The Christmas pageants at each centre had the same story but the participants made each one different and special.

Two centres also had candlelight services with a handbell choir from a Christian girls' high school. A family community worship service was held at a neighbouring Christian girls' school with Aki as the speaker.

Every year, Aki and I invited all the KSSSC directors to our home for a Christmas turkey dinner with all the trimmings in appreciation for their commitment and hard work. It was well worth the effort because they looked forward to what became an annual event.

Our tradition immediately after Christmas was to drive to Tokyo to spend time with Okasan, my mother-in-law, to prepare for the new year. As soon as we arrived in Tokyo, we were put to work shopping for vegetables, seafood, etc. before supplies ran out, which always happened. After the food was prepared, it was placed in stacking boxes, called jubako, and put in the cold back room until New Year's Day, when we enjoyed them with ozoni soup, made with specific vegetables, chicken, and rice cakes.

We all watched the TV program that rang in the new year as we ate soba noodles to connect the old year to the new. I also had to do the last cleaning of the house around eleven p.m. because one must not clean on New Year's Day: that would bring bad luck and mean that one would spend the next year cleaning!

After celebrating a few days with Okasan, we returned to Kobe. I was always totally exhausted because my job as the eldest son's wife was to serve the family. At this time, when I was feeling low, worn out and in bed one afternoon with a migraine headache, the telephone rang. It was the school counsellor from Canadian Academy. Apparently, a senior student who was living in the dormitory had been bullied and had attempted suicide. Due to the school policy, she could no longer reside there: the school was looking for accommodation for her so she could complete the school term. The school had immediately thought of our family because we lived at a convenient location so she could walk to school. My first response was that I just couldn't handle any more responsibility. That didn't work, so my second line of defense was that on our salary we ate a Japanese diet. Well, that didn't work either because the student had a Japanese mother and American father and was accustomed to an Asian diet! Could the student come down to meet me? I responded that I would need to discuss this with Aki.

Less than ten minutes later, the front doorbell rang. When I opened the front door, there stood the student. She was a clone of my first cousin who spent every school holiday with my family and was like a sister to me. My shock must have registered. I invited her in to see where she would stay if she lived with us. I said that Aki and I would make a decision that evening and inform the school the next day.

How could we say no? We couldn't! Her parents, who were residing in Beijing and assigned to the American Embassy, were notified of the situation and flew to Kobe immediately. They came to our home on Sunday. Because their daughter was comfortable with the prospect of living with us, the parents were relieved to have a family willing to accept their daughter for the school term ending in June.

The daughter did her best to fit in and even help in the kitchen, which she had never done before. She was so much like my cousin that I felt we had made the right decision. She also began to feel comfortable around our international guests with disabilities.

In the spring of 1988, when I finally completed my formal part-time language study, a Thai couple stayed with us for ten days. Martin, who was blind, was a professional pianist in Thailand and worked as a typist and secretary at the Australian Embassy. His wife, Suthida, was a social worker at the School for the Blind in Bangkok. He hit it off with the student living with us. She played a tune on the piano that Martin had never heard before. After she played it the second time, Martin sat down to play what she had just played. She was mesmerized by him. Martin performed beautifully at our centres, in the community, and Canadian Academy. We always tried to share our talented guests with Canadian Academy to teach our students that a disability can also be a blessing.

June 5 was the last day of school. Our boarder successfully completed her school year with no difficulties so was informed that she could live in the dormitory in September, which was good news. Because our children attended an international school, many of their classmates would leave the country as soon as school was out for the summer. The school followed the American curriculum, so the school year ended in early June, compared to Canada at the end of June. This made for long summers. Melody volunteered to help with summer school at Canadian Academy until early July.

Because we had a cottage at Lake Nojiri, in Nagano Prefecture, Western Japan, I tried to spend much of the summer there with the children. The Nojiri Lake Association was established by the missionary community for their summer vacation, based on volunteers running their programs. Our children had the time, so we went to Nojiri in mid-July to set up the First Aid station: I was a camp nurse for the season, until toward the end of August.

With our family being active volunteers, I could justify spending that much time at the camp. The children assumed other jobs, like painting the house signs for new owners with their name and cottage number. Cottages were scattered across the mountainside, so house signs were essential. The children took swimming classes registered with the American Red Cross, attended summer Bible School, made crafts, and participated in various sport activities. Aki joined us for about two to three weeks as his schedule allowed.

Then, in August, Aki organized an international seminar with the DPI AP in Bangkok, Thailand, in which agencies such as United Nations Economic and Social Commission for the Asia-Pacific region (UNESCAP), WHO, ILO, UNESCO and UNICEF participated as resources. The theme was "Full Participation and Equality of Disabled People." The issues were refugees with disabilities, persons in refugee camps, those who have less accessibility to various services, community-based inclusive development in rural areas, and women with disabilities because many Asian countries denied the human rights of persons with disabilities.

The Christian Church of Thailand organized their first seminar: "The Church and the Disabled." Aki was their keynote speaker, which resulted in the Christian Association of Thailand sending two exchangees, full-time staff at McKean Rehabilitation Centre, and a leprosarium to KSSSC for two months.

Because the incidence of leprosy had decreased in Thailand, they consulted with Aki about the feasibility of developing a community-based inclusive program for persons with other disabilities to maximize the use of their facilities. The exchangees were stunned to discover that Japan, a technologically advanced society, was still forcing persons with leprosy to live isolated from their families and community on a small island or in a very isolated mountain area. Thailand had had an open-door system for twenty years already that allowed persons with leprosy to live with their families in the community. They spoke in Japanese churches and social agencies to encourage the Japanese people to accept leprosy patients in the community. Many Japanese were shocked to discover how they were dehumanizing persons with disabilities in their own country.

In September, we enjoyed the visit of my mother and Aunt Agnes. The children always looked forward to the opening of suitcases from Canada. To date, every summer sausage has successfully been smuggled into Japan due to skillful packing: again, this time. Because it was Aunt Agnes's first visit to Japan, she and I took the Shinkansen to Hiroshima so she could see the Hiroshima Peace Memorial Museum. The museum effectively communicates the horrific experiences of the atom bomb on the citizens of Hiroshima. Even though my aunt was a nurse and had experienced much in her career, she had to leave in the middle of one presentation.

In October, Aki organized a national study conference on leprosy and invited Rev. Tsushima, a person recovered from leprosy, as the keynote speaker. When the hotel staff found out that he was scheduled to stay at their hotel, they refused, saying if people discovered he had stayed there, they would refuse to use their facilities. This attitude continues to this day.

In spring 1988, I was approached by the Parents' Association of KSSSC to consider organizing a tour to Canada, combining orientation to some social services with sightseeing because they could not travel as a family with a regular tour. People with disabilities took much planning and orientation. One hiccup arose when applying for visas to the US. A question on the form was, "Do you have a disability and/or are you on drugs?" which Aki felt was discriminatory and told parents to answer "no" when, in fact, their adult child did have a disability. It worked!

What an excited group we were checking in at the airport in June. I embarked on a nine-day tour with thirty-three persons: each person with a disability was accompanied by a family member. The group included three persons in wheelchairs (seven at airports) and eight intellectually challenged persons, of which three were autistic. It did not take long for me to second guess my decision to accompany this group. We had a tight schedule, which included Niagara Falls, St. Mary's, and Kitchener in Ontario, Banff and Lake Louise in the Canadian Rockies, Alberta and Disneyland in Los Angeles, USA. The Independent Living Centre in Kitchener and the puppets in the "Kids on the Block Program" were a hit. The Rockies were magnificent with the beautiful clear weather. Some black bears, deer, and one moose made an appearance, much to the delight of the group when we took a bus trip to the Columbia Icefields.

This trip was a once-in-a-lifetime opportunity for everyone, and we had a wonderful time. These families had the common bond of being discriminated against because they had an adult child with a disability. On this trip, they had nothing to hide. Everyone soon knew who carried what or who needed help: we boarded and unloaded buses in record time. Everyone was impressed with the services and attitudes in Canada. When we had a reunion in October, mothers repeated how much this trip changed their lives. One client looked at his video of the trip every day! This trip also fostered fellowship between our institutions.

In the fall, Aki was invited as keynote speaker by the Midwestern Japan Conference of the United Church of Christ of Japan to establish a Christian association with persons with disabilities. Rev. Kanekiyo, who had a disability and was a co-worker of the Hyogo Conference Mission Department Committee, stated that he was so pleased that the conference had become active and supportive and was involving persons with disabilities in the church.

After five years, we no longer heard criticism from Japanese ministers who had been rather vocal about their views that working with persons with disabilities in the Christian social work field was not mission work. Now the same ministers had become positive and were participating in Christian social work! The most difficult task was to have people change their attitudes. Modern society had been excluding people with disabilities.

Many persons with disabilities were institutionalized in isolated areas, away from society and family, thinking isolation eliminated discrimination. Discrimination was also experienced by families in their neighbourhoods, employment and schools if they had a family member with a disability. The Buddhist belief that a disability is the result of one's own sins or their ancestors' sins was not much different from those in Christ's time. Our social service community embraced the philosophy of integration and encouraged the families of persons with disabilities to continue to live together as families while we tried to find employment. This was a challenge. Parents were aging, which made it difficult to keep our clients in their homes. Our next goal was to set up group homes in the community.

We opened two day-care centres in the community, each to accommodate a small number of persons with disabilities, rather than a large centre in an isolated place. This was pioneer work with no government or church support at the time. It took time for society to fully comprehend the meaning of this movement.

I began participating in their worship services twice a month with Rev. Tabuchi, who played the guitar and taught songs with actions. Clients loved this, and it was good exercise for them. The parents so enjoyed the opportunity to worship with these delightful clients. Most were unable to communicate verbally, but they knew when they were accepted for who they were.

Around this time, we discovered our son, Timothy, had developed a rare type of tumour of the thyroid, which, thankfully, was discovered early. His surgery, scheduled for January 1989, confirmed that the tumour had been successfully removed with follow up for only two years being necessary. We later discovered that Tim had the most qualified doctor in Japan.

In May, we were stunned when one of our clients, age twenty, had been killed by his father. His father, forced to retire at age fifty-seven, had to get a second-class job in order to support the family. Unfortunately, he became ill and was hospitalized with a deteriorating illness. Depressed and concerned about who would look after his son when he passed away, he escaped from the hospital at noon one day, went home and killed his son by stabbing him with a kitchen knife. Koji, a quadriplegic, was unable to protect himself. This incident was most upsetting for our clients, who could identify with this situation.

I was again approached to plan a second tour group to visit Canada and the USA because the first group talked so much about their positive experience. I agreed to do so because there had not been any major problems on the first tour. It was easy to plan the itinerary, but a major roadblock was the applications for visas to the US.

The travel agent called me in desperation: he had explored all possible avenues to get the visas but had been unsuccessful. Would I please try? My phone call to US Immigration Services in Osaka was also negative and our tour was scheduled to leave in four days! In desperation, I called the father of Melody's classmate, who was working in the American Consulate. He agreed to approve all the applications for visas, but he needed to have all the information before eleven a.m. the next day because the applications had to be sent to Korea for approval. Miraculously, the visas were issued one day before our departure! I received a phone call from an irate staff person in Osaka who had been bypassed, saying he would never issue visas to me again (he had been the person who had initially told me that the visas could not be issued).

The next day, I flew with thirty-two persons from our organization: half had disabilities, four used wheelchairs. What an experience to keep everyone together. We were an excited group that boarded before everyone else and got settled in our seats for the long flight to Washington, DC. Flying was a new experience for everyone. Our itinerary included Niagara Falls and Kitchener, Ontario, the Canadian Rockies, and Disneyland in Los Angeles, similar to the first tour.

Everyone marvelled at Niagara Falls and enjoyed the Maid of the Mist tour on a boat that went very near the falls. In Kitchener, the Independent Living Movement and the "Kids on the Block" puppets impressed everyone again. This was part of our grassroots movement to educate the families.

In the Rockies, we stayed at the famous Chateau Lake Louise. Everyone was having a wonderful time until one minute before we were scheduled to go into the dining hall for the evening meal. I had just arrived in time to see one intellectually challenged person collapse on the floor in front of me. I found no vital signs, started CPR and called for emergency help, which promptly arrived, followed by a local doctor fifteen minutes later. He started an IV and called for an ambulance to take us to a hospital in Banff, a forty-minute drive away. The travel agent decided that the group would continue as scheduled and fly to Los Angeles early the next morning, and we would seek the fastest way for the patient to return to Japan when able.

When in ICU in Banff, the doctors, unable to find a cause for the patient's collapse, discharged him the next day. Unfortunately, all flights via Vancouver were booked solid. Our only option was to continue as scheduled to Los Angeles, which we did the next morning.

On arrival in Los Angeles, there was a Cadillac limousine taxi waiting for us that had been arranged by our travel agent. The mother decided to take her son to the washroom before getting into the vehicle. I waited and waited and, finally, they appeared. Her son had had diarrhea, which had run down his legs and into his shoes. His mother had done her best to clean him up in the washroom but the smell permeated the air. It struck my funny bone when we got in the Cadillac limousine, smelling like "shit," certainly not the type of passengers that would normally be riding in such an extravagant limousine—but who cared! We had arrived safely in Los Angeles and were with the rest of the group, which was all that mattered!

The group had been very concerned and were elated that we were together again. The mother joined the group for the evening dinner, while I stayed with her son who was exhausted.

The next morning, the client was alert and smiled. He joined the group for breakfast and went to Disneyland with them in a wheelchair to conserve his energy. I will never forget this trip, nor has the client who had a cardiac arrest. Whenever he sees me to this day, he stands directly in front of me with a big grin on his face, unable to verbally communicate. He seems to understand that I saved his life. His smile melts me every time I meet him.

Then it was back to Kobe to prepare for our family to go to Canada in July for home assignment and a school year. The United Church of Canada's policy was that we could go for a three-month home assignment every three years or for a school year every five years. We opted for the latter after listening to long term missionaries' stories. Each family had one child who had developed a psychosocial disability when they went to the US after completing high school in Japan. Having grown up in Japan, their social and cultural way of life was different from their parents' American way of life. In the US, they appeared to be Americans and were not treated as foreigners. They experienced much stress while trying to adjust to their parents' culture. Their families had only taken three-month assignments in their home country so their adult children had never spent a full year 'at home' in North America. For me, this was a yellow flag, so we opted for one school year in Canada for our children.

Melody attended Rockway Mennonite Collegiate in Kitchener for Grade 9 and was active in sports and music; Tim, enrolled in Grade 5, was much healthier since his surgery and enjoyed soccer and volleyball; Matthew, in Grade 1, enjoyed being able to ride a bicycle to school. They all adjusted well to their classes and made friends, as well as finding their own identity with relatives in the area.

Aki was studying full-time at the Waterloo Lutheran Seminary for his M.Th in Christian Ethics, focusing on social work and Christian ethics. I studied Ministry with Persons with a Developmental Disability at Emmanuel Bible College. Weekends were spent speaking in churches related to our ministry in Japan. The end of March 1990, Aki returned to

Japan due to the academic year beginning in April. Because he felt strongly about having one foot in field practice and the other in education, he continued to teach at two universities, Kwansei Gakuin (KG) and Seiwa one day per week, teaching Christian Social Work with Disabled Persons and Pastoral Counselling at KG Seminary Graduate School.

With the Japanese senior citizen population increasing, KSSSC was also focusing on social services for seniors. Three years before, a seniors' day care centre was opened in Wadayama Township with a population of 60,000, 120 km north of Kobe. Six hundred people registered! For that reason, we planned to build a nursing care home in the near future with the aim to have our facility also act as a nuclear centre, coordinating services for homebound senior citizens. The second major centre was a nursing care home for persons with severe mental disabilities. We began with sheltered workshops, vocational training, and day care centres for intellectually challenged persons, but parents were now keen to have a residential service because they were aging and were unable to support their children any longer.

Our three children and I returned to Japan in early July after they had completed their school year in Canada. Our time there had been a time of renewal both physically and spiritually, but we were all eager to return to Japan.

I fell back into my role as homemaker and provider of accommodation for guests associated with our work. Our first exchangee arrived from Sri Lanka at the end of October. I accepted the role of secretary for the Canadian Academy as well as for the Kobe Union Church. Board members included representatives of several international corporations such as Nestle, Proctor and Gamble, etc. who taught me much about management and taking minutes. Both institutions had monthly meetings.

The church had sold its property in downtown Kobe and built a new church on Mount Rokko, beside what had been Canadian Academy. The school had sold its property on Mount Rokko and moved to the man-made island of Rokko. Considering all this, writing the minutes was a challenge. The children returned to Japan to attend the new CA on Rokko Island, which meant getting up earlier to take the school bus.

In October, the director of Seisei-en attended a workshop in Kanazawa Prefecture, famous for making lacquerware. He decided to visit a sheltered workshop for intellectually challenged persons in the same prefecture struggling to find a market for their production of lacquerware because the prefecture was known for lacquerware made by professionals. Our director brought several samples to show Aki and wondered whether we could help. I agreed to try. Two of the beautiful small soup bowls had several little bubbles in the lacquer, so I told Aki. He said, "Send them back and tell them why. They are not asking for charity but business." It hurt to do this, but I did. They replaced them with perfect bowls. Several years later they credited me for motivating them to try harder, which is why they could now produce quality lacquerware.

I started selling their lacquerware at church, international schools, and at special events. I would load up the van and soon became known as the lacquerware lady. My orders rescued Kotokuen, the sheltered workshop. At one point, my sales were equivalent to $17,000 Canadian. My moderate prices created a significant profit, which enabled me to forward funds to the sheltered workshop to be shared with the clients, who were thrilled.

Terminal Care for Okasan

In November 1990, Aki and I brought my mother-in-law to Kobe from Tokyo to live with us due to ongoing difficulties with caregivers in her home. She was unable to walk on her own and was drugged with medication. Using a wheelchair, we managed to bring her, half conscious, to Kobe via the Shinkansen bullet train. Later, she couldn't figure out how she got to Kobe! After seeing the amount of prescribed medications she was taking, we gave her the option of cutting back, becoming more alert, and having a shorter life or continuing on her present medications, which were leaving her so drugged that she was too weak to walk and not fully conscious much of the time: basically, a choice between quality or quantity of life.

She opted for quality of life and soon became more alert and could interact with her grandchildren. She also became strong enough to take some steps. I would drive her down the mountainside to a shopping arcade, and then wheel her to a small restaurant whose specialty was okonomiyaki, a Japanese pancake made with cabbage, onion, and pork on top, which she eagerly looked forward to. She sat in her wheelchair at the counter, watching the okonomiyaki being made, and then served on the same grill. Okasan could still enjoy eating!

At the end of January 1991, she went into a coma and passed away in the hospital. The hospital would not release her body without a prayer by a priest, so Aki ended up being the priest to release her to our home. We held a wake service for her that evening and had a Christian funeral at Kobe Union Church the following day.

The cremation was an unforgettable experience. All family members waited while the body was being cremated: when cremation was completed, everyone was given a long pair of chopsticks to pick up the bones. When a person picked up a bone, he was expected to pass the bone to the next person, both using their own chopsticks. This was the only time in Japanese culture when you were allowed to use chopsticks to pass something from one person to another. The bones were then deposited in an urn. There was an order to it, with the thyroid put in the urn last because the shape of the thyroid was like the image of Buddha. I found this whole process repulsive from beginning to end. Her ashes were then taken to Tokyo for a Buddhist funeral two weeks later.

Japan continued to prioritize economic development, focusing on productivity. Persons with disabilities, the sick, and the elderly were regarded as unproductive citizens unable to work, therefore were not entitled to eat. For ten years, we had been working for mainstreaming and the human rights of such persons.

The medical profession exercised great control over clients' lives. Clients had no right to ask questions regarding their illness or care. The Christian community had been silent; ministers untrained and unaware of the medical, social, and psychological aspects of people's lives. Meanwhile ministers faced the dilemma of 13 percent of the population being over the age of sixty-five. It was predicted that by the year 2020, one in four persons would be a senior citizen. The life expectancy was eighty for females and seventy-seven for males, but the current retirement age was fifty-five to sixty. Companies wanted young graduates with up-to-date technological training who started at a lower wage. Employees were encouraged to retire at about fifty-eight years of age and live on very inadequate pensions.

Industrialization had broken the family system. Seniors were no longer cared for by their families, and they died alone in the hospital. Persons with dementia were often confined to bed twenty-four hours a day due to a shortage of care workers and staff. Family doctors did not exist. Public health services were poor. There was a big gap between the perception of Japan as an economic superpower and the reality of life for the average person.

The Japanese government tried to introduce a licensed medical social worker system which would enhance medical doctors' power. Some sensitive Christian medical professionals organized a national campaign and formed the Medical Social Workers Academy. Aki was invited to give the opening lecture and clearly indicated the patients' rights as consumers and defined the social worker's role as restoring humanity for the patients. Though much of this came from a biblical background, and the majority of members were non-Christians, they agreed with the need to focus on the patient's rights.

In June 1991, Aki was able to establish the Holistic Social Service Research Institute that focused on basic Christian values in medical and social services. This was to provide supervisory training courses for Christian and non-Christian social workers in institutions. In the next decade, the working population would decrease and the numbers of elderly persons receiving social services would increase. Already the suicide rate for senior citizens was the highest in the world. For these reasons, KSSSC decided to also focus on senior citizens and was completing a seventy-bed nursing care facility. Six hundred and fifty persons had already registered in the day care service, which began four years before in Wadayama. Our work with persons with disabilities continued to grow, with three major centres and five day-care centres for those with an intellectual disability, and five centres and one factory for those with physical disabilities.

1992 was a year of growth, challenge, work, fun, and change. Our social work ministry with persons with disabilities and senior citizens continued. Ephesians 2:15 says, "Christ's purpose was to create in himself one new humanity out of two, thus making peace" and so, we worked to create understanding and peace between able-bodied persons and persons with disabilities. In Japan, we had two groups, the kenjosha, meaning healthy or 'normal' persons, and shogaisha, referring to persons who are considered 'obstacles' and are discriminated against. For ten years, we had been working for the integration of shogaisha based on a human rights approach. Many persons with disabilities lived in isolated institutions, away from their families and community.

Because Aki's research on the aging of persons with intellectual disabilities was submitted to the local government, and published, we hoped for changes for the betterment of these people. The research results, which revealed dehumanized situations, were depressing. We were promoting family type group homes for five or six members with intellectual disabilities with an attendant care worker to live together in residential areas. At that time, there was no government support or community understanding of that approach. We now had three parents' groups (180 families) of persons with intellectual disabilities, studying group homes and the concept of the mainstreaming movement. Jesus Christ, our great teacher, talked about the grassroots movement in the Bible. He never built institutions, but, rather, after healing persons with disabilities, he asked people to return to their homes and communities.

I was approached again to accompany a group of thirty from KSSSC, fifteen clients and their parents to Hawaii in June for six days. In Hawaii, the parents wanted their adult children to enjoy swimming at the beach which they loved, saying, "It is such a big ofuro!" (An ofuro is a Japanese bath.) Fortunately, there was no medical emergency this time! The challenge was worth it when I saw the clients' smiling faces.

We had a client at Aisei-en, Keigo Ueda, with cerebral palsy, who was very spastic and only able to use his right big toe. He was totally dependent on all activities for daily living, such as eating, bathing, etc. One day, when Aki visited him, he told Aki that he was going to marry, which seemed unbelievable. Aki asked who he was marrying, and after he told Aki it was one of his support workers, Aki went to ask her if she planned to marry Keigo, and she said yes. He asked if she would be able to feed, bath, and look after Keigo, and again, she said yes.

The director of Aisei-en opposed the marriage, as did Keigo's mother, who said it was irresponsible with no income. Aki said he would support their marriage, believing that persons with severe disabilities had the right to marry, but they needed to organize a support system for daily activities.

The couple applied for government housing and got a unit, so they married. Aisei-en staff volunteered twice a week to help with bathing Keigo. They lived on welfare along with their daughter, Ayumi. Keigo's mother had reconciled with him after their daughter was born. His wife had been helping Keigo with his distance learning through a Buddhist university where he eventually got his BA of Social Work. One day, when his wife was riding her bicycle to get their welfare cheque, she was hit by a truck and killed. Such a tragedy! His mother then moved in with Keigo and her granddaughter, Ayumi, who continued to live on welfare and paid for a support worker.

Fortunately, Keigo's wife had taken out a life insurance policy that benefitted him at this difficult time. Several years later, when we visited his mother in the hospital—she was terminally ill with cancer—she asked us to please look after her granddaughter because the support worker could not look after her too. We promised to do so.

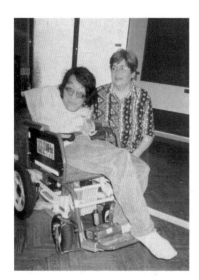

Rev. Keigo Ueda with Marcy.

Ayumi moved in with our family while Keigo had a support worker. Keigo said that he wanted to become a church minister. He had studied theology with local ministers for three years and had been commissioned two years ago as Reverend Ueda. It was very difficult to find a church that would accept his services due to difficulty in understanding his speech caused by spasticity and the accessibility issue. One church accepted a one-year contract only. His contract with the second church, which he was serving, stated that he was to come to the church on Sundays only. Fortunately, a third church accepted Rev. Ueda as an assistant minister for one year. There was still a big wall between kengo-sha and shogaisha in the church, as well as in the community. Christ was asking us to be a bridge between the two groups to make peace. We are all God's children.

Keigo was one of the persons who joined my second tour group to the US and Canada. Ayumi continued to live with us until the spring of 2000. She then lived with her aunt because it was not yet considered appropriate for her to live with her father and a support worker. We later learned that after Ayumi married, she looked after her father until he passed away in 2019.

As chairperson of the International Committee for the Japan Christian Social Work League (JCSWL), Aki promoted involvement with the Church of North India. Reverend Amal De, a guest of JCSWL, who came to Japan to discuss cooperation between the two countries, proposed that Japanese churches and JCSWL support their children's program. The Church of North India was deeply concerned about the plight of the children of tribespeople who had been forced to leave their land and were discriminated against by the Hindus. Because they had a dismal future without education, the Church of North India needed additional funds for a school they had started for these children. However, Japanese churches were slow to respond. Most ministers were theologically oriented and reluctant about any community involvement and social justice issues.

An age wave was rapidly approaching Japan. The past fall, our organization had opened a seventy bed senior citizens home. With beds immediately filled, we had a long waiting list.

We had finally established a church at one centre in Kobe, called Aisei Church, which means "Living with Love." We had six members and a retired pastor, Reverend Mukai. One Aisei-en resident was baptized and several more dearly wanted to be, but their families strongly opposed.

We were so spiritually blessed by Mr. Miyota, a wheelchair user, unable to talk, who used a keyboard to communicate. When his whole body moved his face looked heavenward and his eyes shone with joy as he sang the hymns with guttural sounds. He had been begging his father to be baptized for a year and a half. Mr. Miyota lived the greatest commandment,

"Love the Lord your God with all your heart, with all your soul, and with all your mind." Matthew 22:37.

Summer 1992 was extremely busy for me, probably because I had overextended myself. One Wednesday, KSSSC had a big all-day bazaar sponsored by three of our largest centres in Kobe. I took three van loads of donated used clothing that I had sorted. Our church congregation had just moved into the new Kobe Union Church for our first worship service on September 6.

As secretary, I was saddled with numerous jobs besides taking the minutes. We had tea on Thursday for anyone interested in seeing the building and/or becoming church members. On Friday, I met with a Vietnamese Japanese girl, who kindly consented to write several letters for me to our Montagnard and Vietnamese friends in Vietnam.

Melody was in her final year of high school at Canadian Academy, filling her time with sports, choir, and playing the trombone in the jazz and performance bands. Timothy, the tallest in the family, in Grade 8, was outgrowing all his clothes and was excited about playing the tenor sax. Matthew, in Grade 5, had to curtail his sports activities due to Osgood-Schlatter Disease causing pain in his left knee. Fortunately, he was diagnosed early and it was not severe: it just required knee support at the time, which eliminated sports activities. The pain decreased with control of activity so we had much to be thankful for.

In October, Aki was honoured to give a speech at the UN chapel in New York during the special general session of the UN Decade of Disabled Persons held by the 47th UN General Assembly, recognized by General Secretary, Boutros Boutros-Ghali. In December, Aki was coordinator for an NGO forum and DPI's Leadership Training Seminar in Beijing, China, resulting in a recommendation for the Asia-Pacific Regional Decade of Disabled Persons 1992-2003 by UNESCAP.

Aki continues to be a catalyst in the church, the community at large and the government. Changes come slowly.

First Visit to Vietnam after the War

Our family spent Christmas 1992 in Vietnam after Aki's and my absence of twenty-two years! We were some of the first tourists from the Western world after the war. We landed at Hanoi airport and were met by a used Kobe city bus. The children were so excited to see a familiar Kobe bus being used in Hanoi. When we went to claim our baggage, we discovered Aki's and my suitcase with all our clothes and gifts for friends never arrived! My carry-on was full with the meds for Tim, so I did not have an extra change of clothes. Aki had his bathing suit and a sarong; he slept in his bathing suit, and I slept in his sarong!

We were required to have an escort during our entire time in Hanoi. A young Vietnamese lady dressed in a white ao dai met us and took us to a Cuban built hotel by the small Hoan Kiem Lake, meaning "Lake of the Restored Sword." After checking in, we asked our guide whether we could visit Ho chi Minh's (Uncle Ho's) mausoleum. She produced a big smile and was obviously delighted to guide us there. She said that it was closed for the day, but she would open it for us. We doubted her: when she took us there the gate was locked. With her order, the guard immediately opened the gate. We began to wonder who this young lady was. She explained the life of Ho Chi Minh, who impressed us with his commitment to strive for independence from Western colonization and his simple way of life.

On December 24, we were scheduled to fly from Hanoi to Nhatrang. When we went to board the plane in Hanoi, we soon understood why other passengers had raced ahead. They knew that there were no assigned seats! We were the last ones to board. I will never forget this flight! I had the luggage of the person next to me under my legs, the front right window of the small plane was boarded up, and the fruit being peeled by the attendant across from me went up to the cockpit.

The airport in Nhatrang had no terminal building, just a small tin roofed shack. Our friends were waiting outside for us. It was an emotional meeting with about fifteen previous hospital staff, including Anh Tin, Yong and his wife from Pleiku, who came to meet us and provide transportation since there was no public transportation allowed at the airport. Our friends planned for each of us to ride on the back of their motorbikes.

Aki and I didn't have all of our luggage, but the children each had their backpacks. The kids were hesitant to get on the motorbikes until they saw Aki and me already on ours and realized they didn't have a choice.

We all stopped at a small restaurant to have a bowl of noodles before checking into our hotel. Our friends asked if we wanted to go to Vinh Phuoc church that evening (my home church) for their special Christmas Eve Service, and we said we did. Anh Tin said that we were welcome to go and five motorcycles would come to pick us up, but we must leave right after the church service. We agreed to do so.

The church was full and overflowing with children hanging in all the open windows. But strangely, there was an empty bench for our family only; none of our friends sat with us or acknowledged our presence. It was so unlike old times. We left right after the service. Anh Tin then said he would pick us up on Christmas morning for the service. After the Christmas service, he invited us to his home for lunch along with Yong and his family. This was when we were told that the pastor at Vinh Phuoc Church had been interrogated for an hour after the Christmas Eve service, asked who we were, who invited us, etc. In the afternoon, we attended the worship service at the leprosarium, fully aware that we were being followed. It was an overwhelming experience to be able to worship again with dear friends, but it was also depressing to learn of the continued suffering of many people.

The fact that I was wearing the same clothes every day was not lost on my friends. When they discovered the reason was that one of our suitcases did not arrive, the next morning, when we visited the home of my friend, her husband, a tailor, immediately started taking my measurements and sewing a pair of pants and a blouse for me. Late that evening, my friend and her husband arrived at our hotel, by bicycle, with the finished pair of pants and blouse. On arrival, the security guard asked whom they wanted to see. After a brief explanation, the guard said, "Oh, the lady with the blue pants." That was all he had ever seen me wear until the next day when I modelled my new clothing. For three days, we shared, ate, laughed, cried, and prayed together.

We were stunned to learn that our ex-hospital staff had been forced to move out of the hospital compound after 1975 and were living in the swampy area just outside the compound. They had not been allowed to enter the hospital compound for the last twenty-two years! Our request to see the hospital was granted, along with an assigned escort. Our previous staff accompanied us and were surprised to see that the facilities were now used for rehabilitation of government officers.

We also learned that graduates from our one-year School of Nursing were not allowed to be employed as nurses. Instead, some were selling rubber thongs, peanuts, and coffee at local markets.

One person we had not expected to meet was Thanh, who had fled Vietnam with his aunt Minh seven years ago. We had sent care packages to them in a refugee camp in the Philippines to aid their survival. This was his first visit to Vietnam since he and his aunt had immigrated to Melbourne, Australia. He shared with us how his aunt Minh had been working part-time at a sewing factory and did alterations at their home to support both of them. Out of respect he did not want to share that she often worked until three to four a.m. with his family in Vietnam. On returning to Australia, he had shared with his aunt about our family, our work, and the fact that our luggage had disappeared. She was so moved that a year later a letter arrived by special delivery, with an international money order equivalent to $500 Canadian. It was hard to accept it knowing the difficult life they had experienced. Thanh had just graduated from high school in Melbourne, Australia in December.

Another unexpected treasure was to meet Yong and his wife. We had learned that he graduated from Saigon University through a Vietnamese refugee couple we had invited to our home in Kelowna, BC. Yong shared the discrimination he was experiencing by the Vietnamese in Pleiku, who would not help him with medical supplies as a nurse practitioner. We decided to give him American dollars for his ministry, which, when exchanged for piasters, filled a shopping bag. He was concerned whether he could get past security. We discovered later that he did return safely with the funds to invest in the needed supplies.

Yong had shared in a letter to Anh Tin how Vietnamese military had entered their church, took pictures off the wall, stamped on them, and then forbade them to worship in their church. Yong said they then met in the corn fields late at night to pray because they were no longer allowed to sing.

Boldly, he had conducted a one-day Christian leadership event for Bahnar Christians. When this was discovered, he was imprisoned for one week. Montagnards continued to be discriminated against. Anh Tin informed us that our correspondence with Yong could jeopardize his safety, so it was best to send our letters to Yong through him.

This whole scenario reminded me of the words of Mizuno Genzo, who spent most of his life confined to bed, unable to verbally communicate.

> Suffering . . .
>> If I had not suffered
>> I would not have known the love of God.
>> If many people had not suffered
>> God's love would not have been passed on.
>> If Jesus had not suffered
>> God's love would not have been made visible.

On January 2, 1993, we safely returned to Kobe after a wonderful trip to Vietnam and soon fell into our routines. We had an American Presbyterian missionary family move in next door: their three children, about the ages of ours, became good friends with our children. We took time to orientate them to the community and the school.

With this being Melody's final year of high school, we began working on applications for University of Waterloo (U of W) and Wilfrid Laurier University (WLU), also in Waterloo, Ontario. Melody wanted to study math and kinesiology.

It became apparent that Japanese society was beginning to suffer from economic depression, with many small companies going bankrupt. Workers were discouraged from working extra hours due to decreased consumer demands. However, fewer were laid off than in Canada. With a family-oriented company system, workers' income was lowered to avoid laying off employees. This was a good experience for the Japanese because they had been working too hard and many long hours to build up economic strength. As a result, their family life and the community support system had been neglected. In spite of the economic depression, we had more hope to encourage people to focus on their own family and neighbours' lives rather than on the company's life.

An age wave was also rapidly approaching with 13.5 percent of the population over age sixty-five at this time. It was predicted to rise to 25 percent in twenty-five years. With community support and family systems broken, and minimal social services, the needs were great.

In 1993, we continued to encourage Japanese churches to change from being intellectual and preaching centred to become a healing, growing neighbourhood church. Many church ministers were trained to be professional preachers but not pastors. Our clients, especially those with intellectual disabilities, did not benefit from the long theological sermons.

Aki finally published his book, *The Theology of Social Work*, which clearly spelled out the needs noted above, as well as a booklet, *Pastoral Guidance with Senior Citizens*, based on liberation theology. Ministers, although surprised, showed an interest in the new theology that encouraged Christian and non-Christian social workers to develop human rights. Aki was asked to have a regular study group, to seek justice regarding brain death, organ transplants, AIDS, disabilities, etc. by a group of committed Christian staff.

We continued to promote a community-centred social service system, rather than institutional service. However, very few services were available in the community, such as a family doctor system or community social workers. With most doctors working in hospitals, and social workers in institutions, mainstreaming had a long way to go.

Aki visited Mongolia in August and Bangladesh in October and November to organize an international leadership training seminar with and for persons with disabilities. In Mongolia, persons with disabilities found it especially enlightening to hear about human rights, independent living, job placement, family life, social security, etc. Interestingly, there were very few severely disabled persons in Mongolia because most never reached adulthood due to the lack of medical care, a social service system, or balanced nutrition.

Aki worked closely with UNESCAP, a UN organization promoting the Asia-Pacific Decade of Persons with Disabilities 1993-2002. Over 60 percent of the world's population lived in the Asia-Pacific region, where developing countries did not have adequate statistics regarding persons with disabilities. In order to do this work, Aki was training persons with disabilities as leaders.

In May, tension was building up for the end of the school year as well as Melody's graduation. She had received acceptance at WLU and CGC (Conrad Grebel College) residence, which we felt was the best of all the options. She would be in a caring supportive Christian environment, have a balanced diet, and peer orientation to Canadian culture. She was looking forward to it.

I made a beautiful prom dress for Melody using some of Okasan's black materials, along with shiny trim from one of her happy coats. I also made her graduation dress.

Melody had played in all the sports throughout the school year and received two most valuable player awards for volleyball and soccer, as well as athlete of the year at the closing sports ceremony. At the high school spring concert, Melody played her trombone in the jazz and performance bands and sang in Interlude and senior choir. She was honoured with the John Philip Sousa Award for band and a Ford scholarship worth $3,500. Her year could not have ended better.

Aki was honoured to deliver the speech for Melody's graduating class. Our family had a graduation tea: all her teachers and some friends were invited for her grand finale in Kobe. Immediately following graduation, Melody was hired to work with the CA Elementary Summer Program, and then as a lifeguard at Lake Nojiri until mid-August.

On August 25, Melody and I flew to Toronto, and I helped her get settled at CGC. It was hard to say goodbye, knowing we as parents would be on the other side of the Pacific Ocean! She was able to meet with classmates from Grade 9 at Rockway one weekend and make onigiri (rice balls) with a Japanese Canadian student living in residence. My parents were also a tremendous support by welcoming Melody on weekends.

I returned to Kobe on September 6, immediately jumping into a full schedule again with CA, KUC, KSSSC, starting a three-year term as council member for Kobe Jogakuin Girls College in Nishinomiya, serving as a council and board member for Toyo Eiwa Jogakuin (kindergarten up to and including university) in Tokyo, as well as Shizuoka Jogakuin, a girls' school in Shizuoka representing the UCC (United Church of Canada): I had monthly meetings in Tokyo as a representative to the Council of Cooperation's Shadan, a legal entity, to act on behalf of the UCC for their properties in Japan. It seemed that all of a sudden, my life was becoming too much like Aki's, with a lot of travelling. I was fulfilling responsibilities on behalf of the UCC but it was not a fulfilling experience to function at this level. I was basically a grassroots person and enjoyed making things happen at that level, leaving administrative decisions to others.

I continued to be involved with KSSSC's centres, especially two sheltered workshops. In March, I accompanied eight persons from KSSSC as coordinator and nurse to a Thai International Christian camp for persons with physical and intellectual disabilities in Chiangmai, Thailand. Each one of our centres had one person represented in the group.

How well I remember my conversation with the client from Seisei-en who had an intellectual disability. He was brilliant and spoke a fair amount of English. He shared how his father had bullied and belittled him, saying that he was stupid and would never be able to do anything. His mother, a great support and advocate for him, taught him English. One day, when we were travelling by van to a Thai tribal village, he started scratching his tummy, then his arms and legs. I looked at him and realized he was having an allergic reaction. The driver of the van spoke no English, but he did understand my urgent sign language for emergency medical care. The driver pointed to his watch meaning in fifteen minutes; meanwhile, I could see that the client could soon go into anaphylactic shock without treatment because the swelling was moving up to his face.

We arrived at a medical clinic in the middle of nowhere, and I pulled the client out of the van, dragged him into the small First Aid station, pulled up his shirt, and, well, they got the message. They immediately gave him an injection of Benadryl. Within a few minutes the swelling went down significantly, much to my relief. Needless to say, we made sure that he never ate mango again!

This client thrived on the trip. We delegated him to give the closing speech on behalf of our group, and it moved everyone to tears. Other participants represented included Myanmar, Korea, Thai, Japan, and Canada. He returned to Japan, empowered by this experience, and he wasted no time in telling everyone how Marcy saved his life, which was humbling for me. What a rich experience and education!

A friend shared the logo of her home church, which we felt captured our purpose there as a family. "We are called to GIVE OURSELVES AWAY in unconditional love to God, one another and others SO THAT WE AND THOSE WE TOUCH MAY KNOW GOD personally and intimately through JESUS CHRIST by the power of the Holy Spirit. All to the glory of God."

In spring 1994, when Aki visited Cambodia to organize a self-help group among persons with disabilities, he discovered that there was no self-organized group of this kind. Most persons with disabilities had become disabled due to civil war, especially from land mines. Millions of mines still lie buried in fields and cause people to lose limbs daily. In Cambodia, a rehabilitation program entailed landmine removal. Many NGOs were helping to provide prosthesis and wheelchair services, but there was no grassroots movement of persons with disabilities. Aki decided to continue to help develop an organization of persons with disabilities.

In the fall, Aki went to Indonesia for the Asia-Pacific Regional Assembly of DPI and presented a paper on "Accessibility for Higher Education." While there, he was appointed as the regional adviser for DPI AP, and continued to work with persons with disabilities in the AP region for the Asia-Pacific Decade for Disabled Persons 1993-2002.

In 1994, JCSWL sponsored international exchangees for a rehabilitation program from India, the Philippines, Thailand, and Korea. Aki organized a national seminar on Christian social work with Aids, with Irene Fellizer, General Director of Kabalikati, a drop-in center for street children and prostitutes in Manila, as the main speaker. Through our Asian exchangees sharing, our staff could see and understand the lives of other Asian cultures looking through new lenses!

Kwansei Gakuin University opened a new department: School of Policy Studies and asked Aki to become full-time faculty to teach international social work with persons with disabilities. He was able to continue to train social workers with KSSSC.

On the home front, Melody was in her second year at WLU, and she was finding her studies a challenge. Timothy, a Grade 10 student at CA, worked hard so he could participate in volleyball and basketball. Matthew, in Grade 7, also enjoyed sports again, as well as his cornet!

The year 1995 marked fifteen years since our arrival in Japan. We had been working in the area on many small tasks, which had begun to grow and bear fruit, making us feel it was the beginning of the harvest and that God was also giving us larger tasks.

Fifteen years was adequate time to lay a foundation for our social work ministry where human relations and long-term commitment were an asset to do God's work. Local pastors were also feeling blessed by participating in this ministry.

The Kobe Earthquake

Little did we know how our lives would be changed on January 17, 1995, at five forty-six a.m.

I was sound asleep on my futon when, suddenly, I was thrown awake vertically, then horizontally with a sound like a bomb exploding and a demon-like sound emanating from deep in the earth. The violent shaking continued for twenty seconds—it had to be an earthquake! I felt like popcorn being popped! I was unable to find the flashlight always kept beside the futon for emergencies. Unable to keep my balance, in a panic I started crawling on all fours down the hall. What a relief to have Matthew appear at his door because I was afraid that his sliding door would jam. Water could be heard running from a broken pipe in the next room; we were unable to find any light.

Thor, a sixteen-year-old student living with us, came bounding out of his room at the front of the house just in time to answer the phone. It was Aki asking us to open the front door because it could become jammed, and not to go outside due to possible falling debris. Then there was another violent tremor for ten seconds. It was pitch dark. I couldn't see anything or understand what was blocking the doorway into the kitchen. I asked Thor to get the lighter for the stove that was always beside the phone. When he finally found it, we couldn't believe what we saw. Our kitchen was rear-ranged: the cupboard contents were well distributed on the floor with soy sauce, cooking oil, broken dishes, and a generous amount of cinnamon sprinkled on top. The aroma was great but what chaos!

Then the phone rang again. It was Aki telling us to get the shortwave radio we kept in the living room.

After finding our shoes and jackets and wrapping blankets around ourselves, we ran out the front door in our pajamas. We were greeted by our next-door missionary neighbours, who had panicked because their house was badly damaged. We decided to evacuate to the old Canadian Academy schoolyard above our home, where we stayed until daylight with others. In the darkness, one could see Kobe aflame with billows of black smoke all across the horizon. Fire had started in many places at the same time. People used kerosene heaters in winter and cooked with gas.

At the time of the earthquake our family was in three places. Aki was at a chaplain's retreat on the other side of Mount Rokko, Tim was hospitalized at Kaisei Hospital across the ravine behind our home due to paralysis of the right side of his face, and Matt and I were at home with Thor. Fortunately, I had returned home the night before with Aki's car, but it left him with no wheels!

As soon as it was light, Thor, Matt, and I returned home to get dressed in warm clothes. It was cold with a little snow on the ground. I was concerned about Tim in the hospital because he spoke little Japanese. I had to drive down the mountainside in Aki's car and up the other side to get to the hospital, even though it was directly below our home at the back. Fortunately, there was an English-speaking Catholic Father as a patient in his ward.

Knowing he was safe, I drove home in Aki's car, incredulous at the destruction. The contents of peoples' homes were on full display, spilling onto the road. Some cars parked at the side of the street were packed with personal belongings, ready to flee the area. Then I met the neighbours living on the other side of our home. We decided to walk up to the church across from the old CA campus where everyone had evacuated to decide what to do. The church was built on a sharp cliff.

By eight a.m., Yamaguchi gumi Mafia, whose headquarters were two blocks down the mountainside, had delivered plastic water containers to the church with the name of their godfather, Watanabe written on each one! They were perfect since we had to carry water from Mount Rokko. The Mafia also had bananas delivered to the church by nine a.m.! All bananas entering Japan came through Kobe port. By the next day, the Mafia had pita bread delivered too! Meanwhile, the government was dysfunctional.

Returning home, we discovered that there was a fault between our house and the neighbour's property. The ground had sunk at least six inches in a straight line across the whole property and down into the ravine. I later learned that if you lived near a fault, you could hear the demon-like sound followed by a tremor one second later. That was what I had heard coming up from the earth early that morning.

We also discovered that the metal rails for our carport were bent in the shape of a Z. Thankfully, we had access to a saw that cut metal so we were able to drive our van out. Our telephone was not working properly: I learned that there was a payphone in the cemetery above the old CA school grounds, so I walked up there only to discover a queue that included my Indian neighbour, Jothi, and had to wait in line. She phoned her husband in Hong Kong telling him in a hysterical voice not to return to Kobe that day because there was no possible way for him to get home except to walk from Osaka.

I needed to inform people in the Tokyo office that our family and the two missionary families on either side of our home were all safe and not injured but our houses were damaged beyond repair. Since our phone was out of order, I walked up to the cemetery and joined the queue to use the public phone. I finally got through to the person in charge of Human Resources and said that I just wanted to let him know that we were all safe. His response was, "Well, you will just have to pull together." I thought, what a strange response, so I confirmed the phone call was to let him know that we were safe. Later, I learned he hadn't heard about the earthquake that morning. When he got off the phone, he had asked his colleagues if something had happened in Kobe. They were stunned that he hadn't heard about the earthquake. When he tried to phone back, of course, he couldn't because our phone was out of order.

A pastor who had attended the chaplain's retreat kindly drove Aki home via the mountain road because the regular road was destroyed. He arrived home around ten-thirty a.m., shocked at the destruction. Where he had been staying, they had felt strong tremors, but there was no destruction; our side of the mountain was unbelievable. Aki then said that we needed to clean up the kitchen. I remember looking at him, thinking, clean up the kitchen? Since he started to do so, I fell in line and started to help him but had to be told what to do. I had panicked and was obviously in a state of shock.

Aki and I started to clean up the kitchen and living room for neighbours, amid the frequent aftershocks. We reset the kerosene stove and made the room warm for about twenty people—most of whom were still in their pajamas.

It was then that we took note of the fact that our piano had moved at least one and a half feet from the wall it was sharing with Aki's office and was now on the carpet, which was still flat. This meant that the piano had literally jumped onto it: it had not slid the distance. We had two decks of CDs and a CD player that were on top of the piano too, but everything was in its place only one and a half feet over from its original position. On the other side of the wall, Aki's office had book shelves from ceiling to floor. Aki discovered that he could not open his office door because it was jammed with books. What a tedious job to remove one book at a time to finally get the door open. Then we discovered that all the *National Geographic* magazines that had been piled on the floor below the book shelves pre-quake were now on the other side of his office.

Fortunately, our electricity soon came on because the best way to help panicked people was to serve a warm drink and hot food. Matthew and Thor walked up to the dam on Mount Rokko for water. We three missionary families decided to pool our resources. We were the only home with electricity at the time: one family had a major supply of seaweed and the other a lot of rice, so we cooked three pots of rice in our home to make onigiri, about thirty rice balls.

At the hospital, Tim was served one rice ball for each meal and half a cup of water. We discovered that families staying at the hospital with their patients had no food and not enough clothes, so, in the evening, we made rice balls to share with them and went back home for towels, toothbrushes, and clothes.

From the hospital one could see fires engulfing the city! This continued for three days, along with fire were ambulance, and police sirens, and helicopters flying over us! There was no water supply due to broken water lines: fire engines met blocked streets from destroyed homes and debris: most of the telephone system as well as the emergency communication systems were also destroyed, so rescue teams outside Kobe city did not arrive until the following day. Ordinary citizens had to rescue people trapped by their broken homes. This earthquake was rather unusual because of the strong vertical movement for several seconds, then strong horizontal movements again. As a result, the first floors of many homes collapsed. Most people who had slept on the first floor were killed. The worst part was persons trapped in debris who could not escape the encroaching fires. One friend related how he struggled to help a person crying for help but was unable to before the fire spread. There were many sad stories.

The wife and children of our Indian neighbours across the street had driven away within hours of the earthquake to join their friends who made a convoy to drive to Osaka. The next day, Jothi phoned me (the phone happened to be working then) from Kansai International Airport, saying that a convoy of six cars of Indian friends had made the trip to Osaka the day before, but it took six hours and the sights were unbelievable. Ordinarily, it would take only forty minutes. She informed us that they were leaving the country: she had given their house keys to another neighbour to give to us so we could access the food in her home. Her last sentence was whispered into the receiver, "Marcy, if you need any gas, please tell Aki that he can siphon gasoline from my car since the tank is full and unlocked." I chuckled to myself that she felt that she had to whisper the message—who would know where she lived?

A badly injured teenage boy was admitted to the bed beside Tim. We noticed his parents were spoon feeding water to their son. We provided rice balls for the parents. His parents slept on the floor beside their son in a state of shock, dressed in their pajamas, unable to speak clearly. On the third day, the father was finally able to talk to us. They had lived in a two-storey company apartment which collapsed at the time of the earthquake. He had tried to get up from the floor but couldn't because the ceiling was only about two feet from his head. Panicking, he managed to kick a hole through the ceiling to escape in total darkness. Then he heard his wife calling for help. He managed to rescue her by making another hole. Their son, who slept in the next room, could be heard calling for help. The father broke the floor with his hands, and after two hours he succeeded in rescuing their son.

They were able to drive to a nearby hospital but realized that there was no entrance! The first floor of the six-storey hospital had completely collapsed so they drove to Kaisei Hospital where Tim was hospitalized. The father started to cry as he related the story of rescuing his family. He had also tried to rescue the family next-door. He could see the parents with their two-year-old daughter between them with a beam across their chests. They did not respond to his call and there was no way he could remove the beam or the debris above them. There was also no response from the four- and six-year-old daughters. His hands and feet were badly injured from rescuing his own family. They did have their son who, they discovered, had become a hemiplegic (paralysis of the left side of his body) due to a spinal cord injury but he was alive!

Radio information said that anyone who had lost their bank book or cash card could withdraw up to ¥100,000 ($800 Canadian) with any ID card, so Aki gave the husband the information. His family had lost all their IDs and they had no money. Fortunately, I had just gone to the bank the day before so we were able to help them.

Joanne, a French-Canadian volunteer with KSSSC, had walked six hours from her apartment to get to our place. By evening, our neighbours and the other missionary families joined us to cook a meal over a bonfire. The husband of the Muir missionary family was to be travelling home from Taiwan so they were expecting him to phone home. With their phone out of order, they expected he would call us because ours was working off and on.

Meanwhile, strong aftershocks continued. We felt God's protection after surveying the damage of the three houses. The house on our left side was totally damaged and, basically, unsafe to venture inside, but the husband finally did go in to get some warm clothes and a few other items. The retaining wall holding their home in place was badly damaged, and it was possible that a landslide could occur with the aftershocks. Our house was off its foundation, not level, and it had broken pipes, etc. The house on the other side, three storeys high and built at least ten feet above us, with a retaining wall surrounding it, had two double barrelled concrete chimneys that broke off; one chimney had hit the retaining wall, took out a piece, bounced, and landed outside Matt's bedroom window. The other chimney fell on the front entrance to their home. Their lives had been spared. Then we noticed that the whole side of their home facing ours had separated from the main house. With all the aftershocks, we were afraid that it would fall down on our house. That was what we were facing when we knew that Mr. Muir would likely be phoning us sometime that evening.

It was decided that Aki and two boys would spend the night at our home on standby for the phone call. Terrified that the side of the house next door would fall, they barricaded themselves under the dining table for protection. At two a.m., Mr. Muir phoned from the airport. We told him that the train station nearest us had collapsed so he should wear walking shoes and walk from Nishinomiya train station, which was about a seven hour walk. He arrived mid-morning exhausted.

The first night, Joanne and I slept in Aki's car in the athletic field of the old CA: Matt and Thor slept in the van beside our car. We had carefully chosen a place to park away from all the major cracks in the field, knowing that everything was held by retaining walls. We put the seats as flat as possible, but, with our bulky winter coats and heavy Japanese covers, there was hardly any space to move, and sleep never came!

Matt, Thor, and I stayed in our area while Aki felt that he had to check with KSSSC and all their centres. Many clients and staff had lost their homes, but no one was killed. Several clients did have family members that were killed. One day care centre was destroyed. Over 300,000 people were displaced and moved into evacuation sites. It was difficult for persons with a hearing impairment because they could not hear instructions: autistic persons panicked and were screaming much of the night, which disturbed others. Others with mobility disabilities couldn't access the evacuation centres or toilets, so many of them opted to return to their unsafe homes until arrangements could be made for them to be moved to Osaka. Even with the difficulties of our clients, it was decided that all our centres in Kobe would collectively receive sixty evacuees with disabilities.

KSSSC had a large field used for sports activities in the same compound as Seisei-en and Aisei-en, which they offered to displaced persons who lost their homes. The government was planning to set up fifty temporary housing units, especially for persons with disabilities and senior citizens because we already had medical and social service facilities on the same compound. Our staff were willing to voluntarily help. In fact, staff were already providing bath service for senior citizens and persons with disabilities who had evacuated to local schools that did not have bath facilities. One of our centres started preparing 200 meals daily for evacuees. It could be compared to a war situation; some staff evacuated to our centres with their dogs; people were constantly coming and going.

Because Aki was also responsible for member agencies of JCSWL, he visited children's homes by bicycle because no public transportation was available. Train lines were broken, the subway partially collapsed, roads were heaved, cracked, and blocked. The residential building of Shinai, a children's home, was badly damaged, necessitating the evacuation of sixty-eight children, including twenty-seven babies to Shinseijuku, another children's home. Aki helped. Many children had panicked, some requiring oxygen for their asthmatic attacks and there was none available. Fortunately, Aki, who had a cellular telephone offered by the Motorola company for persons involved with rescue, was able to get oxygen at one of our centres after biking across the burned area of Kobe for two hours, then back again! He was also able to deliver food to evacuees along with John Schmidt, another missionary.

At the end of the day, Aki decided to stop at every Kyodan Church (United Church of Christ in Japan) en route to a missionary's home where he was staying and have prayer with the ministers. Aki said it was a very spiritual experience—one of sincere joy with tears. He found them alive, safe, and with joy amidst tragedy. The first church minister could not meet Aki because he was having prayer with a family that had lost a member. Three to four blocks later, the minister came running, calling Aki's name. They held hands in the middle of the street and prayed with tears. Aki felt Christ's presence working strongly through this tragedy.

He arrived at the last church after ten p.m. Kobe Heian Church building and the manse were badly damaged: the family had evacuated to a kindergarten room on the same compound. Reverend Harano's family, with three daughters, and two church members, who had also lost their houses, were sitting together in a small room. Rev. Harano had just returned from helping a church member. It was almost midnight when Aki reached Lardner and Mollie Moore's home in Mikage, two train stations distance from our home. Aki found them trying to sleep in their front doorway, fully dressed so they could escape if necessary. He was able to reset their kerosene stove, so they could have heat again! When walking home, several people cooking with bonfires offered Aki some food, which he declined thinking it's only for displaced people. What was he?

Everyone slept dressed with their shoes on. Aki wore a pouch equipped with a flashlight, first aid medicines, gloves, and money. Aftershocks were still frequent, twenty-four hours a day.

While Aki was gone most of the time, I visited Tim several times a day. I continued to sleep in the car. The street en route to the hospital was lined with parked cars that were filled with family belongings. Three days after the earthquake, the doctor discharged Tim from the hospital. We had inquired about our centres in Wadayama, about 100 km away, regarding temporary housing for us. They had one empty unit that we could use so we drove there: the Muir family, with their four boys, followed the next day because evacuation centres were crowded and we had nowhere else to go.

It was good to have Tim at home. Half his face was still paralyzed, but he was slowly improving. We two families slept like peas in a pod for about one week. Life was simple, instant ramen because we didn't have anything else, and we recycled the disposable bowls. We did have TV. We had experienced so many aftershocks that we could guess at the strength before it was posted on TV. Generally, we were correct. After one week, Aki made further temporary arrangements for our family, so we returned to Kobe. Matt and Tim stayed with the Schmidt family, Presbyterian missionaries, and Aki and I stayed next door with Mollie and Lardner Moore, also Presbyterian missionaries. Their homes were damaged but livable: nobody had water or gas, which people needed for cooking.

We were so impressed and amazed one day when Senator Yashiro's wife and her friend arrived at the Moore's home (Aki worked with Senator Yashiro who was the DPI AP Chairperson). They had driven all the way from Tokyo with a van load of donations of food, clothing, and blankets. They, too, slept with us at the Moore's home, fully dressed due to the frequent aftershocks.

In the city, there were basically three types of cars everywhere. The Self Defence Army vehicles and army, which we had never seen in Kobe before; fire engines and ambulances from all over Japan, including Sapporo, Hokkaido; and police cars—a state of emergency comparable to WWII according to Aki. From statistics made available later, we learned that 7,000 homes were completely destroyed, 149,000 homes were partially destroyed, 4,800 houses were completely burnt, and there had been 300 fires: 300,000 persons were displaced, 43,800 injured and 6,434 persons died, most in the debris. The fifth floor of Kobe City Hospital had collapsed as well as the fourth floor of Kobe city's office.

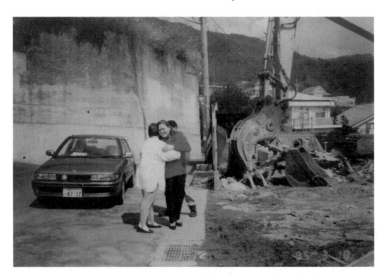

Marcy greeting a neighbour in front of our former house.

The government had begun building temporary housing, with a goal of 40,000 units. At this time, every single park and schoolyard was occupied with temporary housing units due to a shortage of land. Evacuees slept in the gyms, auditoriums, school classrooms, etc. with no privacy, a little like sardines in a tin can. Toilet facilities were limited, the heating systems could not be used since they were a fire hazard: people had been eating cold rice balls and bread for about a month. In the first month, many senior citizens passed away from pneumonia and/or PTSD (post-traumatic stress disorder). Chronic diseases were becoming more serious due to stress, the coldness, lack of a balanced diet, and medical care.

We were concerned about people moving to temporary housing because there were no plans for social or medical services at those locations. At that time, the schools had volunteers and emergency medical personnel, but these people were unable to move to temporary housing. In fact, on March 15, emergency medical personnel left with no local medical personnel filling the gap. The majority of volunteers had been students from across Japan, and they had to return home because the new school year began in early April.

Evacuees had no freedom to choose their site of temporary housing. The government used a lottery to decide the site, which meant that people would not be living with their friends or community anymore. Social work volunteer organizations and NGOs were discussing whether to terminate work or continue. It was a very crucial time and prayers were needed.

There were many Kyodan churches in the Kobe-Nishinomiya area affected by the earthquake. Four churches were completely destroyed. The majority sustained some damage. There were no clergy casualties but an unknown number of members were killed. Two Christian children's homes needed to be totally rebuilt. Several day care centres and schools were damaged.

One month after the earthquake, there still was no water or gas! Our civilized home was totally dysfunctional. With no water to flush the toilets, you ate and drank less! Our children carried water from the river every morning. The Self Defence Army provided drinking water. We used a small camp stove to cook very basic meals. We ate so many bananas and pita bread— compliments of the Mafia—that we often joked that if we never saw another banana or pita bread, that would be fine. We were thankful, though, that we had our basic needs met.

CA realized the importance for students to return to school. There were many obstacles to address before that was possible. The school located on the man-made Rokko island was dependent on public transportation such as the monorail and buses, but, at the time, they were dysfunctional: one lane for cars to drive on and off the island was open, so a modified school day was organized whereby vans would pick up students at several places in Kobe. Because the majority of students lived too far away, teachers living on the island had students move in with them. Fortunately, our sons were able to be picked up by van near Schmidt's home where they were staying. The school day started at ten a.m. due to the horrific traffic situation and returned around two-thirty p.m.: being able to go to school and regain some sense of normality was therapeutic for the students. They had to take their lunch and drinks with them because there was no food or drink available at school. Toilets were not usable due to no water, so deep holes were dug in the athletic field with some temporary privacy constructed.

About two weeks after the earthquake, Toyo Eiwa School in Tokyo held their scheduled board meeting. I decided to attend. Aki drove me to the nearest functioning train station, where I transferred to the Shinkansen train for Tokyo. En route we passed so much devastation. Cars were crushed by homes, houses with their contents had fallen out onto the streets, houses stood at precarious angles. Then, further down the street, houses were standing straight up and people were going about their daily lives as usual. It looked strange.

We had been wearing our clothes until they almost stood up on their own before they were laundered. It was amazing how one's priorities change when it meant survival.

Within a month after the earthquake, KGU found an older home for us in Takarazuka city, three cities' distance from Kobe that was close to the university's campus, where there was minimal damage to homes. This meant we had to empty our home in Kobe of our personal belongings and furniture. Because most dishes had been broken, there was much less to pack. Driving back and forth between the cities to get the task accomplished was time consuming and frustrating because private cars were still not allowed to use the main roads, which were designated for essential service vehicles only. Back roads were narrow, impossible for two-way traffic at places; on the same roads, trucks were demolishing homes and hauling the debris away. Unfortunately, that was the only road one could take. I resorted to playing music tapes for sanity's sake because I spent hours to commute short distances.

Soon after we moved, two large boxes arrived by delivery from Mr. and Mrs. Saito. One box was full of a variety of fresh seafood on dry ice, the second contained a set of beautiful dishes.

My parents, very concerned, had decided to come and help us in early March, just after we had moved into the old house that needed some tender loving care. How Dad ever got through customs with his suitcase that contained a crowbar, hammer, and other carpenter tools we never understood! The occasional hardware store was now beginning to open, so Dad was able to access some supplies to replace the bathroom floor and do many other small jobs. Mom helped with meals and with getting us organized in our new setting, drapes for a little privacy, etc.

The night my parents came was the first night we slept in our pajamas again. The aftershocks were less, but they still jolted my parents during their sleep, which was a shock for them. It was great news when Route 2, a major road, was finally officially opened for general traffic—but only from nine p.m. until early morning.

Cherry blossom time at the end of March, early April, was always exquisite to see. Everyone enjoyed eating, singing, and dancing under the blossoms. This year, it rained and rained so nobody was celebrating: it was like the country was in mourning with us.

A church in Nishinomiya asked me to speak on Mother's Day! Tim, who had just returned from the Philippines, was excited about his Habitat for Humanity experience during spring break. He had met the Filipino doctor with a disability, who had stayed in our home the last spring, when he was on the same flight from up country to Manila.

There was only two more months of school left for the boys and to live with the Schmidt family. It had been harder for them to live away from home than I realized. Matt called home most evenings.

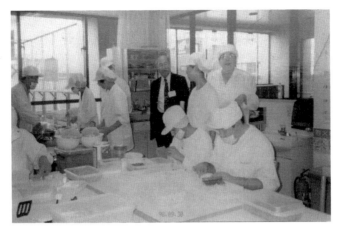

Baking workshop.

Wakamatsu Bunjo Baking Project

Nagata Ward, in the west central part of Kobe, had been most severely damaged by fires during the earthquake. Firefighters had tried to control the fires but water pumps were dysfunctional due to no water. Streets were impassable. Fire trucks from neighbouring cities had been unable to get to Nagata Ward due to major roads being blocked with broken homes and debris. Blocks of homes were burnt to the ground, with family members trapped and unable to escape. With more than 60 percent of the residents displaced, there were not enough families left with young children to enroll in the day care centre for preschoolers run by Kobe City, which was on the fourth floor of Daimaru Department Store.

KSSSC, aware of the vacant space, approached Kobe City, requesting to use the facilities for senior citizens who had been displaced in Nagata Ward and a cookie-baking project for intellectually challenged young adults. Kobe City readily agreed.

My prayer for the last fourteen years was coming to fruition. God had moved the mountains to make it a reality, but what I had not expected was to be told that I was to start the project! I began to ask myself, "God, what did I ever ask for? I can't do this." The KSSSC chairperson didn't ask me if I would do it, but it was said in such a way that there was no option.

I had never worked directly with intellectually challenged persons and did not have the confidence to do so, not to mention my concern regarding fluency in the Japanese language. My Vietnamese was still better! When I was introduced to the fifteen clients excited with the thought of baking cookies, I began to second guess my ability. The clients were not high functioning enough to mainstream but could still be productive: seven persons were autistic, eight had other intellectual challenges. Most could not carry on a conversation. This project brought hope and life to these young adults and their families after the stress of the earthquake. The kanji characters for danger and opportunity, when written together, spelled crisis. So, as a positive thinker, I saw this baking project as an opportunity, an outcome of our "crisis," the Kobe earthquake! Again, God had worked in a miraculous way to answer my prayer; but I hadn't asked to be responsible for it!

It was a miracle to begin the cookie-baking project just three months after the earthquake. I did not have confidence, but I stepped forward: two staff assigned to the project and I shopped for needed equipment, and we were fortunate to buy a large commercial gas oven from a bakery that had been destroyed by the earthquake. The simplest cookie recipes that did not require refrigeration seemed the best way to start. After two weeks, we had assessed the strengths of each client and began training them for a specific job in the process of making cookies.

Mr. Kanatsuki, KSSSC Board of Trustee Chairperson, decided that the logo for our cookies would be "Holy Friends." What could I say! The name of our organization was Kobe Seirei, meaning Holy Servant, so it appeared that we had to fall in line and be "Holy Friends" working together!

It didn't take long to discover how much energy and patience was needed to produce a few simple cookies from nine-thirty a.m. to three p.m. Our work space became our lunch place, so everything had to be cleared by eleven-thirty to set the table. It became apparent that there was a definite way that the dishes had to be arranged. The soup bowl was placed on the right, the rice bowl on the left, with the other dishes in precise order at the back. It was so strictly enforced that I continue to do so to this day when serving a Japanese meal.

Our cookie menu included chocolate chip, ranger, oatmeal, cinnamon, chocolate, and coconut. The clients would pick up the dough and want to play with it like play dough, so I decided that's how we would make the cookies: little round balls and flatten them a little. Cookies were bite size in Japan. I let them taste a sample of each kind so they knew what their cookies tasted like.

After three to four months, I questioned whether the project would fly. Then, suddenly, around six months after starting the project, everyone seemed to have caught on! The repetitive action of shaping the cookies seemed to have a calming effect with the autistic clients and the others now knew the routine. Actions speak louder than words would aptly apply to this situation. Some of the clients were talkative, the other half never talked. The key was basically to demonstrate how to do the task at hand and accept them for who they were. The project designed to provide a job opportunity and generate income was being realized! Now to seek a market.

We began selling our cookies at local public events sponsored by various social service centres, as well as in a small shop in the nearby community. Two big events were held in September about six months after starting our baking project: one was at our centre in Shiawase-no-mura, Village of Happiness, a residential centre for intellectually challenged adults, and the other was at the big compound of Aisei-en, Seisei-en and Yusei-en. These public events were held annually to generate funds for KSSSC. We sold our cookies in a booth and also took turns walking around the compound selling them. This was also part of their training. At the second event, we sold cookies valued at 40,000 yen, equivalent to $500 Canadian. It was an exhilarating and empowering experience for everyone. The profit was shared with the fifteen clients. Parents of the clients proudly took orders and were great advocates for us.

Word spread rapidly with orders coming from different cities, much to the delight of the clients and staff. A Christian friend had introduced our cookies to the Royal Family, who was impressed with the tasty cookies and the post-quake project. Princess Akishinomiya placed a significant order for her daughter's birthday. We felt most honoured with the subsequent orders for more family birthdays.

About a year after beginning the project, I was still feeling inadequate to communicate effectively with the persons with autism. There were two persons that I would not dare to have eye contact with or they would panic. One was Miyashige kun. He always avoided being near me and seemed afraid of me, or so I thought. Then, due to a family crisis in Canada, I was absent for three weeks. On my first day back at our morning meeting, Miyashige kun came up to me, knelt directly in front of me and kept staring at my face. Not daring to make eye contact, I struggled to keep my emotions in check because he had never come this close to me before. After ten minutes or so, he said, "You have wrinkles on your face," then got up and walked away. I wanted to cry because, to me, he was saying that he had missed me. Maybe my presence was making a difference in his life after all. The clients could feel that they were accepted and valued for who they were.

Another memorable experience happened about a year after we had started the baking project. One afternoon, when we were sitting around the tables shaping cookies, Naka san was sitting beside me. She considered herself my sidekick because we always mixed cookie dough together. She was strong and very verbal. On the other side of the table, Nakamura kun, with Down's Syndrome, was also shaping cookies. This was a relaxing time when we could enjoy talking as we worked.

Nakamura kun started the conversation with, "Ano ne, ano ne. Marcy san wa Ninomiya Sensei no Okusan" (You know, you know, Marcy is Reverend Ninomiya's wife). All the clients knew my husband well—he was known as Ninomiya Sensei to them— because he had held simple thirty-minute worship services at their centres over the years, and they were very fond of him.

I could sense that Naka san was becoming agitated when she suddenly shouted, "Chigau, chigau! Marcy san wa Ninomiya Sensei no okusan ja nai! Ninomiya Sensei wa Marcy san no goshujin. Marcy san wa watashi no tomodachi desu." (It's not that way. That's wrong. Marcy is not Rev. Ninomiya's wife. Rev. Ninomiya is Marcy san's husband. Marcy san is my friend). Wow! I thought to myself, who said that Naka san was intellectually challenged!

These two experiences gave me confidence that one need not be totally fluent in a language to be effective. I was their friend, which was all that mattered.

My days were long because I had to take the train from Takarazuka to Nishinomiya, then transfer to go to Nagata Ward on the other side of Kobe, which took more than an hour from door to door. This became my routine Monday to Friday.

I was beginning to feel like an octopus leading a nomadic lifestyle. Besides the baking project and other involvement with KSSSC, I continued to serve the community and church in numerous capacities. Plans also needed to be finalized to build a prefab house for us on the property next door to where we had lived pre-quake.

Post-Earthquake Life

Aki was on another merry-go-round teaching full time at KGU's new Policy Studies Department, overseeing two of the eleven sites of temporary housing in Kobe for persons with disabilities and senior citizens, and coordinating volunteers from JCSWL to support those in temporary housing: KSSSC had two full-time staff and the Social Work League had sent two volunteers regularly for about 150 persons. They looked after daily needs such as meals, shopping, bathing, etc. The dormitory-style housing designated for seniors and persons with disabilities was inadequate, with no sink, toilet, kitchen, or heating in their rooms. They had to use public facilities, and it was cold outside. One third of the residents, having no family contact, felt completely isolated and had no hope for the future. Many had chronic illnesses. Spiritually, financially, and socially they had lost their hope and potential. There were still 90,000 senior citizens and persons with disabilities living in temporary housing.

Our boys continued to live on Rokko Island with a teacher until our new house was scheduled to be completed in February 1996.

Aki's uncle, a professional photographer, and his wife, who had lived on the east side of Kobe, were finally able to locate us and share their story. He had a photo shop in an arcade with their living quarters on the second floor, their bedroom facing the arcade. After the earthquake, they found themselves still in their bed on the ground floor of the arcade, looking up at the sky and wondering how they got there! Their greatest concern was to find the eye glasses and dentures that they always placed beside their bed. It was rather humorous listening to their tale—it was laugh or cry! Much to their relief, they eventually did find their eye glasses and dentures!

Christmas was extra special that year: we were all survivors with painful memories of 1995 to put behind us to celebrate the wonder of Christmas. We shared a celebration with the senior citizens' day care at Wakamatsu, where our cookie baking project shared the same facility. The seniors liked getting to know our "baking gang," and most of our clients enjoyed the special attention they got from the seniors. Every centre had its own Christmas program, which was so special. Music was always a highlight that everyone could enjoy, along with a special treat.

Our boys were delighted to be together as a family over the holidays. After Christmas, we planned to spend some time at our cottage at Lake Nojiri but weren't sure if we would be able to get away, as all major roads were closed due to a most unusual heavy snowfall. In fact, our departure was delayed for twenty-four hours because we had no access to any major road. We were packed, ready to hit the road for Nojiri as soon as the roads would open.

Finally, on the morning of December 27, an announcement came on the radio that roads were open. We got on the Chugoku Expressway in Takarazuka without a hitch, only to come to a complete standstill within minutes. We sat in the same place for hours, not even inching our way! Fortunately, we were stopped near a monorail station, so we had access to a toilet after a challenging hike over a guardrail and a short walk. Aki was intending to travel to Nojiri with us to help set up the cottage, and then hightail it to Tokyo on an early evening train to sleep at Senator Yashiro's house so they could travel to the airport together and fly to Indonesia early the next morning. His plans never got off the ground! At two p.m. we were still sitting at the same place as we had been at ten a.m., so Aki jumped the guard rail with his suitcase, got on the monorail, and started his journey to Tokyo.

We sat and sat. By four-thirty p.m., we had moved a few car lengths: truck drivers had to be awakened because they had been caught in the backup more than twenty-four hours earlier. Finally, by six p.m., we were on the Meishin Expressway, inching along, then came to a standstill! The boys were hungry, and I needed a washroom.

Fortunately, I had bought breakfast before our departure so Matthew made us delicious strawberry jelly sandwiches. The boys and I had decided earlier that when we had a chance to exit, we would do so for the use of facilities. I couldn't have the car running or we would run out of gasoline, so it was very cold! Finally, at nine-thirty p.m., we took the first exit for South Kyoto to get gas, eat supper at McDonalds beside the gas stand, and phone Aki. He apparently had tried phoning our home numerous times, thinking that we had either gone back home or were at Nojiri. He was shocked to learn that, nine hours later, we were only about forty-five minutes away from our home! We then drove to the first service centre for the night after thirteen hours on the road to get some sleep.

After a light sleep, we started driving again at three a.m., hoping the backup would have cleared considerably and the morning rush hour would not have started. Everyone was on the road: it was the end of the year and New Year's celebrations are the biggest event of the year in Japan. We moved ever so slowly for a while and then finally picked up, arriving at Nojiri at eleven-thirty a.m. on December 28!

Akiie had taught the boys how to put the new chains on the tires because people did not have snow tires. The boys were confident that they could do it, which they did while I did the grocery shopping in the nearest town to Nojiri. We were able to make it to the caretakers' hill, where I had difficulty executing a sharp turn upward: I backed up a little in order to cut hard, only to discover the wheels didn't grip, just spun! Behind was a guardrail and a steep drop off, so I didn't want to back up so far that there would not be enough space for someone to push. I asked the boys to get out and push. Initially they thought that I was kidding, but then they realized that we were in serious trouble. After another try, both boys hollered at the same time, "Mom, the chains are gone!" We retraced our steps only to discover we couldn't make it up the hill we had come down earlier. After returning to the caretaker's home, a friend happened to come along and was going to the grocery store where we had put on the chains. I hitched a ride with her while the boys started moving our supplies by sled to the cottage. The chains were never found, so I bought new ones that the caretaker kindly put on for us.

What a relief to finally get settled in the cottage in the afternoon. We started the kerosene stoves immediately, hooked up the gas, and went out for supper because I was too pooped to cook yet. After returning from supper, we hit the sack!

We learned that our next-door neighbours had also taken twenty-seven hours to get there. Thankfully, the return journey was uneventful. I will never forget that trip!

The Kobe earthquake destroyed many churches. The United Church of Christ in Japan (Kyodan), a sister church of the UCC, had thirteen churches completely destroyed. With an average membership of thirty to sixty, they could not afford to rebuild, plus, many members had sustained heavy personal losses. Many people suffered spiritually as a result of the earthquake. The stress level of church ministers was phenomenal! One young minister had a stroke, another a heart attack, several others required hospitalization, and some lost hope and left the ministry due to deep distress and illness. Church members moved away, and the church community affected by the earthquake almost disappeared.

On January 17, 1996, we had the moving experience of participating in a one-year memorial service with a congregation, standing in the open where their church once stood.

We shared this prayer:

> *God, we learned again that at your breath the mountains move and the earth quakes. Lord, even in this suffering, we seek to rise again. In the path of hardship, we sometimes falter. It is not just buildings that have been destroyed but relationships that were cherished. Yet, through the earthquake we came to see wonderful things in people. Many people knew the joy of helping others and the marvel of encouraging each other. We, having lost our church building, thank you for the encouragement and help of many others. For those still distressed and in difficulty, we ask for your comfort, encouragement, and strength.*

It was a moving experience to begin the service on a plot of land where the church building had stood a year earlier.

Kobe, our home for thirteen years, witnessed the complete destruction of 300,000 homes and the death of 6,500 victims. Twenty years earlier, when a specialist on earthquakes assessed Kobe, city officials had ridiculed his report, which recommended preparation for an earthquake with a magnitude of seven on the Richter scale. The city opted to set up a safety standard to five for economic priorities. The major developments of the last quarter century were destroyed in the "twenty-second big shake," with the 7.3 earthquake on the Richter scale. After the quake, there were no community-based systems because the city had emphasized economic growth rather than quality of life. The human disaster was amplified when many victims died within two days under collapsed debris because there were no rescue squads, fire department, medical care, etc.

In March 1996, the city of Kobe acknowledged that at least 20 percent of the 1.4 million population had deserted the city. However, 45,000 persons, mostly the elderly and persons with disabilities, were still forced to live in temporary housing. The Japanese government had not offered one yen for the victims, but they spent money on reconstructing the harbour and roads and planned to build a new airport to recover economic power.

In February 1996, we moved into our new prefab home in Kobe, next door to where our previous home stood. It was built with retaining walls all around and had an amazing view of the city. We looked down on the property where we had lived for fourteen years and on our former neighbours' properties that were now a playground for the wild boars in the evening.

It was wonderful to be a family again and back on Mount Rokko, which eliminated hours of travelling for all of us. The boys could walk down the hill and catch the school bus. Tim was challenged with his studies in Grade 11 and thrived on playing his sax in the performance and jazz bands: Matt, in Grade 9, enjoyed his classes, sports, music, and socializing. He was a real helper around home because he saw that his parents were more involved with the community and he wanted to help out. In June, Melody returned to teach in summer school at CA and lifeguard at Nojiri before returning to WLU for her final year, majoring in math and physical education: she planned to apply to Teacher's College for the fall of '97.

There were two major family events in 1996. Aki and I celebrated twenty-five years of wedded life! Reflecting on our years together, we were grateful for companionship, expanded viewpoints, and challenges. The other major event was Timothy's move to Ontario to live with his grandparents in Conestogo for Grade 12 at Elmira Secondary High School, where he enjoyed discovering his family's roots. This was a difficult decision to make, but it was made with Tim's future in mind.

In 1996, I continued to serve in various capacities in the home, church, and community in addition to supervising the cookie-making project at Wakamatsu Bunjo. In October, we were privileged to have Kin Eun Ju from Wonju Christian Hospital Vocational Rehabilitation Centre, Korea for orientation to our program. Clint and Sandra Rohr from St. Jacobs, Ontario, where Clint was the Director of the Woolwich Community Health Centre, spent a month based in our home while he conducted workshops on community-based health care at the invitation of JCSWL.

In Japan, the hospital represented the main health care service. There was no general practitioner system. It was important to develop a community-based health care system for senior citizens due to the rapidly aging population to meet their needs. Clint Rohr shared how a community-based health care system could promote health through diet, exercise, recreation, and sports by seniors initiating such a program themselves by collaborating with the local government. The purpose was to promote good health not to be treatment focused only.

Clint then explained how the community-based health care system project extended to develop a community-based senior citizens' housing corporation, creating a senior citizen's condo corporation, also managed by the residents themselves. It included community activities, exercise classes, horticulture, and a neighbourhood watch system. It was a pioneer project in Canada, one of a kind, known as the St. Jacobs Meadows Residential Community where we now find ourselves living twenty-five years later!

The year 1997, brought new and rewarding challenges. Aki organized student volunteer groups to build homes for the homeless in the Philippines during their spring and summer breaks. They worked for victims of the Mount Pinatubo eruption in Luzon Island and for families living in the slums in Mindanao and the Negros islands. Four Habitat for Humanity university chapters were established that year. Even though there were very few volunteer movements in Japan, we found that the younger generation was willing to devote itself to others through volunteer service. Aki also sent seven students to South India to do volunteer work for a group home and day care centre for mentally challenged persons, run by Mr. Abraham in Kerala, South India, whom we continued to mentor.

We saw mission work as having a multilateral approach: we could educate and train the younger Japanese generation to work with other Asian countries such as India, the Philippines, and Thailand, rather than just representing an "economic animal" in Asia—just like Saint Paul went to Rome, which became a centre for mission in Europe.

I continued to help develop Wakamatsu Bunjo, the income generating baking project that produced cookies, as well as chocolate, maple nut, and oatmeal muffins. It was exciting to watch the clients' skills develop each year.

Melody graduated from WLU in April, and then set out to cross Canada by bicycle to raise funds for Habitat for Humanity. Much to our disbelief, she completed the trip by the end of July. She was currently enrolled at Queens Teachers' College and planned to be married on June 13, 1998 to Scott Morton, who had also cycled across Canada with her. Timothy was in his last year at Elmira District Secondary School, and he continued to live with his grandparents and adjust to the Canadian way of life. He was wondering about his future plans. Matt was in Grade 10 at CA with jazz band and soccer as his first loves.

A dream of ours since 1982 actually became a reality in 1998. I never imagined that the group home for five intellectually challenged adults would be located on the site where we lived until the 1995 Kobe earthquake—thanks to the United Methodist Church of USA! With the prohibitive cost of land in Japan, the UMC made this miracle possible by making the land available to KSSSC for twenty years at no cost. The blueprint was finalized, and, when the building permit was received, construction began. Hallelujah!

The Parents' Association was equally excited about this project, having saved funds for ten years. Their contributions were then matched by KSSSC, leaving a shortfall of seven million yen ($87,500 Canadian).

Nagamine Group Home officially opened on April 28, 1998 for five intellectually challenged adults and house parents. I was busy coordinating schedules of volunteers, who played a critical role in achieving our goal. Parents of students at CA came daily for painting in the interior: students from KGU also helped with the painting and yard work. Due to the generosity and volunteer manpower of many committed people, community, churches, and schools, the home was paid for with just a few yen to spare. Truly a second miracle! The third miracle was the changes in the lives of the volunteers! "Ask and it will be given to you; seek and you will find; knock and the door will be opened to you." Luke 11: 9

Christ met many people with disabilities, healed them, and encouraged them to return to their families and community. Because many people had been involved in the construction of the group home, our neighbourhood accepted the residence as part of its community. Neighbours, including their children, frequently visited the group home, which made the fourth miracle!

Our family left for home assignment in the summer of 1998. Our first destination was Vancouver, where we rented a car and drove to the Okanagan Valley to meet members from Aki's previous seven-point charge, the Okanagan Japanese United Church, the majority of whom had been interned during WWII. Most were now over eighty years of age, and still isolated from family and community.

Our final destination was Waterloo for our daughter's wedding. Melody was marrying Scott Morton, whom she had met at a Habitat for Humanity work camp. The wedding was beautiful, with the bride wearing my wedding gown made in Bangkok, Thailand in 1971.

Melody was now teaching at Rockway Mennonite Collegiate in Kitchener, and Scott was enrolled in the Graduate School of Social Work at WLU in Waterloo.

Tim, recently graduated from Elmira District Secondary School, had enrolled in the Biological Research Technology program at Seneca College in Toronto, which he was enjoying. He was fortunate to share living accommodation with a friend from Elmira. Matt continued his studies in Gr. 11 at Canadian Academy in Kobe.

In October, Ayumi, age twelve, the daughter of Reverend Keigo Ueda joined our family. You will recall that we had an understanding that when Rev. Keigo's mother passed away, our family would be responsible to meet Ayumi's needs. Due to difficult living circumstances, Ayumi became our family member but stayed in close contact with her father.

Besides teaching full time at university, Aki continued to work with earthquake victims who were resettling back into society from temporary shelters. He had been researching NPOs (non-profit organizations) and management to empower the residents and promote a healthy environment to live in the community. The Japanese aging society had increased rapidly in the previous twenty-five years. Company workers were forced to retire at the age of sixty and expected to live to the age of eighty-five. After retirement they had no social status, little income, and no community involvement. As a result, many lived in isolation, loneliness, and poverty. For these reasons, Aki had been encouraging the residents to support each other through networking. Unfortunately, many elderly persons, who had lost hope living in an affluent industrial society, died by suicide.

Aki had invested much energy in organizing and establishing community-based social service projects. Two were working efficiently and effectively: one urban in west Kobe and the other in a rural setting, were both providing day care services for senior citizens. Both projects involved Aki's university students as part of their field placement requirement.

The Japanese social welfare system was drastically changing from a welfare state to a social service state. Until now, the national government had centred on welfare service, but, due to the rapidly increasing population of senior citizens, was unable to continue providing the same service. Many senior citizens and their families had great anxiety about their future. We saw our mission as encouraging residential people to organize self-help groups within the community and share resources in terms of personnel, material, information, and professional skills. We had modelled this social service approach after Canada, especially Waterloo, Ontario.

Aki published many articles on community-based social service systems and two books. One is a translation of *Voluntary NPO Management* (non-profit organization), and the other is *Asians with Disabilities and International NGOs* (non-government organizations).

Aki had been trying to promote a Christian social work model on Japanese soil. Matthew 4:23-25 tells how Jesus healed those who were oppressed, isolated, sick and disabled: he healed them and let them be self-supporting and able to contribute to society. What a challenge!

I continued to be based in Kobe and was excited about the additional business at Wakamatsu Bunjo—a new coffee shop called Angel Wings began serving our cookies as part of their menu, resulting in a tremendous boost to our sales.

Our group home next door was deeply appreciated by the five residents with live-in houseparents. Two residents had jobs in the community, one worked at the cookie project, one attended a day care program, and another was in our training program for intellectually challenged adults. It was our hope to see the group home develop stronger ties with the community because it had a keen interest in the home from the beginning.

Another highlight of the year 2000 included Aki receiving a Distinguished Graduate Award at Waterloo Lutheran Seminary at the conference by the Eastern Lutheran Synod in Waterloo in July. It was a humbling experience.

Aki and I then drove to Virginia to participate in a reunion for personnel who served in Vietnam with MCC, the Mennonite Mission Board or VNCS. There were 170 persons registered, including the first person who served in Vietnam in 1954! We felt bound together as a family as we shared our many stories with laughter and tears.

Melody continued to teach at RMC, and her husband, Scott, graduated from WLU's Graduate School of Social Work and was working in the K-W area with new immigrants, especially related to their housing. Scott was also a member of the Peacemakers and spent two weeks at Burnt Church, New Brunswick where there was much unrest that summer between the native fisherman and federal fisheries' officers: the heart of the dispute was about aboriginal rights to natural resources.

Timothy continued studying at Seneca College in North York, Toronto. In the summer months, he worked in a furniture factory.

Matthew graduated from Canadian Academy in June 2000 and was the proud recipient of the Ford Motor Company Scholarship and Music Award. He was now attending Rockway Mennonite Collegiate for one year.

Return to Canada

The biggest news for 2000 was our move back to Canada in December. It was very painful to say goodbye to "family" and many friends made over the years and the multiple projects that we had been involved with in Japan and Asia. When we reflected on our time in Japan, it hardly seemed possible that it had been that long. We had felt challenged, encouraged, discouraged, and fulfilled over the years. Our application to the DWO of UCC, twenty-one years earlier, had stated that the only country in Asia we did not want to serve in was Japan. God had worked in mysterious ways. We cherished the memories and friendships.

Aki and I found ourselves on another journey, this time with an unknown destination. Persons with KSSSC and JCSWL wanted to continue to stay connected with us even though we were no longer in Japan. We sensed God's presence with us, knowing he would guide us, but we were uncertain which way to step forward.

In January 2001, Hamilton Japanese United Church, without a bilingual pastor, approached Aki to ask if he would agree to be an interim pastor for five months, which was arranged. Their stories touched our hearts. Post WWII, the Canadian government released Japanese Canadians from internment camps in British Columbia, with the stipulation that they not return to the west coast but, rather, were forced to resettle further east. Members of the Hamilton congregation still carried memories of their move to Ontario with nothing more than they could carry. We became fond of the members, who wanted Aki to stay on as pastor, but God had other plans.

In March, ten of Aki's former students from KGU came for a ten days' visit. Aki had a reputation for being a challenging but caring professor who gave his students every learning opportunity, including the Habitat for Humanity experience in the Philippines, which changed the lives of the participants. They wanted to come to Canada because they had just graduated and had time to visit before joining the workforce.

During our time in Japan, Aki had written a series of ten articles in a medical magazine about the quality of life in the medical field. These articles caught the attention of a doctor in Shinanomachi, near Nojiri, who became a good friend through my volunteer work as camp nurse in the summer months. Many seniors were living alone in the area after their adult children had moved to the city. We later learned that the doctor was so empathetic with his patients that he even looked after their dogs during their hospitalization. Through this connection, Aki was invited to be the main speaker for the National Conference for the Association of Government Hospitals, to be held in Nagano, October 2001.

Aki insisted that I accompany him because he felt strongly that God would give a sign for the next step in our mission. We had no idea what it would be, but when it came, he wanted to be able to consult with me knowing we were partners in mission.

Our non-refundable travel tickets included ongoing travel to Bangkok, Thailand and Phnom Penh, Cambodia, for DPI AP's conference scheduled in November. Unfortunately, we received word that it had been postponed due to the September 11 terrorist attacks incident in the US. We flew to Bangkok on October 21, as scheduled, to help Mr. Topong, the DPI AP Development Officer.

Unexpectedly, we were able to participate in an international conference on landmines in Bangkok in early November, organized by Handicap International (HI), recipient of the Nobel Peace Prize. This was an overwhelming three days of learning about all the unexploded explosive ordnance (UXO) in Laos, Cambodia, and Vietnam, making it unsafe for farmers to work in their fields. Many citizens had lost limbs due to hitting a land mine while farming, and it would take years and years to make their land safe again.

Because the DPI AP workshop in Phnom Penh was postponed indefinitely, Aki thought we should use this time to travel to Vietnam, although we had no way of communicating with our friends about our travel plans at this late date. He felt strongly that we would meet Yong, who was living in Pleiku, but foreigners were not allowed to travel to Pleiku at that time. He insisted that God had told him to prepare a $500 US bill to give to Yong.

We flew to Saigon (renamed Ho Chi Minh City, but it will always be Saigon to me) and took a train to Nhatrang, arriving around midnight. The next day we rode bicycles several kilometres to Anh Tin's home. He was stunned to see us. We invited him to a local restaurant for dinner that evening to get caught up on the latest news about our friends and the current situation. We asked him when he had last met Yong, and he said about two years ago. After dinner, we rode our bicycles back to our hotel in Nhatrang. As we entered the hotel lobby, the receptionist said there was a phone call for us. It was Anh Tin, with whom we had just had dinner. He was so excited that it was difficult to initially understand his message. Apparently, when he returned home from the restaurant, Yong was sitting on his doorstep! Aki was right, we would be able to meet Yong after all!

Anh Tin invited us to his home for the noon meal the next day so we could talk with Yong. What a wonderful reunion! Yong and a friend had driven their motorbikes all day, 300 km through the mountains from Pleiku to Nhatrang. Tribal persons required permission from the government to travel out of town, which Yong did not do because he had felt led to go to Nhatrang immediately. We discovered that Yong had translated the New Testament into his Bahnar language and wanted to have it printed. He had checked the cost to do so in Pleiku but found that the cost was too expensive, which was why he decided to check the cost in Nhatrang. That morning he had already gone into town to get an estimate. Aki passed the envelope with the $500 US bill to Yong, then asked him the cost of printing in Nhatrang. Before Yong opened it, his response was $500 US!

It was a miracle to meet Yong, who did not know we were going to Vietnam, and it was the exact amount he needed! We all celebrated later that day along with other friends. Yes, I had to admit, God had spoken to Aki! We could not have arranged this if we had tried. God had performed a miracle!

We returned to Bangkok in November where we met with Naoko Ito, JICA expert (Japan International Cooperation Agency), who was assigned to explore the possibility of establishing APCD (Asia-Pacific Development Centre on Disability) and Yuki Nakanishi, a former United Nations Economic and Social Commission in Asia-Pacific (UNESCAP) officer on disability and development. Naoko asked Aki if he would be available to take the Chief Advisor's position if approved by the Tokyo office. Aki mentioned that he might not be qualified because he no longer had Japanese citizenship. Naoko's research showed that citizenship was not an issue, but noted that JICA had never hired anyone without Japanese citizenship. We returned to Canada on November nineteen, feeling that a door might be opening for us in Bangkok.

CHAPTER 6

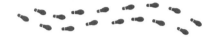

New Call from God

At a regional UNESCAP meeting on disability it was decided that the APCD project was to be established in Bangkok. Because the Royal Thai Government and Japan agreed to jointly establish APCD, JICA was actively seeking a candidate for the position of Chief Advisor of APCD.

Mr. Yutaka, UNESCAP Expert on Disability, and Mr. Topong, DPI AP Regional Development Officer on Disability, strongly recommended Aki as a candidate: Japanese Senator Yashiro, wheelchair user and close friend of Aki, founder and Honourable Chairperson of DPI AP, also recommended Aki to JICA Headquarters, as well as other international organizations of persons with disabilities in the Asia-Pacific region.

In January 2002, Aki and I flew to Asia for the DPI AP Biannual Regional Conference and Leadership Training Program in Phnom Penh, Cambodia. On the last day of the leadership training, we were taken to the Tuol Sieng Genocide Museum that chronicled the Cambodian genocide. The site was a former secondary school that had been used as a security prison by the S-21 and as an interrogation and detention centre of the Khmer Rouge, well known as the Pol Pot regime. The tour was so grue-some that fellow Cambodians refused to go with us, except for one young woman who had survived her experience there. As a child, her one hand had been nailed to a piece of wood so she could not escape. She related her story by sign language because the torture had left her deaf.

We then were taken to the Killing Fields, a number of sites where 1.5 to 2 million Cambodians were systematically persecuted and killed. A large see-through container was full of skulls. We were shown the tree where babies were beaten to death as their mothers were forced to watch.

We returned to Bangkok on January 14 for one day before leaving for Yangon, Myanmar to visit organizations that Aki became acquainted with through DPI AP, such as Eden Centre for Disabled Children, a non-profit organization established in 2000 to provide necessary basic services such as rehabilitation, education, and social services for physically and intellectually challenged children; the Christian School for Blind Persons and the Mary Knoll School for Deaf Persons; as well as Association for Aid and Relief Japan (AAR0, an international NGO running a vocational training centre in tailoring, hairstyling, and computers. Most of the trainees had physical disabilities resulting from landmine accidents and polio.

Our return to Canada was via Tokyo for several days, where we introduced ourselves to persons at JICA headquarters. We arrived in Toronto, Canada in time for Aki to do the worship service at Hamilton Japanese United Church the last Sunday in January. Aki and I needed to pray that a decision would soon be reached regarding an assignment to Bangkok.

Finally, Aki was notified that JICA would like to interview him in Tokyo on February 27 and 28 for the position of JICA Chief Advisor for the APCD project. They had basically already decided that he was the man for the job.

Aki learned that, in 1998, JICA had conducted a project formulation study for the welfare of persons with disabilities in Thailand and Indonesia. This study had been conducted by a group of experts in prosthetics, medical rehabilitation, and other disability fields, but did not include one person with disabilities: it called for a project that focused on services for persons with disabilities by non-disabled experts. Then, in 1999, JICA asked Yuki Oka, a wheelchair user and an ex UNESCAP officer on disability, and Aki, as an academic researcher, to do extensive research on disability and research in Thailand, based on human rights and the disability movement.

JICA was considering specific project components in reference to their study, when an event occurred that greatly changed the nature of the project.

Persons with disabilities in wheelchairs, who had been staging an independent living movement in Tokyo, visited JICA headquarters. They noted that JICA's assistance so far had centred on service provision by disability-related experts, regarding persons with disabilities as service recipients: they had not been placed at the centre of its activities. This turned the conceived project into one centred on persons with disabilities that would actually benefit them.

In 1999, further research by a JICA advisor to Thailand noted that Thailand was ahead of many countries in the region in regards to disability-related policies and organizations with activities by NGOs and DPOs. In addition, many NGOs and UN organizations had branch offices in Bangkok covering the Asia-Pacific region. Because many Thai persons with disabilities were highly educated, they could act as resource persons for JICA's third-country training programs. Visits to Cambodia, Laos, Myanmar, and Vietnam revealed the need to train persons with disabilities as leaders to strengthen DPOs, improve accessibility of the built environment, guarantee access to communication and develop networking, and cooperation amongst regional DPOs.

At the same time, in Thailand, in January 1999, the Ministry of Labour and Social Welfare had set up a task force that included experts with disabilities to accommodate the needs of persons with disabilities. It was agreed that the project, Asia-Pacific Development Centre on Disability, should be implemented by persons with disabilities themselves. They called for "a barrier-free society and empowerment of persons with disabilities as a means of preventing their marginalization and promoting their integration into society under the concept of achieving full participation and equality of persons with disabilities." It was important to promote independent living and relevant skills at a community level, as well as to support community-based rehabilitation (CBR). The proposed project was required to benefit persons with disabilities in their communities.

In October 2000, the Thai government submitted a concept paper to their Japanese counterpart, JICA, asking for a technical cooperation project and grant aid. It set the policy to establish the Asia-Pacific Development Centre on Disability project to empower persons with disabilities in the region through human resource development, information support, networking, collaboration, and the promotion of full participation and equality of persons with disabilities. After accepting the proposal in April 2001, JICA assigned an expert to the Department of Public Welfare and the Ministry of Labour and Social Welfare of Thailand.

Many studies in 2001 included severely disabled persons to help formulate this technical cooperative project. Their participation and commitment had a tremendous impact on the formulation process. Mr. Suporntum Mongkolsawadi, Redemptorist Vocational School for the Disabled Principal, and a wheelchair user, said to a Japanese study team, "For us, disability is life itself, our way of living. If the APCD is for persons with disabilities, what can we do for this project?" The stakeholders were greatly impressed that this project would be for and by persons with disabilities.

JICA requested that Aki spend approximately six weeks in Asia, from April to May 2002, based in Bangkok: he was to accompany Naoko Ito, JICA expert, and a JICA representative to Cambodia, to conduct pre-research to ascertain the feasibility of their collaboration with APCD related to persons with disabilities. This was in preparation for discussion with the Royal Thai Government and the Government of Japan to establish the APCD project as an international organization. After the two groups agreed to proceed in May 2002, JICA dispatched a project team, including Aki, to Thailand in late July to establish the APCD project.

While in Bangkok in May, Aki had checked the possibilities for our housing. He narrowed it down to three that were very different. One was a condo in an elite area with all the amenities, which I would not be comfortable living in because we were to work with the less fortunate: another condo was within easy walking distance of APCD but not accessible for persons with disabilities, so that was not an option. Then there was an old Thai house within a compound of ten houses in the Thai community. The owner and her relatives occupied seven of the ten houses. The remaining three were rented by personnel working at UNESCAP. I opted for this old house with old furniture that had a kitchen out back and an outdoor laundry area, along with a small flower garden begging for attention. One could walk to APCD in forty minutes or take a bus: it was private, but, at the same time, in a Thai community, so we agreed to rent this house on returning to Bangkok in July.

On July 7, Aki and I flew to Tokyo for ten days of orientation with JICA, and then took a six-hour flight to Bangkok for what we understood to be a two-year term.

Our Thai friend, Suthida, was familiar with the Ratchawat area where we lived because it was near the School for the Blind, where she had worked as a social worker for many years. We walked to the local market just five minutes away that reminded me of the Nhatrang market in Vietnam. There was an abundance of tropical fruit and fresh vegetables, with the fish and meat sections at the back with the flies. Fresh fish were on ice with some shrimp still jumping, and the meat had cuts on the table with large pieces suspended on hooks. Because fish and meat were cleaned and cut on the spot, water drained from the tables into a trough along the front of the table. One had to be careful not to fall on the slippery greasy floor. Markets had always fascinated me: they were where I practiced learning a new language.

Suthida also introduced us to two "famous" restaurants on our one and only street: by Western standards, they were just two "holes in the wall," not really sanitary, but I had learned years ago that these "holes in the wall" often served the most delicious food! We feasted on pad Thai, the famous noodle dish, while Suthida enjoyed her fried oysters. In the evening, we went to the second shop famous for its lad na, another noodle dish of wide flat rice noodles, bok choy with pork, and a thick gravy sauce poured on top (translated it meant "pour on the face"). We soon learned that one could buy nutritious meals on the street for a little over a dollar. Another one of our favourites was a noodle soup similar to the Vietnamese.

Initially, I spent a significant amount of time in the market, bargaining and surfing their goods. They never expected you to pay their first price. It was a game that I had perfected in Vietnam, and I enjoyed haggling with them. When they discovered I knew the prices and understood what they were saying, there was no more bargaining. One was expected to choose the item one wanted to buy to avoid being disappointed in what was sold. I soon learned my preferred vendors and they gave me the same price as their Thai customers. We really appreciated Suthida's orientation to Thailand and our area specifically.

Suthida also taught us how to greet people in Thailand. Men were to say Sawadee-krap and women were to say Sawadee-kha. When saying the greeting, one was to "wai": place the palms of one's hands together, with fingers extended at chest level close to the body, and bow slightly. The higher the hands were placed, more respect was shown. Subordinates might raise their fingers as high as their nose, but the tips of their fingers should never be above eye level. A wai was not used to greet children, servants, or street vendors. That just required a nod and smile.

A wai could mean "Hello," "Thank you," "I'm sorry," or "Goodbye." It was goodbye to bowing in greeting, as we had done in Japan, and I no longer had to wonder how low and long I had to bow to be polite. This was so much simpler.

Our landlady did her best to make us feel welcome and have our needs met. Because everyone had a maid to do the laundry and cleaning, I felt obligated to accept the offer of her maids to do those services for us at a cost. Shortly after moving in, Aki and I returned home one day to find the landowner's maids going through our garbage. No secrets here.

I also enjoyed exploring. Within five minutes walking distance from our house, one could access the bank, market, flower shop, hairdresser, restaurants, photocopy machine, etc. The post office was about a fifteen-minute walk. I bought a city map but still had to learn how to use public transportation to get around, so I got on a local bus with my map in hand and followed its route until I came back to where I started. It worked!

Asia-Pacific Development Centre on Disability (APCD)

When the APCD project opened on August 1, 2002, we had our first international visitor. We were honoured to have Henry Enns from Winnipeg, Canada, the first general secretary for DPI, whom Aki had met in Singapore in 1981 when DPI was born.

Aki was very excited about his challenge at APCD because it stood for all the things he had tried to work toward in Japan to empower persons with disabilities to live in and be part of their communities. He could finally apply his theory, vision, and dreams! Aki had always needed a challenge to be content, so he dug in his heels immediately. Having worked with persons with disabilities for over twenty years in Japan and with international NGOs for eighteen years through DPI AP, he already had a network with many Asian countries. His first major and unique challenge was to have thirty Asian countries sign a memorandum of understanding in the first two years of the APCD project. This meant Aki was travelling to one or two countries per month. An MOU, a bilateral agreement between the respective countries' governments, had to be signed so a country's persons with disabilities could qualify to participate in the training programs offered by APCD.

With Aki travelling so frequently, I filled my time exploring, helping behind the scenes, editing English correspondence for APCD, and continuing language study with the landowner who spoke good English and wanted to help me adjust to the rhythm of the Thai way of life. Of course, she was pleased that her overrun flower garden now had a new face!

On October 16, my birthday, I flew to Toronto to visit my mother due to her deteriorating health. With the time change, it was the first and only thirty-six-hour birthday I had ever experienced!

Aki didn't really miss me during my three weeks absence because he was travelling too. He had been invited to Manila, Philippines for a four-day regional workshop by the Asia Development Bank as one of the major speakers, representing APCD to share his vision, mission, and five-year plan of action. That was followed by travelling to Shanghai, China to participate in a five-day DPI AP conference.

After Shanghai, Aki flew to Tokyo to debrief JICA on the development of the APCD project. From October 24-28, 2002, he participated in the UNESCAP Conference in Otsu, Japan, where the Biwako Millennium Framework for Action Toward an Inclusive, Barrier-Free, and Rights-Based Society for Persons with Disabilities in Asia and the Pacific, known as the BMF, was adopted, recognizing another decade of persons with disabilities 2003-2012. It included a regional policy by the UNESCAP with recommendations for action by governments and concerned stakeholders and identified APCD as the regional agency to provide leadership training and empower organizations of persons with disabilities. Aki was honoured to be recognized as a representative of APCD for 2003-2012. It is to be noted that Madame San Yuenwah, the UNESCAP officer in charge of disability, proposed the concept of establishing a decade for persons with disabilities from 1993-2002 jointly to Dr. Sang, representing China Disabled Peoples' Organization (CDPO) and the Chinese government, and Aki, representing Japan at the UNESCAP General Assembly in Beijing in 1992. Aki travelled to Japan and met with Senator Eita Yashiro. They then travelled to Beijing and met with Mr. Deng Phu Fan, CDPO President and the son of Deng Xiaoping, leader of the Peoples' Republic of China. As a result, the Japanese and Chinese governments jointly proposed to have an Asia-Pacific Regional Decade for Persons with Disabilities (1993-2002).

The APCD project began to step forward and establish an intergovernmental organization managed by an autonomous public agency and endorsed by UNESCAP that recognized APCD as an intergovernmental agency, enabling it to sign agreements with other government ministries concerned with disability.

On December 3, United Nations Day on Disability, the official opening ceremony for the APCD project was held at the UNESCAP Conference Centre with many VIPs attending.

After the official events, Aki and I decided to invite all the staff of APCD to our home for a Canadian Christmas dinner with turkey and the trimmings for six-thirty p.m. This proved to be a lesson in Thai culture that related to the concept of time. The first persons came before seven, and some of them were leaving when the last ones arrived. Needless to say, I never made another hot meal for future events. Instead, they enjoyed sushi.

Aki continued his ongoing travels to one to two countries per month to have MOUs signed. While he travelled to India over the new year, his Japanese office coordinator invited me to join him, his wife, and a Japanese friend to go on a vacation (I think that he was feeling sorry for me). He had forewarned me that it was a very basic camping experience and, if I was comfortable with that, I was welcome to join them. He was fluent in Thai and known for being game to do anything, and so was I, I thought!

Well, his description of the vacation was spot on! We drove about two hours toward Kanchanaburi, which shares a border with Myanmar, where we left our car and boarded a motor boat waiting for us, already full with other passengers and supplies for an overnight stay on a floating campsite. I was sandwiched in an aisle seat, holding supplies for the one-hour ride on a massive reservoir, which was the result of the Srinagarind Dam being built to collect flood water.

What a shock to discover how I had unknowingly agreed to bring in the new year of 2003! The whole camp, with fifty plus campers, was floating on water with only primitive washrooms on solid ground! After orientation in what was our dining area, we were directed to our sleeping quarters. We had to walk on slats of bamboo tied together on several walkways until we reached our respective rooms. I shared mine with another Japanese friend. Much to my shock and horror, the floor was of split bamboo with small spaces in between which meant we were looking down at deep water until we unfolded our plastic mats. Frankly, I was petrified that the bamboo slats might break under my weight and that would be the end of me. I couldn't swim and was terrified of deep water. Thin bamboo walls separated us from campers on all sides but made us privy to all activity on the other sides of the walls. We were given free time to rent boats, swim, and bathe in the lake in front of our rooms. This was a new learning curve for me too. The Thai ladies each had a sarong wrapped around their bodies for bathing in public but never exposed themselves. We didn't have sarongs so they must have thought we were quite dirty.

We had assigned seats at dinner, and at our table we enjoyed the company of a baker and his wife from Victory Monument, twenty minutes walking distance from APCD. After the tables were cleared, we were to entertain ourselves for the evening. Everyone was free to participate in any way. It was the funniest evening. Thai have an innate ability to turn everything into a joke. Some people sang, but it was their pantomimes that had everyone in stitches for three hours. The next day, we loaded up because the other vacationers had to join the full tour, which took them to the other end of the reservoir, near the Thai-Burmese border. We had to accompany their group to their meeting place, then return to the opposite end of the reservoir where we had left our car: we then drove to Erawan National

Park. Our day ended at a three-star hotel near the Thai-Burmese border that was overbooked, so we were assigned tents pitched on the backside of the building. The loud music and activity until the wee hours and the cold kept me awake. The one heavy blanket and pillow were not enough to keep me warm even with my clothes on! The next day was elephant trekking for a half day through the forest and rivers. It was an experience not to be forgotten!

January 2003 proved to be a busy month for me, with Melody's second child due and, at the same time, my mother's health continued to deteriorate. On January 17, I flew from Bangkok to St. John's, Newfoundland to be with Melody and Scott who had moved there in 2002. Their second child was due soon after my arrival. Aidan, a healthy baby boy, made an appearance on January 25. Unfortunately, two days later, Mom passed away in Ontario. God gives life and He takes it away. After a quick trip back home for the funeral, I flew back to St. John's to help as needed. Then, on February 18, I flew from St. John's to Toronto, Tokyo, and Bangkok, a thirty-six-hour day from cold blustery weather to a tropical temperature!

Aki was very busy in Bangkok when he wasn't travelling overseas. He visited organizations in Thailand that were working with persons with disabilities to inquire if they wanted to become associate members of APCD. One organization was the Redemptorist Technological College for Persons with Disabilities in Pattaya, established by Father Ray Brennan, an American priest of the Redemptorist Order. In 1987, the school accepted its first full-time students for vocational training, offering free accommodation, food, and medical help to young adults living with disabilities. Courses offered included Information Technology, Computer Business Management in English, Elementary English, and Electronic Repair. After three to four years, Father Ray asked their graduates to run the school. Aajaan Suporntum, a graduate from the first graduating class, became headmaster of the school and his colleagues became teachers and managers. The school was well known for having persons with disabilities actually running the school for persons with disabilities.

When Aki met Aajaan Suporntum to ask if the Redemptorist Foundation wanted to become an associate member of APCD, he was in charge of the department seeking employment for graduates of the school. They had a reputation for finding employment for all their graduates: if graduates lost their jobs, they continued to help them find employment.

Aki felt strongly about empowering persons with disabilities and sought to employ graduates from the Redemptorist School. The first graduate Aki employed was Khun Saowalak, a wheelchair user, as secretary for APCD's coordinator: soon after, he employed two young men, also wheelchair users, as computer technicians, and a young lady with one hand for clerical work. They all had an amazing command of the English language, which was the working language for APCD.

In March, Aki wanted to visit the Thai Autism Vocational Centre in Taling Chan, an NGO in a suburb of Bangkok, to inquire if they, too, wanted to become associate members of APCD. I asked if I could tag along because I was interested in their activities. After the meeting adjourned, I asked the director, Aajaan Chusak, and a member of their Parents' Association what plans they had for their graduates. They both said that they wanted to start a cookie-baking project. Aki's immediate response was, "I know someone who has done that before." They were all ears as he looked at me.

Aki explained that I had started a cookie-baking project for seven autistic young adults and eight intellectually challenged persons after the 1995 earthquake in Kobe, Japan. They said that they were definitely interested in starting a project like this but needed several months to prepare for it. This excited me because, as much as I thought that I never wanted to work with intellectually challenged persons, in Japan I had discovered that they empowered me!

Meanwhile, I worked as a volunteer in the background for APCD with English correspondence and helped Mr. Topong Kulkhanchit, the DPI AP Regional Development Officer, who occasionally requested my help compiling English reports for him. Aki had known Mr. Topong for several years from his involvement with DPI AP. I first met him in November 2001 in Bangkok when he enlisted my help to write English reports.

Mr. Topong was a colourful character with a charismatic personality, who endeared himself to everyone. He had been a member of the Royal Thai Army with the rank of lieutenant colonel when he had an accident, resulting in a cervical spinal cord injury. He was confined to bed in a military rehabilitation hospital in Bangkok when Mr. Narong, president of the Association of the Physically Handicapped in Thailand, encouraged him to participate in the DPI AP Regional Conference to be held in Bangkok in 1987. Mr. Topong went to the Conference in his bed, where he met Shoji Nakanishi, who had the same cervical spinal cord injury. Mr. Topong was stunned to see Mr. Shoji active in a motorized wheelchair. He was determined to become active too, and he got a motorized wheelchair to become somewhat independent. Then, several years later, Mr. Shoji invited Mr. Topong to a wheelchair marathon in Nagoya, Japan. Mr. Topong was met at the airport by Shoji, who had driven to the airport in his own car that had been modified for paraplegic persons.

Mr. Topong couldn't believe it! He returned home, decided to terminate his hospital life, and began to live in a local community. He became an advocate for persons with disabilities in Bangkok and throughout Thailand, saying that there was nothing that persons with disabilities could not do. His appeal to all persons with disabilities made an impact. He became the president of the Association of the Physically Handicapped of Thailand, which grew from a small group in Bangkok to a national organization. In 1991, Mr. Topong visited a centre of the independent living movement (IL) in the United States. This experience made him an IL activist. He had lobbied the government for the enactment of the Rehabilitation of Disabled Persons Act in 1991. He advocated for wheelchair users, who were calling for better accessibility to the sky train station or the new airport.

As a disabled person whose empowerment by a peer had completely changed his life, Mr. Topong put forward the idea of peer empowerment by which persons with disabilities could empower other persons with disabilities to establish the APCD project. He had an open mind, listened to others, and touched the hearts of persons with any kind of disability. Mr. Topong did not hesitate to contact me for assistance.

In April 2003, Mr. Topong organized a Women with Disabilities Workshop for a week in Nonthaburi, Thailand. He had invited Ms. Pavina Vongsouvanh, a powerful advocate in Thailand for women's rights, who later became the country's Minister of Social Development and Human Security.

The Thai New Year, Songkran, a national holiday, always falls on April 13. It coincides with the rising of Aries on the astrological chart and with the new year of many calendars of South and Southeast Asia, in keeping with the Buddhist calendar. It is the hottest month of the year, with everyone joining in the fun of splashing water on everyone they meet. I had been riding the bus one day when someone with a water gun sprayed me. Windows on the bus are only closed if it rains or if they no longer open. One time, I had ice water poured down my back when walking to the market. Until then, I had assumed nobody would splash water on me as a foreigner.

In May, Aki and I decided we were ready for a vacation together. We flew to Chiang Rai in northern Thailand, where Myanmar, Laos, and Thailand share borders. It is known as the Golden Triangle because it was originally the opium-growing region of Northern Thailand, Eastern Myanmar, and Western Laos. We toured the Opium Museum, a cultural museum, and several tribal villages. Chiang Rai was a melting pot for ethnic minority groups such as the Karen, Akha, Hmong, Lahu, Lisu, Palong, and Mien (Yao). It was the perfect place to discover authentic hill tribe culture and traditional hill tribe life. A few of the hill tribal villages, set up for tourists to provide an income for the villagers, also served as a way to preserve their ethnic traditions and culture.

In August, Aki and I were able to participate in the Phuket Autism Conference organized by Mr. Chusak, the director of the Thai Autism Vocational Centre in Bangkok. He was a strong advocate for persons with autism and wanted to establish a chapter in each prefecture to promote awareness.

Baking Project at the Thai Autism Vocational Centre

In late September 2003, Mr. Chusak contacted me to inquire whether I was still committed to beginning a cookie-baking project with autistic students at his vocational centre in Taling Chan, a suburb of Bangkok. I assured him that I was able to begin at their convenience. The first challenge was to navigate the public transportation system to get to his centre. It required about a fifteen-minute walk from our home to get a bus going to Bang Khun Si market, where I was instructed to walk through the market, and then cross the street to board a truck with "red letters" because the "blue lettered" truck went another direction (the truck was like an army vehicle with two long benches on either side). I was told at what point to press a buzzer so the truck would stop at the end of their long laneway. If I was lucky, it took an hour and a half one way to travel because no bus schedule existed: they came at irregular times and only stopped when they were flagged down out in the country. What a relief to arrive at my destination!

Fortunately, my brother-in-law Murray Calder, who was coming to Bangkok as a representative of the Canadian government for an APEC (Asia-Pacific Economic Cooperation) meeting, kindly agreed to bring my cookie recipe books.

October 1, 2003, I met with Khun Ning, who was in charge of the baking program, at the Thai Autism Vocational Centre, to begin preparation. I shared my suggested recipes, and, when we went to buy supplies, she informed me that a friend was temporarily allowing them to use her facility and baking equipment. Mr. Chusak wanted to have a trial run of baking for six weeks to determine whether he should consider investing in baking equipment for the centre.

Khun Ning took me to the facility where we would be baking temporarily. What a surprise! We unlocked the metal gate and discovered layers of dust and dirt covering everything. The walls were built to waist level with the remainder consisting of wire netting to the ceiling, which kept the birds out. Traffic on the road running directly in front of the building created dirt and pollution. We decided that we would just clean half of the building that we would use.

The gas oven was unlike any I had seen. It was considered a commercial gas oven, wide enough to have five burners that had to be lit by hand. This oven frightened me because it was also hard to control the temperature. Outside the front entrance gate was a sink that was not connected to any pipe, and it needed to have water carried from a barrel that was halfway back near a pit privy.

And so, on our first baking day, Khun Ning, another staff person, three autistic clients, and I cleaned our working space and equipment and unpacked our supplies. We did eventually get the gas oven to work and produced one recipe of sesame cookies! The clients were so proud of their accomplishment! I was exhausted! Then it was another ninety minutes of public transportation to get home: I was thankful that healthy meals could be bought on the street for a price cheaper than if you made them yourself!

It was agreed that we would bake cookies three times a week in the afternoon so the clients could continue with their other activities. If, after six weeks, it looked like the project would succeed, Mr. Chusak would decide whether to make it part of their curriculum.

After six weeks, the clients were so excited about their baking. Mr. Chusak was so impressed with the results that he authorized Khun Ning and me to buy an oven and the necessary equipment to begin baking at his centre. He had a flyer printed in Thai and English and decided on a logo with a lady with short curly hair and glasses, with "Aunty Marcy, Natural Cookies" written underneath. When deciding on the colours for the logo, they wanted to have the hair coloured grey, I guess to reflect my hair colour. My response was, "Grey? Why not yellow?" Their response was, "Yellow?" I thought for marketing, eye appeal was important. Well, the hair became yellow!

The English flyer said,

> *Try Your Aunty Marcy Cookies Now!*
>
> *The Aunty Marcy Cookies are joyfully made by trainees at the Thai Autism Vocational Centre, who take pride in producing quality healthy cookies made without additives or preservatives for you to enjoy.*
>
> *The intent of the project is to empower persons with autism by participating in a social activity, building self-esteem and confidence, generating income, and promoting independent living.*
>
> *The delicious homemade cookies include, chocolate, chocolate chip, coconut, coffee, healthy, oatmeal/coconut,*

*organic poppy seed, peanut, sesame, tamarind, and sun-
dried tomato.*

*The logo honours Marcy Ninomiya, a volunteer from
Ontario, Canada who helped develop this project and
supervises the trainees making the cookies.*

Information about ordering cookies followed.

Because I had already learned much from having started a baking
project in Japan with persons with autism and intellectual disabilities, this
project was not difficult after assessing the abilities of the "bakers."

We baked cookies three days a week. I focused on teaching the weigh-
ing of the ingredients and mixing with several bakers. I had discovered
long ago that their one cup of flour and my one cup were different, so we
always used a digital scale. One hundred grams was a hundred grams!

Two clients had the strength to mix the dough and learned to do it
well. One day, I caught one of the mixers drooling a little because he was
working so hard mixing the batter. Needless to say, a mask was added to
his uniform.

They were very proud of their achievements and made the best sales
reps. Parents were approached by some of the bakers to buy a small bag of
five cookies when they came to pick up their children.

Our market soon expanded to include a local supermarket that gave us
a stand inside the main entrance to sell our baking, which generated some
regular customers. This was another opportunity to teach the clients how
to greet customers, accept payment, and put orders into bags. We also went
to the UNESCAP in Bangkok twice a month, but the Parents' Association
continued to be our strongest supporter.

Hospitality was another one of "my caps." When our personal guests
came, Aki and I did our best to be knowledgeable tour guides: having guests
was an opportunity for us to learn about the most informative and interesting tourist attractions in the Bangkok area and elsewhere in Thailand.
In October, Moriyama Khun, his wife, Aki's former students from Japan,
and Dr. Mike Shimpo from our house church in Canada visited us.

In November, the visit of Melody, Scott, and their children, Maya and
Aidan was very timely. They celebrated the Loi Krathong festival, known

as the Thai Festival of Lights, with us. Traditionally, a slice of a banana tree trunk is decorated with flowers, banana leaves, and incense sticks and set afloat in water, with a prayer later in the day. It is seen as a time to wave goodbye to misfortune, wash away sins of the past year, and make wishes for the coming year.

Because we felt it was important to also include orientation to missionary work being done in Thailand, we took Melody's family to visit the McKean Rehab Centre in Chiang Mai. It had an interesting history. In 1907, an American missionary, Dr. McKean, officially asked the ruler of Thailand to donate a piece of land to found a leper colony for the socially unacceptable disease, which was fairly common at that time. As a donation, he received an island in the Ping River, Chiang Mai, where rulers had kept their elephants and where locals didn't like to venture for fear of the spirits of white elephants. So, in 1908, it became the McKean Leper Asylum, which started with six patients but soon expanded to include thousands of residents in the future.

There was no cure for leprosy until the early 1980s, but patients at McKean received care, support, food, comfort, compassion and, most importantly, shelter from the stigma of society. They developed their own well-organized community, established schools, shops, gardens, and community centres. After the cure for leprosy was widely available, the number of cases had significantly dwindled so McKean became a rehabilitation centre. A small bridge takes one across onto the island to this day.

There was vocational training, education, and many kinds of support for residents in need. Their gift shop was a wonderful place to support their vocational training, especially with the purchase of greeting cards, lacquerware, woodwork, and sewing. Some elderly residents cured of leprosy, but with no family left or willing to take them in, continued to live on the island.

Aki and I spent the Christmas holidays in Ontario with Timothy, Matt, and Katie, then flew to St. John's for the 2004 New Year's holiday with Melody, Scott, Maya, and Aidan. We learned much about the history of St. John's. This was where Terry Fox, who became a national hero, began his Marathon of Hope, a cross-country run to raise money for cancer research. The cold weather was a shock for us though.

In mid-January 2004, we were back in Bangkok. Work as usual continued for Aki, and I resumed making cookies with my autistic friends. They looked forward to my coming, and I had missed them. They stood watching at the locked gate to their compound. When they saw me walking down the lane, I heard them shout, "Khun Marcy maa leo" (Marcy has come already). Their time in the baking project was "hands on," and they knew that I had accepted them for who they were. I never asked more of them than I knew they were capable of doing. To set them up for failure would defeat the purpose. It was a joy to see them become more self-confident as they became more skilled in producing cookies.

Whenever guests came, they participated in my activities. So, when Dad, my sister, Susan, my brother, Robert, and sister-in-law, Helen, came for a visit in February, they also donned caps and aprons to bake cookies for the day. Dad was a good sport and was admired by all the staff for participating. No Thai man at the age of eighty-six would be found helping to bake!

I enjoyed introducing my family to the local market, giving their taste buds a workout. The tropical fruits, especially the different kinds of bananas, papaya, cactus fruit, custard apple, mangoes, guava, rambutan, etc., were enjoyed. We flew to Chiang Mai, where they visited McKean Rehabilitation Centre. Dad enjoyed touring their wheelchair manufacturing project run by persons who were cured of their leprosy. Ethnic tribal villages were fascinating, with their handicrafts and the famous night bazaar. We also enjoyed a "khantoke" dinner and a cultural show at the Old Chiangmai Cultural Centre. A khantoke is a pedestal tray used as a small dining table by the Lanna people, Laotians, and by people from northeastern Thailand that can be made from wood, bamboo, or rattan. Our dinner was served on a red khantoke with various Northern Thai dishes that one traditionally ate with the right hand: a hill tribal dance show followed, which was fascinating and educational: each ethnic tribal group performed a dance from their culture.

While Aki was busy, I took the family on a day trip to Pattaya, a two-hour bus ride from Bangkok, and introduced them to the Redemptorist Centre, which provided educational services for persons with disabilities who were excluded from the regular educational system. We also took a speedboat to a small island, where my four family members took a wild ride on an inflated banana, then were dumped in the sea closer to shore. Dad had forgotten to take his hearing aids out before going on this ride. Miraculously, they were still in his ears after being dumped in the sea, and they still worked!

Their visit was over Valentine's Day. Why do I remember? Apparently, Dad had been courting Anna Shantz, unknown to our family. She had sent a valentine card along with Susan to give to Dad on February 14. Robert was stunned one day when Dad said that on this trip, he needed to decide whether to marry again or not at the age of eighty-six. It was news to all of us! He decided to marry Anna, and I found myself on a flight to Toronto for Dad and Anna's wedding on May 8, 2004.

Whenever Aki needed to hire staff, he communicated with Aajaan Suporntum at the Redemptorist Foundation to see if there was a graduate needing employment. Yes, there was a young lady, Khun Jam, who was graduating and was the only one in her class who had not been employed. The reason was that she was born without hands. Everyone who had interviewed her felt that, without hands, she was unable to be a productive employee. Aki employed her and found she spoke excellent English and had good computer skills.

Finding accommodation for her was a challenge. If you've ever used a bus in Bangkok, you would understand how dangerously most buses were driven—speeding, switching lanes, and frequent sudden use of brakes. If you are able-bodied and could hang on to something, it is not a serious problem. But if you have to stand and have no hands to hang onto a seat or bar, it is dangerous. After two falls on the bus, we knew we had to seek accommodation closer to APCD for Khun Jam. Fortunately, she was not injured.

Khun Jam had been a conscientious, capable employee for approximately two years when the Thai director of APCD informed Aki that Khun Jam could no longer be employed because Thai employees working for the government must have a minimum of high school education, which Khun Jam did not have. All of Aki's persuasive power could not reverse the decision of the Thai government director, which hurt him deeply. Khun Jam had to leave. She returned to Pattaya to enlist the help of the

Redemptorist Foundation to help find employment. Finally, she was hired by an American tourist agency based in Pattaya.

All was well for about eight months when serious sexual harassment began, so she left the agency and began looking for employment again. She was at a decided disadvantage because nobody wanted to employ a person with no hands. Khun Jam came from a poor area in Northeastern Thailand. Her parents, wanting the best for their daughter, had been at a loss of what to do when they heard of the Redemptorist Foundation that provided a free education for persons with disabilities. This was an answer to their concerns. Now that Khun Jam was again unemployed, Aki and I kept in contact with her and encouraged her to study toward getting her high school diploma because she was so bright. She got her diploma and Aki hired her back.

APCD Project Activities

I audited some of APCD's workshops on community-based rehabilitation, non-handicapping environment, and independent living to be knowledgeable and updated for our work.

Because APCD did not yet have its own facilities, workshops were held at different venues. One workshop, Training of Initiators for SHG (self-help groups) of Persons with Disabilities Toward a Rights-Based and Sustainable Community Development, was held at the Redemptorist Conference facilities in Pattaya. Participants were all persons with disabilities from Cambodia, Laos, Myanmar, Vietnam, and Thailand. The facilitator was Venky, an amazing blind man from India, who had established self-help groups in poverty-stricken villages in the Aranya Pradesh area of India. His efforts resulted in establishing self-help groups, using microfinancing to generate income to support their families. They were now registered as a self-help organization and still growing. It was empowering to listen to his story.

I was able to participate in his workshop in August 2004. Venky did not use any notes as he conducted the three-week workshop. Due to cultural differences in communication styles, his strong straightforward way of communicating was stressful for participants, who were unaccustomed to being addressed in this way. I sat between two participants from Myanmar. The lady on my right was reduced to tears one day since she felt belittled in front of the group. A young Cambodian man refused to answer any more questions after feeling humiliated. Because my husband was the Chief Advisor for APCD, I felt eyes turn on me to handle the situation. Venky, being blind, was unable to see how he hurt others.

Our participants were divided into four groups for field trips. My group visited a young man, about eighteen years of age, who became a quadriplegic after a drunken driver hit his motorcycle. His life had been changed in the flash of a second to being confined to bed and totally dependent on his mother for care. It was so sad to hear his story and know that he did not have access to needed services that patients have in Canada.

On the second last day of our workshop, Nay Lin Soe, from Myanmar, asked me to give him a tour of the chapel on the Redemptorist compound. It was built in Thai style, with murals on all the walls depicting Christ's life and other Biblical stories. A magnificent work of art.

Nay Lin Soe continued to communicate with me after returning to Myanmar. He was a very bright young man who had an orthopedic disability due to polio at a young age. He felt so empowered after the workshop that on return to Myanmar he went from door to door in his community, inquiring if there was a person with a physical disability in the home. He then organized a small group, then another until there were about sixty persons with disabilities identified. About this time, Nay Lin Soe was accepted as an exchangee for a one-year Duskin Exchange Program in Japan that provided leadership training for persons with disabilities. He returned to Myanmar a year later and organized a self-help organization called MILI, Myanmar Independent Living Initiatives, which offered training to empower persons with physical disabilities. He has continued to communicate with me to this day, always addressing his correspondence "Dear Mom."

An event that Aki and I were eagerly looking forward to was the celebration of MCC's fifty years of service in Vietnam in Hanoi, September 24-25, 2004, where we hoped to meet some familiar faces. MCC began its work in Vietnam in 1954 after the Geneva Accords brought hope for peace and reconciliation for many. There was great expectation that independence from colonial rule was near for the Vietnamese people. A collection of displaced people in South Vietnam was a side effect of the Accords that divided the country into North and South at the 17th parallel. MCC began its presence with the intent of aiding these displaced people. The first MCC director was to assess the needs of these displaced people and begin a program.

MCC's presence in Vietnam could be divided into five distinct periods:

1. 1954-1965: Displaced people's assistance and program buildup
2. 1966-1972: Cooperation through Vietnam Christian Service
3. 1973-1979: Presence in the transition to a unified Vietnam
4. 1980-1989: Working through Vietnam's difficult years
5. 1990-2004: Establishing a representing office and increasing grassroots activities

In my era (65-71) the focus was on the medical needs in Nhatrang and Pleiku.

Besides the official ceremony, former MCC and CWS personnel shared their experiences. One of the first MCCers in 1954 also attended and entertained us with many humorous experiences. There was a significant number attending from my era of service.

A field trip to outlying villages helped us realize how much had been done in the field of agriculture, health, education, and economic development. This was the first time for most participants to visit North Vietnam. It was a wonderful feeling to sit on small low chairs and sip the famous Vietnamese coffee and savour a Vietnamese sandwich, which consisted of a small baguette with meat and veggies, sold early in the morning by women plying the streets with a tray balanced on their heads. We were all billeted in the "Old Quarter" with its rich history and culture. We enjoyed a water puppet show with the puppets acting out an historical event, with a narrator supplying the facts. After the event, Aki returned to Bangkok, and I stayed on.

I had arranged for six persons to travel to places where we had worked, as well as more sightseeing. The group included Alan Hostetler, a MCCer who had helped build the hospital in Nhatrang in 1962; Pat Niska, a social worker from Saigon with CWS: Carol Dahl, whose husband had served in the office in Saigon; Katy Dyck, who worked with me in Nhatrang and Jake, her husband, and me. We flew to Hue, toured the old walled city, and then hired a van to drive to Danang, two hours south; we stopped briefly at a shop that sold items from Marble Mountain near Danang, then continued on to Hoi An, our destination for two nights. The drive from Hue to Danang was breathtaking, looking down to the sea from high up in the mountains.

Hoi An was an UNESCO World Heritage Site: the old town of Hoi An was the city's historic district, a Southeast Asian trading port dating from the fifteenth to nineteenth centuries. Its buildings and street plan reflected a blend of indigenous and foreign influences. Its iconic attraction was a Japanese covered bridge that dated back to the eighteenth century, created by Japanese living in Hoi An as a way to reach the Chinese quarter across the water. It continues to stand as a symbol of Hoi An.

I introduced the group to Mr. Binh, a wheelchair user who had enrolled in APCD's Information and Communication Technology program as well as a web management workshop in July 2003. He returned to Hoi An and began a computer class for persons with disabilities. What I discovered on our visit was that Mr. Binh had already developed a project called Reaching Out, a fair-trade gift shop with quality handmade gifts by people with different abilities. His pamphlet stated, "The shop was founded in 2000 by a group of 'disAbled' craftspeople in Hoi An to teach young disabled persons marketable skills in a friendly, supportive environment, to earn a fair wage, and become self-reliant. It brought talented disAbled artisans from all over Vietnam." Mr. Binh had married and had a young son who loved to sit on his father's lap as they went zipping down the street in a motorized wheelchair. He extended hospitality to our group by inviting us to a local Vietnamese restaurant for a simple meal, which we all enjoyed.

After three days, we drove back to Danang and caught a two-hour flight to Nhatrang, which was Katy's and my home stomping ground for our three-year terms. We had arranged to meet the director of the hospital for a tour, in which our former staff joined because they had not been allowed to enter the hospital compound. The hospital was now a rehabilitation facility for the elite military.

I organized a surprise birthday party for Katy at our hotel near the hospital, while the rest of the group took an island boat tour. Former hospital staff were delighted to attend. The Vietnamese language had come back for Katy and me: we had so much fun that time just evaporated!

I was on a high returning to Bangkok and getting back to making more cookies. The most popular was the chocolate cookie made with cocoa, chocolate chips, and cashew nuts; I had modified the legendary Neiman Marcus cookie recipe forwarded by VJ, a nursing classmate.

In November, we had guests from Japan: Yuki Ohara, a former student of Aki's; Sawada San, a neighbour in Kobe; Nagase San, and Yokoi San. Yokoi San and I had worked together at the Wakamatsu Bunjo baking project after the earthquake in 1995. I will always remember her as the only person that I had ever worked with naturally synchronized without talking. Our working style as a team had been calming for the clients.

APCD's new buildings were finally completed. The administration building had three floors: the second floor was office space with a meeting room: the third floor had office space available for NGOs to rent. The main floor included an outdoor but undercover cafeteria, a hairdressing salon, and a craft room all designated for vocational training of young girls under the care of the Ministry of Social Development and Human Security in the same compound.

The second APCD building was for training and workshops. The main floor was classrooms and IT facilities: the second floor included the dining area and state-of-the art accommodation for thirty persons with all types of disabilities. Because orientation had to be available for all persons in English, I was designated to record instructions for use of the building. Braille was posted throughout the building so participants with a visual impairment could find their way around. If you would visit today, you would still hear my voice! All rooms were equipped with flashing lights for hearing impaired persons in an emergency.

The International Day on Disability, on December 3, was always a major event for us and persons with disabilities. Since Aki would be in Hanoi, Vietnam until just before Christmas, we hosted the staff Christmas party in early December. It was sushi this time, with fresh fruit and some home baking.

I was eagerly looking forward to our sons, Timothy and Matthew, coming for a visit. People "back home" think it is so exciting to do all kinds of travel when living overseas but don't realize how much family time and how many events one misses.

Tim and Matt arrived on December 23. On Christmas Day, we invited our close Thai friends, Suthida and Martin, a blind pianist, for a Christmas turkey dinner, which Martin stills raves about today. He thought turkey meat was always dry but discovered it didn't need to be. In the evening, we were honoured to be invited by Mr. Sato, JICA's representative to Thailand, for a delicious Japanese meal.

We wanted to do some sightseeing with the boys, so we decided to travel to Koh Chang Island, Thailand's most eastern province that borders Cambodia. It was known as an unspoiled island with many beautiful beaches, fishing villages on one side, and lush jungle-like mountains on the other. This entailed a five-hour bus ride from Bangkok, taking a tuk-tuk ride to the ferry, an hour ferry ride, then another tuk-tuk ride to our bungalow, right by the sea. The scene and beach made the travel time worth the effort. The next day, we took a tour and rode elephants through a jungle setting and some deep water. When the water level reached my feet while on the elephant, I panicked.

After four days, we returned to Bangkok to prepare for the next segment of our vacation. Aki and I thought that the boys should see Angkor Wat in Cambodia while in Asia, so we left Bangkok by train on January 2, 2005 for Aranyaprathet, the Thai town closest to the Thai-Cambodian border to enter Cambodia. The train was packed, with people going home for New Year's. We stood for the five-hour ride and decided it was best to spend the night there. The next morning, we took local transport to the border at Poipet, Cambodia and joined the queue for immigration. We could not believe all the labourers pulling heavily loaded carts of used clothing into Thailand. Now we understood where all the used clothing at Bangkok's weekend market came from!

Aki always researched travel information before taking any trip, so he knew that the best way for us to continue was to take a taxi from Poipet to Siem Reap, the closest town to Angkor Wat. A hard bargainer, he got a taxi for $35 US for the 150 km drive. We were not prepared for the huge potholes: the taxi frequently left the road to avoid falling into a pothole. "Gas stations" were barrels of gasoline at the roadside with a pump attached, sold in one litre bottles. In the rainy season, this trip would be impossible. The trip took most of the day to reach our hotel that was full of Korean tourists. We were privileged to have water on the tap because 80 percent of Cambodians living in Siem Reap did not have running water or washroom facilities at home.

The next day we took a tour of the famous Angkor Wat, an enormous Buddhist temple complex made of sandstone and built in the twelfth century. It was rediscovered in the 1840s by a French explorer Henri Mouhot, who wrote that the site was "grander than anything left to us by Greece or Rome." A fifteen-foot-high wall, surrounded by a 100-meter-wide moat, protected Angkor City and the temple from invasion. The sandstone causeway served as the main access point for the temple. Tim and Matt climbed the steps to the top of the temple, which proved simple compared to descending: they couldn't believe how high they had climbed and there was only one way down, to descend the well-worn narrow steep steps made for smaller feet.

We then went to see another one of the Angkor Thom temples where there was a person with disabilities selling his artwork in pictures and greeting cards. Because there were few customers, we spent considerable time talking with him through our guide. We wondered if he would consider studying art in Japan if sponsored. This wasn't an option because he was homeless with no fixed address. We noted his old wheelchair chained to a banyan tree beside him. He wrote his name for us, and we promised to get a new used wheelchair for him. Whether he really believed us, we didn't know.

On returning to Bangkok, we discovered our neighbour who worked at UNESCAP was soon planning to go to Angkor Wat on vacation. They kindly agreed to take a wheelchair for the artist. They did find him and delivered the wheelchair to him! When they went to visit him the following day he was not there. He must have been riding on his new wheels!

During our travels, we were unaware of the terrible tragedy that hit Thailand on December 26, 2004. There had been an earthquake, 9.1 on the Richter scale, beneath the Indian Ocean, off the coast of Sumatra, Indonesia, resulting in tsunami waves over 100 feet high along the Indonesian coast lasting one and a half hours and killing 170,000 persons. The tsunami waves also hit beaches in Southern Thailand, in the Andaman Sea islands, during the peak season for tourists. There were six big waves: the Thai officials sent out a warning, but only after the first deadly wave. Five thousand four hundred people died, of whom 2,000 were foreign tourists. We learned that Khun Poom, the adult autistic son of Princess Ubolratana, was one of the victims. The marine security boat for the princess was washed a kilometre and a half inland, where it stands today as a testament to the tsunami.

We heard the story of a ten-year-old British girl who had been vacationing with her family at Khao Lak at the time of the tsunami. She had been standing on the beach and noticed the water level rapidly receding, and hollered, "A tsunami is coming! A tsunami is coming! Run for higher ground!" She had just studied about tsunamis before vacationing. Her action saved the lives of many people.

Our boys left Thailand on January 5, 2005, for Canada after a full vacation learning more about Asia. Unfortunately, they missed the visit of Lill and Neville Muir and their son, Ian, who had been our next-door neighbours in Kobe before the 1995 earthquake. They were now based in Melbourne, Australia and couldn't resist taking a tour in Thailand. Such a fun time in their two-day visit with us!

Aki and I were active members of the Evangelical Church of Bangkok (ECB). The church was very concerned about areas destroyed by the devastating tsunami; homes, schools, and businesses had been destroyed; many children had lost their homes and parents and were being raised by surrogate grandmothers. Aware of the psychological impact on the children, our church decided to have a one-week camp in mid-April, during the Thai New Year, for the children in the Khao Lak area who had been most affected by the tsunami. I volunteered to be the camp nurse. We filled a bus with volunteers and drove fifteen hours south to Khao Lak, where we stayed at a very simple bed and breakfast. I shared a bed with a volunteer from Myanmar and an army of ants.

Children appeared from everywhere and seemed to thoroughly enjoy our morning camp. Reading about the damage and seeing it were very different. Children had painted artwork on several remaining walls of buildings. Most showed a huge tsunami wave rolling high above the palm trees and a small insignificant child in the distance: others showed their homes demolished.

Our leader could make any situation humorous, so the children kept asking us if we would come again next year. We were given a tour of the area and saw numerous large fishing vessels that had been washed ashore and were perched in the middle of the village. In the evening, several of us walked down to the seashore. Personal effects, clothing, etc., were embedded in the soil: there were posters in English nailed to trees with a description of a missing person: if found please contact so and so. One notice was for a two-year-old Swiss child. It was so sad, and this was four months after the tsunami. We left, moved by what these people had experienced and would have to cope with long term.

About this time, APCD needed to hire another staff person and was introduced to Sam, a graduate from the Redemptorist Foundation's School for Computer Business Management in English. Sam was in Pattaya, currently unemployed. One of APCD staff who knew Sam and his situation said that he had no resources to rent a room, but he was willing to work for APCD if living arrangements could be made. Aki and I decided that he could live with us for several months until he would be able to rent a room on his own, which is what he did.

With Aki travelling so much I had lots of time to get to know Sam. He'd had polio as an infant, which left his legs paralyzed. His parents, at a loss of what to do with their son, had left him on the doorsteps of an American missionary family in Northern Thailand. He lived with them until the age of eighteen when the missionary family returned to the States. Because

Sam was legally an adult and not registered as a family member, he could not leave with them. That was when he heard about the Redemptorist Foundation's educational program and registered. We did our best to help him rent a room near our home four months later. In time, Sam married and had a healthy little boy called Sammy.

In June, our son Tim graduated from Conestoga College in Chemical Engineering Technology and was looking for work. Matt graduated in Civil Engineering at University of Waterloo. Melody and Scott continued to work in restorative justice with MCC in St. John's, Newfoundland.

Many guests graced our home over the years. Dad, Anna, and Aunt Lena came for two weeks. Dad always enjoyed travelling, exploring, and learning new things. Fully aware that he would not get Anna's permission to go on a six-week trip for both of them and his sister, Lena, he decided to just make the travel plans. The itinerary included two weeks in New Zealand because Aunt Lena's daughter was living there; two weeks in Australia that included visiting a couple who had been stranded at Mom and Dad's in Conestogo during a severe winter storm; then the final two weeks were with Aki and myself in Bangkok. Although the three of them were in their late eighties, they were troopers.

By now, I qualified as an official tour guide! I knew that foreigners visiting the Grand Palace had to have their upper arms covered and wear shoes covering their toes and heels: no shorts were allowed, so skirts were available for unknowing tourists. Aunt Lena had fairly lengthy capris that I thought would pass, but the ticket master had a measurement chart attached to his booth that showed that her capris fell about an inch too short. Aunt Lena didn't miss a beat, she pulled her capris down just enough to meet the requirement, then looked him in the eye and asked, "Is this ok?" He responded with, "If you don't pull them up again." We had a good laugh.

Of course, Dad, Anna, and Aunt Lena wanted to see APCD and hear about Aki's work. The office staff could not believe that three seniors over the age of eighty were travelling unaccompanied. Dad could have passed for fifteen years younger. The three of them also visited the cookie project at the Thai Autism Vocational Centre and met the director. Aunt Lena, who had never travelled to Asia before, was fascinated by the market's tropical fruits and seafood. She was out to learn as much as she could. I travelled with them to Chiang Mai and gave them the usual "Marcy tour" to McKean Rehab to see the businesses run by persons recovered from Hansen's Disease (leprosy). The wheelchair factory fascinated Dad, who tried riding several different types. The khantoke Northern Thai dinner and folk dances were a hit, as was a boat tour up the Ping River to a fruit farm where we enjoyed a plate of fresh fruit from their fruit trees. Another highlight was the Mae Sa Elephant Camp and a show where elephants even did art painting. Aunt Lena and I enjoyed walking around our hotel area and surfing the night bazaar, a must for tourists who want to buy Thai handicrafts.

Pakistan and Kashmir Earthquake

From September 22-26, 2005, APCD organized the Asia-Pacific Regional Workshop on Capacity-Building of Self-Help Organizations of Persons with Disabilities in Islamabad, Pakistan. During the workshop, Aki decided to make a courtesy call to Mr. Haq, Minister of Religion. Aki shared his experience of meeting with Mr. Haq's father, the late President Zia-ul-Haq, who had attended the DPI AP Conference in Islamabad in 1988. His father's opening speech had been, "I am standing here not only as president but also as the father of my daughter with an intellectual disability," who was standing with him on the podium. He added, "I am proud of my daughter." This so moved Mr. Haq that he offered to attend the closing ceremony. Because he was so popular, many participants were excited to have him make a speech at the closing ceremony, which empowered the various organizations of persons with disabilities to collaborate and work together.

This workshop was the first time that major DPOs in Pakistan could meet together, so they organized a national network of DPOs in Pakistan. Then, on October 8 at eight-fifty a.m., a 7.6 magnitude earthquake struck northern Pakistan and Kashmir. Fortunately, persons with disabilities had just established a national network at the workshop twelve days earlier. So, when the persons with disabilities in Kashmir asked DPOs in other cities to help, groups in Islamabad, Lahore, and Karachi got organized to do so.

The IL Centre in Lahore rented a school bus, filled it with food, water, medicines, blankets, and clothes and persons with disabilities drove the bus to Kashmir. STEP, Special Talent Exchange Program in Islamabad, committed to mainstreaming disability through empowering individuals and organizations, organized an evacuation centre for persons with disabilities and persons who had just become disabled due to the earthquake. The death toll was over 100,000, with approximately 38,000 people injured and 3.5 million made homeless; 19,000 children died, many due to their schools collapsing: 17,000 school buildings and most major hospitals close to the epicentre were destroyed or severely damaged. Numerous vital roads and highways were closed due to landslides. Some villages and towns no longer existed. Besides the landslides, there were rock falls involving large rocks or boulders, which caused considerable damage and resulted in significant fatalities. Many homes, built of rocks, collapsed on the women working in their kitchens, causing spinal cord injuries. At least ninety women became paraplegics.

In Lahore, within a week of the earthquake, an independent living group received funds from the World Bank to build ten centres in different locations. They also began a wheelchair company to produce wheelchairs.

Aki's experience with the 1995 earthquake in Kobe, Japan, proved helpful at this time. Within a month after the earthquake, Aki travelled to Pakistan to ascertain the needs. His good working relationship with the government and persons with disabilities made it easy to be productive. Victims did not have enough blankets to keep warm, so I encouraged Aki to go to the market and personally buy a huge supply of blankets, which he did. Three months later, Aki, with a team from APCD and JICA personnel from Tokyo headquarters, went to visit the new IL centres and returned to Islamabad on another road. They encountered a huge hole, which the driver said was impassible. Aki got out of the car and told everyone to start throwing rocks into the hole. Two hours later, they were able to continue driving.

Six months after the earthquake, JICA had dispatched a reconstruction team to Pakistan via Bangkok, so Aki was able to meet with them and promote construction of accessible schools and medical facilities. He was able to dispatch resource persons to the National Workshop on the Reconstruction of Buildings and the Universal Design organized by APCD in collaboration with the Ministry of Social Welfare and Women of Pakistan. Participants included trained policy makers, architects, and leaders of persons with disabilities. Aki also asked Mr. Topong to run a national disaster management workshop because he had been involved with the reconstruction of the area destroyed by the tsunami in Thailand earlier that year.

Six months after the earthquake, March/April 2006, APCD organized a ten-day Workshop for Women with Paraplegic Disabilities and Peer Counselling Training in Bangkok, inviting Pakistani women using wheelchairs. They returned to Pakistan to conduct peer counselling with women who had become paraplegic due to the earthquake. The outcome was the Association for Women with Disabilities!

I continued to be involved with the DPI AP office, as needed, with Mr. Topong, who was active in many projects, one of which was to distribute used wheelchairs sent from Japan. Mr. Topong asked me if I would be interested to accompany him, with his friend, Mr. Anuson, a high school teacher, and twelve of his high school students, to Laos to distribute used wheelchairs to persons with disabilities. He added that six Japanese high school students and their chaperone would be joining us at Nong Khai, the closest Thai city to the Thai/Lao border, to be part of our caravan to Vientiane, the capital of Laos. Of course, I was interested. I assumed he wanted me to go along as a bridge between the Japanese group and the Thai participants.

I learned that the used wheelchair project in Japan was the result of Mr. Yamaha, a wheelchair user himself, who had attended the first DPI meeting in Singapore in 1981. He had returned to Japan and established an independent living centre in Nagoya called Aino Jiritsu Undo. Over time, the residents began a campaign to recycle good used wheelchairs, called Asian Persons with Disabilities Support Project. They involved high school students as volunteers to clean the used wheelchairs. In 2002, they sent 400 used wheelchairs to Afghanistan with Mr. Ogura, also a wheelchair user, who was responsible for the project.

With access to so many good used wheelchairs, Mr. Ogura contacted Mr. Topong to work in partnership to distribute wheelchairs in Asia. After distribution in Thailand, Mr. Topong's wife organized distribution to Laos, which was when he contacted me.

Our two vans left Nonthaburi (thirty minutes from Bangkok) with excited high school students: Mr. Topong driving one van and his friend, Mr. Anusong, driving the other. After driving all day, we spent the night at Nong Khai, near the airport, where we were meeting the Japanese group of six high school students and their chaperone the next morning to drive to Vientiane, Laos. I joined their vehicle so they did not feel so isolated. After lunch, we went to a Laotian high school where some of their students joined us as volunteers to clean wheelchairs in their athletic field that had been shipped ahead of us. What an experience with so many excited high school students and an assortment of local people watching this international group working together. Later in the afternoon, we delivered two wheelchairs to their recipients. One was a seven-year-old boy with cerebral palsy who was getting too heavy for his mother to carry, so his days were spent on a bamboo bed under their home built on stilts, which was the coolest place for him. We helped put him in the wheelchair and showed his mother how to use it. She was as excited as her son when she pushed him down the street!

The second wheelchair went to a seventeen-year-old young man who had been homebound, unable to go to school due to his disability. I wish everyone could have seen his face after sitting in the wheelchair and being mobile on his own for the first time. Before we left, he poured out his heart by singing a song he had composed while playing his guitar. What a wonderful way to express his appreciation and share his talent with us.

This trip was an eye-opening cultural experience for all the students but even more so for the Japanese. Life was very simple and basic here with poor sanitation. The Japanese group did a little more sightseeing before returning to Japan and we left the next morning for a long day of driving back to Nonthaburi.

This project continued to develop with wheelchairs being sent to Cambodia and Myanmar. Fundraising was done in Japan, but the distribution was arranged through Mr. Topong's DPI AP office until his death in 2007. Then Mr. Ogura, who ran the project in Japan, oversaw the distribution of approximately 100 wheelchairs annually, utilizing the late Mr. Topong's wife as an assistant.

When Aki and I reflected on the year 2005, we gave thanks for our many blessings. Thousands had perished in the Thai tsunami and the earthquake in Pakistan: much suffering continued in South-East Asia due to natural disasters. Our hearts went out to those who experienced the loss of family members, loss of income, and became disabled.

We were fortunate to be flying to Ontario, Canada to spend the Christmas and New Year holidays with our family and friends.

I reflected on a poem written by Genzo Mizuno, a Japanese man who became paralyzed at the age of ten, unable to move or speak. He developed a means of communicating with his mother by blinking his eyelids. Genzo has left a legacy of poetry which has inspired many people with the witness of his life.

> Not once have I sung aloud
> a joyful Christmas hymn,
> Not once have I used my voice
> to speak Christmas greetings,
> Not once have I written Merry Christmas
> . . . but . . . but
> In my room which is buffeted by snow and wind
> I sing in my heart
> I speak greetings within myself
> behind my eyelids I write cards
> I rejoice and give thanks
> For the birth of my Saviour.

Genzo's "voice" coming from impossible circumstances was a shining light of hope and peace in this Christmas season.

Aki and I returned to Bangkok safely on January 5, 2006. My cookie-baking project was blossoming with the trainees at the Thai Autism Vocational Centre. "Aunty Marcy" cookies were on the market with eight different kinds. Her Royal Highness Princess Ubolratana, who lost

Khun Poom, her son with autism in the tsunami, had taken an interest in the project.

Another volunteer job I held in 2006 was to serve as chairperson on the Missions Committee at ECB, the Evangelical Church of Bangkok. The church had been supporting twelve mission projects, several involving children, Christian tribal groups, the Far East Broadcasting Corporation that had a weekly Christian radio program broadcast in seventeen languages, and three projects with women who were trafficked. I decided to visit each project, which meant travelling to northern Thailand for two projects. One, for tribal children to go to school, was deep in the mountains; another, for trafficked tribal girls, was closer to the Golden Triangle. It was a privilege to be able to support and minister to those in need. I learned so much and felt empowered.

In April, I enjoyed being a camp nurse for 350 children for a week at Khao Lak again with a bus load of eager volunteers. The previous year's camp had been a highlight for the volunteers as much as for the children at Khao Lak.

Immediately after summer camp, Aki and I looked forward to the three-week visit of our son, Matthew and his fiancée Kate Driedger. This was an excellent opportunity for her to visit Asia and for us to get to know her. Their first weekend in Thailand, Mr. Topong extended an invitation to go to Cha Am with him, his wife, sister, two more ladies in wheelchairs, and Ken, a blind Japanese young man. He said that his military friend had a lovely beach house at the waterfront and we could use his facilities free of charge for the weekend.

Cha Am was well known as a quiet, safe beach with silvery sand, 180 km south west of Bangkok. We travelled in two vans that were open in the back, arriving in Cha Am early afternoon. Much to our surprise, the beach house we were allowed to use was old and had not been used for some time. We did a quick survey of our setting. There was a communal open area with a large table that could also be used to recline on, a hammock, and a small kitchen on the main floor, as well as washroom facilities: all the sleeping quarters were upstairs. It was covered with dirt and dust: we had not expected to have to do a major cleaning job.

While the able-bodied set about cleaning, one of the girls in a wheelchair went down to the beach with Ken. Ken went swimming alone, and the girl in a wheelchair lost sight of him and came back to inform us. We were all very concerned and went down to the beach to look for him. He was nowhere to be seen. We inquired of other swimmers and combed the long beach area, but no Ken! Finally, about an hour later, someone brought him to our beachfront wondering if anyone knew him. He had drifted downstream with the current and of course couldn't tell anyone where he was staying because he didn't know, plus he could not speak Thai. Needless to say, he was reprimanded by everyone.

Ying, Mr. Topong's wife, invited us to go to the local seafood market with her to buy fresh food for our dinner. We returned with a live lobster, fresh crabs, shrimp, and fish to grill. I hadn't realized that Katie had never eaten any seafood. Watching a live lobster being immersed into a pot of boiling water and Ying stabbing fresh crabs was a new experience for her. My memory of the evening meal was Katie eating little more than rice.

Then we needed to decide where everyone would sleep. Able-bodied persons were assigned to two rooms upstairs. Katie and I slept on a bed of boards with our towels as pillows: Aki and Matt slept on the floor of the same room using the only fan to keep the mosquitoes away. Ken slept on the floor in the room next door. He got up in the morning after a sleepless night, having fought with the mosquitoes all night. We then learned that the washroom facilities on the main floor were not wheelchair accessible, so the two girls in wheelchairs had contacted a local friend late that night and stayed at their home. Mr. Topong had slept on the table in the open area below our room. This was our life in Thailand—you just went with the flow.

Matt and Katie's itinerary with us included flying to Chiang Mai where we rented a car, so we were free to organize our days. Of course, it included McKean Rehab, a khantoke dinner with traditional tribal dances, and driving to Pai, a town in Mae Hong Son Province in Northern Thailand, where Bong, Mr. Topong's sister, lived and worked in community development, especially with various ethnic tribes. She had arranged for us to travel in the back of her friend's pickup truck to a tribal village that she was working with. While navigating the steep winding mountain roads, up and down, dodging big potholes, it was no surprise when we got a flat tire in the middle of nowhere. Because there was no jack, Matt and Bong's friend struggled to get rocks placed to function as a jack, while Katie and I roasted in the hot sun. Finally, we arrived in a Hmong village where villagers were delighted to have foreign visitors. We watched them weave on simple looms attached to the outside of their homes. They generated income by selling their weaving. We bought two beautiful handwoven blankets dyed in a natural mint green colour.

Pai was known for its hot springs, nearby gorges, and handicraft shops. We also visited a traditional Chinese village with clay houses and enjoyed their Yunnan cuisine and tea. The two-hour return trip to Chiang Mai would challenge anyone with motion sickness because it was constant curves, climbing, descending, and crossing forty bridges to reach our destination.

Bangkok served as home base for our travels with Matt and Katie. After visiting APCD, we toured Khao Lak, the area devastated by the 2004 tsunami. They also enjoyed sites around Bangkok such as the Grand Palace. One benefit of having guests is you learn much about interesting places for tourists.

Matt and Katie returned to Canada to prepare for their wedding on August 5, 2006. It was a beautiful day and a lovely wedding at Avon Mennonite Church in Stratford, Ontario. Melody, Scott, Maya, and Aidan flew in from St. John's for the occasion. We had some quality time with family before returning to Bangkok.

In early November, Dad sold the homestead in Conestogo. I was glad that I could not be there because it would have hurt to say goodbye to it all.

Our years based in Bangkok seemed to fly by with so much constant activity. Anyone who has had a garden understands the process of planting a seed, waiting for it to germinate, watching it grow and mature, and then produce fruit. APCD completed its fifth-year program in 2006 that focused on persons with physical disabilities and blind persons and was due for its evaluation by JICA. They witnessed many outcomes due to the commitment of persons with disabilities, who previously were deprived of opportunities in society and were now making waves because they had become empowered.

Several of the outstanding projects in 2006 related to independent living for persons with disabilities. Judy Heumann, an American human rights activist and strong supporter of independent living, gave the keynote speech for an IL workshop. Two resource persons for the training were women from Japan and Thailand, both quadriplegics. They inspired other persons with disabilities from Malaysia, the Philippines, and Pakistan with severe disabilities to never give up. Persons with severe disabilities taught peer counselling, IL management, and skills to form small groups of people with disabilities in order to support each other. Today, there are three independent living centres in Thailand, two in Malaysia, three in the Philippines, and five in Pakistan. In Malaysia, one is named "The Beautiful Gate" (Acts Chapter 3) and another in the Philippines is called HAC IL Centre which stands for "Handicap's Anchor is Christ."

It was at the IL workshop at APCD when I first met Khun Earth, who was interpreting for Judy Heumann. She struck me as a bright humble young lady with a positive attitude and a good sense of humour. Over time, our paths crossed and we became good friends. When I visited Khun Earth in her condo, she willingly shared her life story.

Khun Earth had been an outstanding student who enjoyed playing sports with her Grade 11 class. After a full day participating in Sports Day, she returned home feeling exhausted, with an ache in her neck, and she immediately fell asleep. When she woke up, she was unable to open the small bottle of smelling salts at her bedside. She discovered that her fingers were weak, and she was experiencing difficulty breathing. She had lost sensation in her body: she could talk but not move and then, no more pain. After Khun Earth was hospitalized for a month, the doctor told her that she had acute transverse myelitis, which was an inflammation of segments of her spinal cord. The doctor shared that some people have near complete recovery in three months, others do not; the only reason she was still alive was that she had been healthy before.

Khun Earth remembers her doctor as an honest humble man who, on her discharge from the hospital, told her to never give up hope! She found it difficult to be dependent on others and confined to bed. About this time, a Christian missionary couple who lived nearby came to visit Khun Earth frequently: the Thai wife had married an American and became a Christian when living in the US. The wife was unfamiliar with religious vocabulary in Thai and Khun Earth was eager to learn English, so their visits became mutually beneficial. She wanted to learn more about Christianity.

Khun Earth began to pray to God. She and her three sisters became Christians. Her mother then became upset that her four daughters had changed their religion, which she thought was confusing the spirits.

Khun Earth apologized to her mother and promised to say goodbye to Christianity, but she still prayed to God. She reflected on this past experience as she lay in bed at home, talking to the walls. She felt that God had given her another chance "to show what a human being can be and an opportunity to live a life that human beings should live." A friend of her mother came and told her that she knew someone who could help her: "You know Jesus is the answer."

Knowing how much Khun Earth wanted to go to a Bible School, her mother's friend knew of friends in Chiang Mai who agreed to voluntarily provide care for Khun Earth while she studied. It was then that her friends discovered her bed sore that needed medical attention. They contacted McKean Rehabilitation Centre where they provided surgical treatment for her pressure sore. The team of doctors, a physical therapist, and an occupational therapist met with her. A doctor said, "Khun Earth, you can do many things. I train many people like you to become independent. You could join our three-month rehabilitation program." She decided to do so. After a month, she was discharged and returned home where her mother had a bed made to accommodate access from a wheelchair.

In 2005 she met Mr. Topong in the DPI AP office and she became an intern there. Mr. Topong taught her many things about the IL movement, with which she became involved. She also became active at church. In fact, Mr. Topong had taken her to Parliament with him, where he had served on a panel several times to help the government formulate policies related to persons with disabilities. It was this experience that taught her, "Our voice is very important. If we (persons with disabilities) do not share, people will never know how much we suffer."

Another eye-opening experience for Khun Earth was in 2007, when she was one of ten persons invited to the US for a month for paralympic sports training. She was amazed at the accessibility options available.

After returning to Thailand, missionary friends visited her and she started attending a church. She translated and interpreted for missionaries as a volunteer until 2005. She then began supporting herself by interpreting for Christian organizations, translating for church services and various government ministries.

Khun Earth was an exemplary role model to me in many ways. She had a strong faith. We continue to communicate and share. She said that her challenge in 2021 is to address her emotional needs through self-awareness. She said, "I know that God loves me and I want to walk in love and truth." She is a gifted, sensitive person who has much to share with others.

Second Term with APCD Project

As a result of JICA's evaluation of the APCD project, they recommended an additional five-year project focused on persons with intellectual and developmental disabilities and hard of hearing and psycho-social groups because they are the least developed in the Asia-Pacific region. They also recommended the continuation of support to the first five-year projects' outcomes for further development.

Thailand continued to have political turmoil. In the last six months of 2006, we experienced instability for the first time due to a bloodless military coup in June. It divided the citizens' loyalty between the ousted government and the military that promised a fair election. It was at this time that people wore yellow-coloured tops in support of their king whose birthday was on a Monday. In Thailand, the days of the week are represented by a specific colour. Monday is yellow, Tuesday pink, Wednesday green, Thursday orange, Friday blue, Saturday purple, and Sunday red. Everyone in Thailand knew what day of the week they were born and their colour. To me this was fascinating because most Westerners do not know what day of the week they were born. The ousted government of Thaksin Shinawatra represented red. Peaceful protests became more frequent and began escalating while people on the street wore yellow. At this time, our friends Marie and Ernie Fretz, came to spend three weeks with us. In our correspondence before they arrived, Marie had written that she would wear a yellow blouse so I could easily identify her at the airport. I laughed because most of Bangkok was wearing yellow!

It was fun planning their itinerary. Aki and I had never taken an overnight train to Chiang Mai before, so this seemed like a good time for the experience. Because we would be travelling at peak time for the New Year, reservations had to be made as soon as tickets were for sale. I stood in line for two hours the morning the wicket opened and got four seats that turned into upper and lower berths for the night. Ernie and Marie arrived on December 28, all pumped for an exciting time of getting acquainted with our work and seeing cultural sights in Thailand.

The evening of December 29, we boarded the train and arrived in Chiang Mai at seven-thirty the next morning. It was an interesting night, trying to sleep while hanging on to one's personal effects, due to possible theft. We gave Ernie and Marie a Chiang Mai Tour and enjoyed a khantoke dinner to celebrate Marie's birthday. While we were there, we received a phone call from APCD staff that two bombs had exploded in Bangkok. We continued travelling but were on alert for any unusual activity.

They enjoyed the Mae Sa Elephant Camp performance and our visit to the Mae Sa Orchid Farm. The variety and colours of the orchids were exquisite. We then hired a driver to travel north through the mountains toward Chiang Rai to the Golden Triangle. We enjoyed a hot spa en route and the beautiful scenery.

In January 2007, returning to Bangkok meant going back to work for Aki. I had Ernie and Marie accompany me to the Thai Autism Vocational Centre to meet my friends and the "cookie gang." there. The students also enjoyed showing them other handmade projects such as silk screen artwork, pottery, and dance performances.

Later, they were awed by the Grand Palace. We found that just riding the Chao Phraya water taxi up the river to the last stop was a relaxing education. The river had been the original means of transportation when the city of Bangkok was established. Now one could still see loaded barges plying the river, tour boats, ethnic communities living at the riverside, poor areas where houses looked unstable, extending into the river, etc. We also took a two-hour bus trip to Pattaya to enjoy the beach there because Thailand has both mountains and beautiful beaches. They left Thailand in January 2007, after a packed three weeks.

One weekend in March 2007, Aki and I decided to visit a Thai Care Ministry project in Northern Thailand because it was a project that our church sponsored, and I was the chairperson of the Missions Committee. We drove our rent-a-car through winding narrow mountain roads for four hours to our destination. Thai Care Ministry had been started by Ralf, a German, who was employed in Bangkok and had donated his income for stateless tribal children to provide an education for them because they were not entitled to a formal education or legal protection by the Royal Thai Government. The children lived in rooms like peas in a pod. The house parents were responsible for overseeing their animal husbandry and gardening.

In the evening, when we joined the children for their devotions, we were asked to share our personal faith. When asked for their favourite Bible passage, they all had one. They knew their scripture! Aki and I had the privilege of sleeping in a tree house overlooking a river that even had a flush toilet! Ralf, an entrepreneur, was an amazing man! We were humbled by the Maenachorn Hostel project.

In March, I flew to Canada to make housing arrangements for Tim. We were able to purchase a small condo in Waterloo, Ontario that seemed ideal for him to live with a friend for quality of life.

After returning to Thailand, I picked up with my usual activities of baking and being a support for APCD and DPI AP as needed. Mr. Topong also served as a resource person for APCD and Aki saw him as a candidate for the executive director's position of APCD. Informally, Mr. Topong had agreed to consider this role after the transfer of Thai government management to the APCD Foundation, which was chaired by Mr. Tanin Kraivixien, Royal Privy Councillor and former Prime Minister of Thailand.

Mr. Topong, a national and international leader in the disability movement, was also a founding member of the APCD project. He frequently was a resource person for missions, especially those related to regional capacity-building and self-help organization training in Papua New Guinea, Central Asia, and Pakistan. It was prior to his scheduled mission to Bangladesh as a resource person for a workshop on self-help organizations at the beginning of June 2007, that he was not feeling well. Aki encouraged him to take a rest, but he refused. Instead, he went to Bangladesh and worked hard to empower many persons with disabilities, even though he was unwell. He returned to Bangkok on June 5, very ill and was immediately hospitalized with a high fever.

Mr. Topong was scheduled to be the keynote speaker the next day at an international conference organized by UNESCAP and APCD on the human rights of persons with disabilities in the Asia-Pacific region for government representatives, international organizations, and UN agencies. Because he didn't make an appearance at the conference site, Aki's secretary inquired where he was and discovered he was very ill in the hospital. Aki ended up giving the keynote speech on Mr. Topong's behalf. Immediately after his speech, Aki asked me to contact Mr. Topong's wife and be a support to her. Thankfully, I went to the army hospital as he was being transferred from a regular ward to an ICU in another building. He was put on life support but by morning on June seventh, our dear friend and colleague had passed away.

When shared at the conference, this news was met with disbelief and shock: many participants knew Mr. Topong as a dynamic person, passionate about empowering persons with disabilities. Several participants had just been with him in Bangladesh a few days earlier. His funeral on June ninth, dovetailed with the closing ceremony of the conference, which enabled many participants to pay their last respects. A rumour started that Mr. Topong staged his passing so he could say farewell to his international friends. He had the saying, "Soldiers in the army die in the field, so I hope to die on the job." He got his last wish! He had never wanted to be in administration, but, rather, be a leader at the grassroots level and an advocate for the disability movement.

It was impossible for anyone to fill Mr. Topong's shoes, but Ms. Saowalak Thongkuay, a graduate from the Redemptorist Centre in Pattaya, whom Aki had hired as secretary to APCD's coordinator, agreed to serve as DPI AP Development Officer. As a wheelchair user, she was also an agent-of-change, a dedicated advocate, and a strong believer in the empowerment of persons with disabilities. Ms. Saowalak is now serving as the UN

Commissioner for the CRPD (Convention on the Rights of Persons with Disability) for the term of 2021-2024.

In September 2007, Aki and I participated in the DPI World Assembly held in Seoul, Korea. It was a great reunion with many friends and international leaders of persons with disabilities. It was amazing and a blessing to see how far the disability human rights movement had developed since 1981.

In October, Aki and I flew to Ho Chi Minh City, primarily to research the situation of children and persons with autism. A family working with Wycliffe Bible Translators had two sons with autism. The wife, concerned about other children with the developmental disability, organized a monthly meeting for mothers of children with autism out of concern that it had not yet been recognized by the Vietnamese government. Thirty mothers came to her monthly meetings. The government policy regarding disability included persons with a physical disability, blind and deaf persons, as well as persons with intellectual disabilities, but did not specifically note a developmental disability such as autism.

To follow up on the matter of autism in Vietnam, APCD visited the Ministry of Social Development and Welfare in Hanoi to encourage the government to recognize autism as a disability. APCD then conducted a workshop on persons with autism for the parents. Later, government officials were invited to Thailand to visit Mr. Chusak's project for persons with autism. They were introduced to the Aunty Marcy cookie project as well.

JICA extended Aki's contract another two years, which meant we would be based in Bangkok until July 2009. To date, thirty-two governments and at least 180 NGOs are collaborating with APCD, and more than 600 trainees from twenty-six countries in the Asia-Pacific region have benefitted from the various training sessions.

Although my life was subject to change without notice, there was some consistency. It primarily revolved around supervising the cookie-baking project. Other "hats" were proofreader for APCD's newsletters, chairperson for the church missions committee, tour guide, and hostess. Friends and Aki's former students from Japan came for brief visits and kept us updated.

Unexpectedly, unusual requests came. One was to do a recording in English of the king's book about his dog, Tong Daeng, the next morning at the School for the Blind. I was assured that it was just a few pages, so I agreed to do it if I could have a copy of the script that night to be prepared—blind people wanted to "read" the king's book. I received a copy at ten p.m. and discovered it was eighty-five pages! I read through and marked words that were new to me with unknown tones.

The Thai language consists of five tones (Vietnamese has six tones): if one uses the wrong tone, the word has a completely different meaning. Some consonants change their pronunciation if they are the last syllable of a word. So as soon as we got to the School for the Blind, they kindly answered my questions, and I quickly marked the tones on my copy. I soon discovered that a well-known radio announcer was also coming to record in Thai, and I was to record in English. At the time of recording, I was not allowed to use my copy! The radio announcer recorded first, and I mimicked her tone. Because blind persons could not see the photos in the book, I had to describe them in English. It took all day to do the whole book.

Doing the recording, I discovered that the king was very fond of dogs. His favourite was Tong Daeng, originally a street dog who sat at his feet every day anticipating his needs. The king was using his favourite dog as a role model to teach morals to Thai children through his book.

I was ready and excited to fly to Canada with Aki on December 22, five minutes before midnight. Living so far from family and friends, we valued our limited time with them. After celebrating Christmas in Ontario with Tim, Matt, and Katie, we flew to St. John's to spend a week with Melody and Scott's family. Because Aki made no secret about how much he enjoyed cooking a Japanese meal, he was delegated to prepare one with Atlantic salmon for Melody and Scott's close friends and colleagues. We enjoyed the puppet shows that Maya and Aidan performed at home, and a sleigh ride with them and Bertha, a cheerful child who endeared herself to everyone she met. Bertha is an ethnic Inu child with special needs that Melody and Scott have been fostering since 2006 when she was six months old.

On January 2, 2008, we flew back to Toronto and Aki continued on to Bangkok for work. I stayed in Ontario for another two weeks. When we returned to Bangkok, our Thai friend Martin, a professional blind pianist, informed me that he had been invited to perform in Phnom Penh, Cambodia in an arts festival featuring persons with disabilities. He really wanted to participate, but his wife, Suthida, had a knee injury, so would I consider accompanying them? Of course, I would! So, from February 28 to March 2, I accompanied Martin for his performances and pushed his wife in a wheelchair.

In August, we celebrated my dad's ninetieth birthday. He continued to do some volunteer work and sing in a male choir. What a wonderful role model!

That same month, APCD conducted a workshop for persons with autism in Hanoi, Vietnam and helped organize a network for the parents. We really wanted to have a national organization for parents of children with autism and have the government recognize it as a disability.

In October, Aki went to Bishkek, the capital of Kyrgyzstan, to set up a regional office for the five Central Asian countries of Kazakhstan, Tajikistan, Turkmenistan, Uzbekistan, and Kyrgyzstan to have a sub-regional network endorsed by UNESCAP.

In October, Aki also went on a mission to Myanmar with Madame Panomwan, Thai Association for Deaf Persons President, who had been communicating with the Deaf Association in Yangon, of whom several were ex-trainees of APCD. Aki invited five deaf persons from Myanmar to accompany Madame Panomwan and himself to JICA's Office in Yangon, where he introduced them and their situation in Myanmar. As a result, JICA and the Ministry of Social Welfare and Resettlement began a new project to develop a national sign language in Myanmar. Deaf persons from Northern Myanmar in Mandalay spoke sign language taught at the government school for deaf persons; in Yangon, deaf persons were using another sign language they had developed themselves. Because deaf leaders from all areas of the region had been ex-trainees of APCD, they were excited to participate in a new project with government officers to develop a national sign language dictionary for deaf persons over the next four years.

In November, APCD was honoured to receive a JICA award as a distinguished model project in humanity development.

The international airport for Bangkok was closed for ten days in December due to the Thai government's conflict, which necessitated APCD to postpone the first Asia-Pacific Congress on Community-Based

Rehabilitation that had more than 600 persons registered from fifty-six countries. It is impossible to describe the unrest and conflict of the political situation in Thailand, which continued to destabilize the country, although we continued to feel safe. We had three prime ministers that year: the opposition group occupied the government house for three months, and the temporary government offices were now in the old airport building. What would 2009 bring?

On December 18, Aki and I flew to Toronto to spend quality time with our family over the holidays, first in Ontario with Tim, Matt and Katie, then a week with Melody, Scott, Maya, Aidan, and Bertha. Tim's work had slowed down with shared time, but he was hanging in, Matt was employed as a civil engineer, and Katie was teaching full time. In Newfoundland, Maya was in Grade 2, Aidan in kindergarten, and Bertha in day care. Scott was working at the Ministry of Justice and Melody was conducting research on gender issues with an eye to further education. We enjoyed and appreciated the brief time together, thinking that by next Christmas we would be living in Ontario.

New Baking Project in Pattaya

January 2009 found Aki and I back in Bangkok. It was the countdown for Aki, knowing his contract with JICA would be completed by the end of July. One day, shortly after returning to Bangkok, I was entering the APCD compound when I saw a parked car with the driver's door open and an empty wheelchair beside it. I naturally assumed someone needed help. It was Aajaan Suporntum, from the Redemptorist Centre in Pattaya. When asked if I could help him, his response was, "Yes, you can. We would like to start a cookie-baking project at the Redemptorist Job Placement Centre for persons with disabilities." I was rather taken aback but said that I would think about it because that would mean terminating my volunteer work at the Thai Autism Vocational Centre. The truth was, I was attached to my bakers, who looked forward to my return, but the reality was there were no further development plans in place. The current staff could continue baking at the present level.

After much consideration and consultation with Aki, I decided that the timing was right to start a project in Pattaya. It was hard to tell Aajaan Chusak that I was terminating my volunteer work there because it was his showcase project at the centre. Aki agreed to support me to take on this new challenge, which meant that I would have to be in Pattaya four days a week, 120 km from Bangkok. Then again, he was constantly travelling too.

I contacted Aajaan Suporntum to say that I was willing to begin a baking project at his centre for persons with cross disabilities next week. Several Catholic sisters had apparently had a baking project there previously, so there was some basic equipment. After cleaning and getting organized, I began teaching how to bake cookies.

My "apprentices" included two deaf girls, one could lip read, two persons with orthopedic disabilities, a young gal of short stature, and a teenage boy from their drop-in centre. Because I did not know sign language and was not proficient in writing Thai, I had to use body language to communicate with the two deaf girls. This was the first time I was not teaching persons with autism or intellectual disabilities, and I was shocked to discover how fast we could produce cookies! It was amazing! They were a delight to work with.

My new routine became taking the five-thirty a.m. bus in Bangkok on Monday morning and arriving in Pattaya in time to begin work. When the bus was nearing Pattaya and I could see the MacDonald's sign, I would telephone Aajaan Decha, and he would be at the bus station waiting to pick me up before seven a.m. Then Thursday late afternoon, I took a bus back to Bangkok, arriving home around nine p.m.

I discovered that the Redemptorist Centre had many international volunteers who were teaching English in the two-year computer program for persons with disabilities. Because the baking project was independent from the school, I only met volunteers in free time in the evenings. While they ate their meals in the hotel dining room, I ate my lunch with the bakers, and then the evening meal with the Thai persons with disabilities and school faculty in the school cafeteria. I felt honoured to be included with the students and the Thai faculty eating a typical Thai diet. It meant they had accepted me as one of them, and we had many interesting conversations.

In the evening, I would walk around in the compound. Often the students would be playing sports on the blacktop. I especially enjoyed watching players in wheelchairs play basketball while others cheered them on. They were amazing. There were dormitories for 180 persons with disabilities in the two-year computer program, a shop for their one-year electrical repair program, a hotel for guests—where I stayed, a conference centre, a church, a swimming pool, and a day program for persons with autism. I enjoyed talking with some of the students in the evening, who liked to practice their English.

Within a short time, Pi Moi, a chef from their hotel kitchen, was assigned to the baking project. She had studied baking previously and was happy to be assigned to the bakery. We made a good team. Shortly after opening the project, we had purchased a large commercial oven and a wooden stand to sell our baking in the compound just outside our building which we named Friends' Cafe. Pi Moi, a professional baker, knew what sweets the Thai enjoyed the most. I learned so much from her, not just baking but also packaging. The Thai knew how to make something simple look so attractive. Staff from other departments and guests soon became regular customers due to our varied menu. Others just dropped by to chat. Bob, an American volunteer, occasionally brought a petit blind lady, who lived in a room at the other end of the compound, to ask questions about baking with her little oven. Maria enjoyed the time to socialize as much as discuss baking!

Soon our bakery was responsible for providing the mid-morning and mid-afternoon snacks for participants at the conference centre. We found an unused tricycle with a cart attached at the back that Khun Orawan, our gal of short stature, could ride around the compound. Late in the afternoon, she

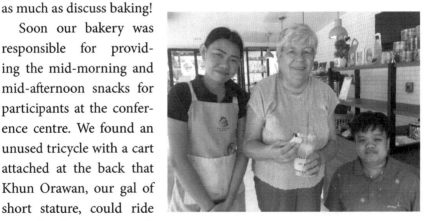

Two trainees, Joy and Orawan, with Marcy at the bakery.

would sell our baking to the students when their classes finished at four—with her smile she could sell anything to anybody! Because Khun Orawan was so short, we assigned her to the Friends' Cafe as our mascot! She soon knew everybody and they knew her!

Orders soon came in from the public or for other events in the compound. The international volunteers just followed their noses and kept popping into the bakery to see what was in the oven. Our baking began with just cookies but soon expanded to include brownies, banana cake, pound cake, deep fried bananas, and steamed pork buns. Because Pi Moi was talented in cake decorating, we also took orders for birthday cakes.

In early February, I was busy finalizing plans for the three-week visit of my Dad, ninety years young, and my sister Brenda. Brenda had travelled to Vietnam in 1971, to Japan several times when we were living there, as well as Thailand in 2006. Because Anna was not keen on travelling, she was relieved that Brenda agreed to travel with Dad.

Dad and Brenda arrived safely on February 5, 2009: Dad, a seasoned traveller, went to bed early and was ready to go the next morning. We were invited to an event in a neighbouring province that was sponsored by persons with disabilities. The festive atmosphere included a band playing, special Thai food, and a twenty-minute foot massage for Dad and Brenda! In the afternoon, when Aki returned to work, the three of us took the Skytrain (monorail) to visit Rahab, one of the mission projects supported by our church that provided vocational training for women who had been trafficked. It was an eye opener for them to see Patpong, an area well known for prostitution. After we purchased some beautiful greetings cards made in their vocational training program, we took a ride up the Chao Phraya River on a water taxi, enjoyed a simple Thai dinner in a restaurant by the riverside, and took a tuk-tuk (three-wheeler) ride home. In the evening, Melinda Maldonado, our niece, arrived with a friend from Korea for the weekend. The next day, I took Melinda and her friend for a tour of the Grand Palace, while Aki took Dad and Brenda to the IT complex in Pratunam for camera equipment: we all met at the Pratunam shopping centre for lunch, and then had a fun time shopping for Thai silk, clothing, and souvenirs. Dad bought a lovely scarf for Anna, while the others emptied their wallets!

Sunday, Melinda and her friend flew back to Seoul, Korea and Dad, Brenda, and I had a two-hour flight to Hanoi, Vietnam. We checked into our hotel in the Old Quarter and enjoyed a leisurely lunch. We were fortunate to get four tickets for the famous water puppet show that afternoon. In the evening, we had dinner with Hiro, who had served with MCC in Vietnam when Aki and I were there. He and his wife were teaching Japanese at a high school in Hanoi.

Monday, February ninth, we were up early for our tour of Halong Bay and were booked to sleep on a junk for one night. This was on my bucket list! Halong Bay is 180 km by car from Hanoi, along the Northeastern coastline of Vietnam. It includes over 1600 islands, most of limestone with lush jungle vegetation: the islands rise on average 50-100 metres from the emerald-coloured waters of the ocean. The translation of "Ha Long" is "descending dragon." It was with great excitement that we left our hotel around seven-thirty a.m., on a tour bus heading for Ha Long Bay. We stopped for a break at a huge sheltered workshop that provided employment for persons with disabilities, who were creating beautiful art with silk threads.

We arrived at our pier at noon, boarded our junk, and were shown our rooms. They were clean and very adequate. After a delicious lunch served on board, the junk plied the waters around the mountains and ended up at a cave. Out of concern for Dad, we asked our tour guide about the number of steps involved. He assured us about fifty. Well, there were more than that just to get to the entrance of the cave, then it was up and down and around inside the cave for one and a half hours. Brenda and I were getting concerned for Dad, but there was no way to backtrack so we kept on going at our own pace (Dad's diary says there were 225 steps). We were relieved to exit the cave and let Dad have a rest. Brenda and I just looked at each other, both nurses, wondering what were we doing to him! After descending yet more steps, we arrived at our junk.

The scenery was breathtaking! Our junk wound around the mountains until we found a scenic spot for the night, where we could see the sunset and sunrise the next morning. After a game of Rook, we were served a sumptuous dinner of homemade recipes with seafood.

The sunrise the next morning was beautiful. After breakfast, our guide said that we would be sea kayaking. Everyone was excited, but fear of deep water haunted me. I was determined not to spoil the fun: Brenda and I were in one kayak, Aki and Dad in the other. To get into the kayak, one had to descend a ladder with small narrow metal rungs attached to the junk. All was fine until we returned and had to climb up that ladder. Dad went first, and it was clear that he was having difficulty gripping the rungs with his right hand. He'd had polio as a teenager, resulting in a weaker hand. Our guide on the junk, who was looking down, was concerned too. In the end, Dad succeeded. What a scare!

After a scenic ride back to the dock, we transferred to a tour bus for Hanoi and tried to rest a little because we were scheduled to take an overnight train ride to Sapa that evening. We arrived at the hotel, where they had kindly kept our luggage while we were on the junk: they allowed us to shower, etc., go out for dinner in the area and return in time to go to the train station. The hotel staff insisted on taking us to the train station at eight-thirty: we soon discovered why. It was pure bedlam. We never could have navigated the system alone.

Sapa, also on my bucket list, was a small mountain town in Lao Cai Province, about 350 km northwest of Hanoi, close to the Chinese border. The overnight train, on which we had rented a compartment with bunks, arrived in Lao Cai at five-thirty a.m., where our tour guide and driver were waiting for us for the forty-five-minute drive to Sapa: we checked in and enjoyed a hearty breakfast before going sightseeing.

The Hong Lien Son range of mountains was a lush green as we travelled a narrow mountain road full of curves. The famous rice terraces were spectacular on the mountainsides, and we stopped for some photos. There were five ethnic groups in Sapa: the Hmong, Dao, Tay, Gray, and Ca Pho.

The Lao Chai and Ta Van villages were interesting to visit. Their ecological and simple way of living was so impressive. Their gardens all had bamboo spikes around them to keep wild animals out. The villagers formed a caravan walking through the villages with us, children giggling as we went. The villages, iconic rice paddies, and forest treks were a few of the main attractions of Sapa.

Aki, Brenda, and I were enjoying the Vietnamese meals, and Dad, never fond of noodles or rice, never complained. After a bowl of pho noodle soup with chicken, our guide took us across a swinging bridge to an outdoor spa, about a forty-five-minute walk over rough terrain. Dad, Brenda, and Aki enjoyed this outdoor natural spa immensely. When it was time to return, we discovered that part of the path had been bulldozed closed, so we had to find another route back to the car. We did, but it taxed Dad's energy.

The next day, we drove to Fansipan mountain, with an altitude of 3,143 metres, located about nine km southwest of Sapa town. We stopped to see a silver waterfall and enjoyed an herbal tea with a snack, served by an elderly lady just waiting for customers. We had lunch at a restaurant that trained disadvantaged youth. We then drove to Ta Phan Village, about seventeen km from Sapa, hidden behind mountain slopes, beside green terraced rice fields. Ta Phan Village, home to Hmong and Dao ethnic groups, was famous for the peaceful natural landscape and the unique culture of the Red Dao people and their handicrafts. Aki enjoyed bargaining with several of the ladies for their weaving. This game was enjoyed by everyone: Aki had it down to a fine art. The day ended with us driving up to the border and looking at China! The sound of the train going down to Hanoi was very different from its huffing and puffing up to Lao Cai!

At five a.m. we were back in Hanoi and checked into our favourite hotel, had a good rest and breakfast, then left for the day. Aki bought some stamps for a collection before our first stop, a visit to an NGO project providing vocational training for deaf persons: after lunch we visited a centre that provided services for intellectually challenged children. Dad enjoyed a rest while the three of us went out shopping for handicrafts. The evening meal was at the historical and famous Cha Ca Thang Long Restaurant that only served fish and fresh vegetables. While we enjoyed a fruit drink on our walk back to the hotel, Aki visited his friends.

Saturday was our last day in Hanoi. Aki flew back to Bangkok in the morning while we toured the Vietnam War Museum. At three pm, Dad, Brenda, and I flew to Nhatrang, where I had left my heart in 1969. Mr. Bu, a Vietnamese friend who owned La Paloma Hotel near the hospital compound, picked us up at the airport. What a great feeling to be back. Sunday morning, we walked to Vinh Phuoc Tin Lanh Church where we met many of my friends and former coworkers. Anh Tin invited us for lunch: another friend gave us a tour of Nhatrang town. We walked to the hospital so Dad could see where I had worked for four years of my life in the late 1960s. Because it was impossible to meet everyone in this short visit, I invited everyone to dinner at La Paloma so Dad and Brenda could meet my friends. One gal, Co Huong, fell in love with Dad and kept hanging onto his waist: he lapped it up. For them, it was unthinkable for a ninety-year-old man to be travelling to Asia.

Monday, Dad, Brenda, and I decided to try out a new mud bath spa on the mountainside. We returned squeaky clean in time to meet again with some friends for dinner. Tuesday, we took a leisurely walk down to the beach for a swim. I remember Dad burnt his feet in the hot tropical sun. Later, Mr. Bu kindly took us for a drive north of Nhatrang through the mountain pass. It had changed so much. The refugee fishing villages with their thatched homes and fishing nets drying out front were gone! The area was developed and the view was spectacular.

Wednesday, we were up at the crack of dawn to begin our drive to Saigon in Mr. Bu's vehicle. Because he was going to Saigon anyway, we took him up on his generous offer. The ride was pleasant. The roads were paved, no old dirt roads full of potholes: a blind person would have known that we passed through Phan Thiet where they made nuoc mam (fish sauce). The beaches and sand dunes were still an attraction, and the area was developing five-star hotels. Mr. Bu also stopped at a pottery shop to check on his order, which gave us an opportunity to see them at work. By five p.m. we finally arrived in Saigon where we stayed at Madame Cuc's B & B, which was conveniently located downtown.

Dad and Brenda were struck by the contrast between North and South Vietnam. They couldn't believe all the motorbikes on the streets that drove en masse: they were afraid to cross the street without traffic signals. They soon learned the secret to crossing was to begin walking across at a slow but steady pace—not hesitating out of fear—because the motorbike drivers paced their speed according to the pedestrians. It was only dangerous if a pedestrian stopped midway crossing the road.

We enjoyed a walk and a delicious meal at a local restaurant. I definitely wanted my family to tour the Vietnam War Memorial Museum the next morning. The photos were a vivid testimony to the horrors of war that needed to be seen and heard. It took several hours to reflect on the sobering facts and history that the Vietnamese had endured. In the afternoon, we walked to the famous Ben Thanh Market, where one could spend hours and hours in all the alleys inside the building and buy everything possible: clothing, jewelry, handicrafts, Vietnamese grown coffee, delicious fruit drinks, and cooked food.

After enjoying ice cream at the famous Pole Nord on the main street, we returned to our B & B, each of us riding in a cyclo: you cannot visit Vietnam and not have a ride in a cyclo. A cyclo has a passenger seat in front with the driver peddling behind. Several Vietnamese could easily fit in one seat; but one Western person fills it!

Friday, we got up early for a day tour to the Mekong Delta, an amazing network of tributaries and coconut groves. A boat ride took us through the groves and farm countryside. We learned how useful and productive the coconut tree is. Coconut milk is delicious to drink, but it is also made into many other byproducts. We watched how coconut toffee and candy is made: coconut oil, palm oil, etc. The coconut shell is also made into fertilizer and handicrafts.

Saturday was our last opportunity to shop before packing and returning to Bangkok late afternoon. Aki was glad to have us back safely. Being in Bangkok on Sunday made it possible for Dad and Brenda to join in our worship services.

After a quiet evening at home, we woke up early Monday morning for a day trip to the Redemptorist Centre in Pattaya. I wanted them to see the baking project recently started there. They donned caps and aprons to help bake for an order of 800 cookies the next day. After lunch, Aajaan Manop kindly offered to give Dad and Brenda a tour of the classrooms at the school for 180 persons with disabilities, a workshop, and the church while I continued to bake. Late afternoon, Aajaan gave us a tour of Pattaya city and the harbour, then dropped us off at the bus station for our return trip.

In Bangkok, I introduced Brenda to a tailor to have the beautiful woven piece of material she had bought in the Red Yao village outside of Sapa made into a suit before she left.

Two special friends that we wanted Dad and Brenda to meet before leaving Thailand were Martin, the blind pianist, and his wife, Suthida. We met at a Japanese restaurant, Akiyoshi, and enjoyed a meal that was cooked as we ate, followed by Dad's favourite—ice cream. Back at home, luggage was packed, ready for their departure to the airport the next morning. It had been a busy packed schedule that would likely be Dad's last Asian trip. It was a highlight for all four of us!

Aki's Termination as JICA Expert

Aki and I were back to our routines, beginning to feel that leaving Thailand was becoming a reality. The end of July, we packed to move back "home" to Canada and to an unknown future after seven years based in Bangkok. Aki had completed his term as JICA Chief Advisor to APCD: I had started two bakeries, and we said goodbye to many dear colleagues and friends. We were humbled by persons with disabilities who told us they had been empowered through our efforts.

En route to Canada, Aki was invited to give an official report at JICA headquarters in Tokyo, Japan. We were so pleased to meet people related to our previous work with persons with disabilities in Japan who had come from Kobe, Nagoya, and Agape, as well as persons working with JICA who valued the APCD project.

We were uncertain where God would be guiding us on our return to Canada but found out soon enough. In early September, the telephone rang. It was His Excellency, Mr. Tanin Kraivixien, APCD Foundation President asking Aki to return as executive director.

Aki said that he would reply after discussing it with me. This meant that he would be hired by the Thai and receive a Thai salary, a third of what he had received under JICA. After discussion, Aki and I agreed that if we did not return, the APCD project would likely not stand, which meant that all the groundwork accomplished in the previous seven years would be lost.

In August and September, we spent quality time with family and friends in Ontario. Tim's work at Art of Time had slowed down: Matt and Katie were both employed in their professions. We flew to St. John's to visit

Melody, Scott, and our grandchildren and do some sightseeing on "The Rock." The end of September, we were back in Bangkok and living in the same house: Aki was executive director of APCD, and I was welcomed back to the bakery at the Redemptorist Centre in Pattaya. I also continued to support APCD with proofreading of the newsletters, documents, etc.

Aki worked toward reorganizing the APCD Foundation from a government organization to an international NGO with effective sustainable management.

Every year brought new challenges and a sense of fulfillment when we saw persons with disabilities that had been empowered. The year 2010 was no different. In January, APCD organized a workshop on the capacity-development of self-help organizations of parents and persons with autism. Members included Brunei Darussalam, Cambodia, Indonesia, Laos, Myanmar, the Philippines, Singapore, Thailand, and Vietnam.

APCD organized the ASEAN Autism Community Network (AAN) as well as the South Asian Disability Forum. Our visit to Vietnam in April incorporated them into the Autism Network. In December, APCD organized a seminar for the inauguration of the AAN. Then, in 2011, the AAN was organized in Bangkok.

The staff in APCD's office included capable persons with visual and hearing impairments and a mobility disability. They were our resources and future leaders.

APCD needed to hire a person to work with the APCD office for Inclusive Community Development. Aki phoned me one morning at the bakery in Pattaya to inform me that the job opening had been posted on the internet, but he was still looking for the right person. Did I know anyone at the Redemptorist Centre who would qualify to apply? The application process would be closing at noon. One staff person said she knew about a young man who was employed in the centre's library doing work on the computer. She said he had a good command of the English language but had experienced difficulty getting a job due to his cerebral palsy, which left him with some spasticity making it difficult for some people to understand his speech. The staff person immediately notified Khun Wacharapol of this opportunity. At eleven a.m. he appeared in the bakery saying he had submitted his application to APCD!

His application to APCD included his life history in which he shared how he had been made to feel inferior and was belittled, but his parents had supported him. He graduated from Korat University with a BA in English. The only job he could get was in the library run by the Redemptorist Foundation, working alone in a back room. Khun Wacharapol was ecstatic when APCD employed him! He was trained to be a team member for Inclusive Community Development and, eventually, in management. Now, years later, he is valued as a capable responsible person in his field, and he empowers persons with disabilities.

Around this time, Aki felt the need to recruit more staff with disabilities. He especially needed someone to fill the role of manager for Inclusive Community Development. He recalled Jasper Rom, a Filipino and wheelchair user, who had been a resource person for one of APCD's workshops. When he asked Jasper if he would consider moving to APCD, he did not say yes. Aki's policy was to show deep respect for persons with disabilities in a humble manner. Because Aki felt that Jasper was the man for the position, he booked the two of us to fly to the Philippines, then transfer to another flight to IloIlo Island to meet Jasper. Jasper was rather surprised to have the executive director of APCD and his wife visit him and his project run by HI (Handicap International).

We toured his project that promoted access to the built environment and organized Self-Help Groups (SHG) of persons with disabilities. His project was excellent. Aki humbly bowed down to Jasper, asking him to come to APCD as manager of community development. He finally accepted. Jasper had graduated from Georgetown University in Washington, USA with a Masters in Administration. His English was at a professional level. We discovered one of his favourite hobbies was playing chess. He was Master of Chess in the Philippines. One month later, he arrived in Bangkok and we looked for accessible accommodation. Later, he joined the Thai chess club and became the Master of Chess in Thailand! Shortly after, Jasper married a colleague from HI in the Philippines and they had a son, Jacob.

In 2015 and 2016, Aki organized ASEAN workshops on accessibility in Jakarta, Indonesia because they were planning to build a new ASEAN building. Jasper was a resource person for the workshops with ASEAN high level representatives and senior officers present. They were so impressed with Jasper that they offered him a job! Today, he is employed by the ASEAN Secretariat in Jakarta, Indonesia as senior officer for community development and is promoting accessibility for a new ASEAN building. Jasper, his wife, and two children are thankful to be agents-of-change.

Aki still wanted to recruit one more person to work with APCD. You will recall how Aki had tried to keep Khun Jam as APCD staff but had been unsuccessful in negotiating with Thai government staff because she had not completed her high school education. We still kept in contact with her and were delighted that she readily agreed to work at APCD because it was now a foundation. Khun Jam had introduced us to her

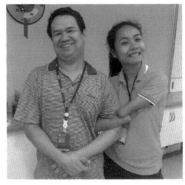

Jam with Wacharapol at APCD.

fiancée at our home, so we knew that she was planning to get married. She found accommodation, but transportation was still an issue. Taking the bus when one has no hands to hang on is dangerous. She invested in a small car and practiced driving without a license for several months. After taking her driving test with no assistive devices, the person testing her, without a comment, just stamped her paper "passed." He probably could not believe what he had just witnessed.

Khun Jam then drove her car to her home in Issan, about twelve hours of driving. Her parents were stunned. When she drove her father to market, he never said a word. Khun Jam has continued to do exemplary work and challenges many things. When she became pregnant, her parents insisted that she was irresponsible and could not possibly raise a child. In tears, she talked with Aki about what to do. He supported her in keeping the pregnancy. She had a beautiful little boy named Tim, unknown to her, the same name as our son.

Aki had invited a deaf gal from Gallaudet University, Washington as an intern for one year. She offered sign language classes for APCD staff. One day, Aki asked her how Khun Jam was doing in the classes. Her response was, "She is one of the best students because of her facial expression and body language." Khun Jam continues to be valued as a regular facilitator for international training at APCD.

Aki authored a book in Japanese, *Kurumaisu ga Iku Asia no Machi-Machi* (wheelchair going around Asia) based on his experiences with APCD and persons with disabilities from 2002-2009.

We always enjoyed having guests and sharing the rich Thai culture. In September 2010, Donna Patterson, a nursing classmate, and her friend, Margie, came for a three-week visit. Donna had hosted my sister Brenda and I for ten days in Bangkok in 1971, when I had finished my work with MCC in Vietnam. She had introduced me to a tailor who had made my wedding dress. Donna, now single, had not been back to Thailand in forty years. This was my time to reciprocate hospitality to Donna and her friend, who was visiting Thailand for the first time.

Of course, Donna wanted to do some exploring in the area where she had lived and eat some authentic Thai food again, namely the famous green papaya salad. She was in heaven seeing the sights of Bangkok again and the unbelievable changes: the highways, the Skytrain (monorail), and the traffic. One day we took the Chao Phraya riverboat taxi to the last stop and rented a long-tail boat to go to Kho Kret Island just north of Bangkok. It was known as a settlement of the Mon people, whose famed terracotta was on display in the Kwan Aman Museum in Bangkok. This traditional earthenware was still produced in potteries along the river.

I had bargained for a fair price for the ride in the long-tail boat to the island: yes, it was long and narrow with two seats. Donna and I managed to squeeze into one seat, and Margie sat behind. All was well until we had to disembark. Donna and I were stuck and needed the help of the helms-man to get us out. We all laughed so hard at this hilarious sight but did manage to extricate ourselves so we could tour the small island. Watching the potters at work with their intricate designs was fascinating. Our boat was waiting for us and our helmsman had a big grin when it came time to get in the boat again. When I went to rent a long-tail boat for other guests years later, much to my chagrin, the helmsman greeted me with a huge grin: he remembered me and gave me a good rental price this time too!

The Redemptorist Centre in Pattaya was always part of my tour package for guests, so Donna and Margie were no exception. I introduced them to the bakery and the school for persons with disabilities, who were enrolled in the computer program. They met several international volunteers while eating lunch in the dining hall. I asked Donna if she had ever considered doing volunteer work before. She admitted that her life felt rather empty: she would think about it. Well, Donna did come for six months as a volunteer to teach English to the students, but, later, they also used her expertise in the medical clinic early in the mornings. This was such a positive experience that Donna came back two more times for three-month stints. We could meet frequently because I was in Pattaya four days a week baking, and Donna occasionally came to Bangkok to stay with us.

The bakery was developing good team spirit. The one deaf baker, a fast learner and competent, informed us one day that she was able to get employment in the bakery of a grocery store in Bangkok, near where we lived: she could stay with relatives until she could live independently. That was wonderful news because the purpose of the bakery was to provide a life skill for persons with disabilities to live independently; we would miss her.

In November, my cousin Ruth from New Zealand also came for a week's visit. We had fun touring around the city of Bangkok, the Grand Palace, and Chinatown too.

Fortieth Wedding Anniversary

When the year 2011 rolled in, we reflected on our lives. God had blessed our marriage for forty years! Forty was also significant in the Bible: Moses and the Israelites wandered in the wilderness for forty years before they reached the land of milk and honey. Maybe we hadn't wandered, but we had covered much territory in our forty years. God had blessed us with three wonderful children and their families, who were well established in Canada. Melody was pursuing her doctorate degree at the School of Medicine, Memorial University in St. John's, focusing on FASD, Fetal Alcohol Spectrum Disorder: Scott was the affordable housing coordinator for the city of St. John's: Maya and Aidan were growing up with Bertha with special needs: her family lived in an Inu village in Labrador. Timothy, living in Waterloo, was struggling to get employment. Matt and Katie were busy in their professions of civil engineering and teaching.

Aki and I decided to recognize our forty years of marriage with our adult children and their families, travelling to Japan in the summer for two weeks. It seemed the perfect place to celebrate because that is where our children lived until their post-secondary education. Aki and I left Bangkok several days in advance to finalize travel arrangements and stayed at the condo of our friends, Donna and Shig Tatsuki, on Rokko Island, Kobe.

We decided to rent two vans to accommodate our family of ten during their stay. Aki set up the GPS in both vans, and I was to follow him to Itami International Airport in Osaka to meet the family on arrival. We had no sooner left for the airport when Aki took a different route than my GPS showed. I started to panic because I had missed the turn off shown on my GPS when I had been so intent on following Aki, so I had no choice but to follow him. His route had us driving through the outskirts of Osaka in rush hour! Aki had no idea of my predicament. When we finally reached the airport, the flight had already arrived thirty minutes earlier. I agreed to stay with both vehicles in a no parking area while Aki went into the terminal. I waited and waited.

Finally, an hour later, Aki appeared, saying our family had not been on the flight. What? Apparently, they had missed their connecting flight from Narita, Tokyo to Osaka due to Air Canada's delay from Toronto, Canada, to Tokyo. While in the terminal, Aki discovered that our family members' names were on the airline's computer screen and were in the process of being rebooked to arrive at the Kansai International Airport on an eleven-p.m. flight. Aki was stunned to learn that our GPS had given different directions, so it was agreed that I would follow him back home again.

What a relief to meet the family on arrival that night. Everyone was excited and wanted to start driving to Lake Nojiri immediately. Melody and Matt enjoyed their first experience of driving in Japan.

This was the first time our adult children had visited Lake Nojiri since they had left Japan years ago for further education. Our family had many special memories from our summer and winter vacations there. For two days, they enjoyed exploring the mountainside again and meeting some friends. One evening, we went to our favourite fish farm, Wakatsuki, to catch our evening meal, which was prepared while we enjoyed the onsen spa. The next day we went to Togakushi, deep in the sacred Shinto mountains, followed by eating the famous Togakushi soba noodles in Japanese style. The Ninja Village nearby was a fun challenge, with everyone renting ninja costumes and exploring the ninja training house, which included crossing the pond ninja style. The grandchildren really enjoyed this experience.

We then drove along the west coast toward Kanazawa city, taking time to stop and put our feet in the Japan Sea. We spent one night visiting our friends Mr. and Mrs. Saito. They took us to see the famous Kanazawa castle, which fascinated the grandchildren, especially because it had been the headquarters for the Maeda clan for fourteen generations. There were many camouflaged hidden doors to escape throughout the castle. The castle's distinctive whitish roof tiles were made of lead, not only to be fireproof, but legend also said that at times of siege the tiles could be melted down and cast into bullets. A system of moats and canals surrounded the castle for extra protection. For even further protection, the castle grounds were split into nine enclosures divided with earthen ramparts, stone walls and fortified gates surrounding the main bailey where the Amanda clan had their main residence. It was fascinating!

The next day, we drove through the mountains to Kobe and checked into a hotel in Shiawase-no-Mura, Village of Happiness, where our organization KSSSC had a residential centre for intellectually challenged adults. Everyone enjoyed sleeping Japanese style on tatami. Aki and I stayed behind while the others took the Shinkansen train to Hiroshima and celebrated Peace Memorial Day with the world on August sixth. Our time in Japan ended with a day visit to Kyoto and a tour of the good old Canadian Academy grounds on the man-made island of Rokko. We parted ways at the airport, our family flying across the Pacific Ocean back to Canada: two days later, Aki and I returned to Thailand.

Mail waiting on our return to Thailand included a letter from Wilfrid Laurier University Alumni Association that was partnering with the school to celebrate 100 years of exceptional education by creating a program to recognize 100 of their exceptional Alumni of Achievement in the past 100 years. Because Aki had been selected to be among Laurier's 100 Alumni of Achievement, he was invited to the program to be held in Waterloo in October. He was being recognized for his contribution to international development work with persons with disabilities, especially in the Asia-Pacific region. Because Aki was unable to attend, Matt and Katie went on his behalf.

Aki and I extended friendship to newcomers at our church. One Sunday in January 2011, we met a young lady from Nepal. We introduced ourselves and, of course, Aki, always focused on food, asked her if she made momo dumplings, one of Nepal's most popular dishes. Yes, she did, so we invited her to come to our home the next Sunday after church along with our Japanese neighbours and watched her make momo. We were fascinated to watch her mix and roll the momo while squatting on the floor. The delicious pork and vegetable filled momo were the beginning of our friendship.

Aki and I soon became good friends with the Nepalese lady. Since we passed her apartment en route to church, it became our custom to pick her up, attend the church service together, and share a meal afterward. After learning more about Christianity, she decided to become a Christian and be baptized. Before her baptism, she shared:

> My family believed in Buddha. When I worshipped Buddha, I didn't feel well. I was still sad. I didn't know what to do. One night I dreamt about a large building with a cross on it. My friend said that it was only a dream, but in my heart, I felt that it was more than that.
>
> Then, I had another dream. I dreamt that I went to many steps and at the top, there was a large round tank of water. Somebody told me to jump into the water, but I didn't see anybody. So, I jumped into the water. I was so afraid that I prayed; after I prayed, I opened my eyes and looked up. A light was shining on me. It was so bright that I couldn't keep my eyes open. Suddenly, I woke up from my dream so afraid that I was shaking. I looked around and saw nothing.
>
> I heard some friends talking about church and decided that I wanted to go too. When I went to the Evangelical

Church of Bangkok (ECB) it was just like my dream. Since then, I have been going every Sunday. My life has changed. I have joy in living.

I joined the 'Experiencing God' class, where everyone shared how God was working in their lives. My English was too poor to share. I was embarrassed, so I decided not to go to church again. But I had another dream, that somebody sent a SMS message on my telephone that said, 'Why don't you go to church?' When I woke up there was no message. So, I decided to go to church again because I was sad and down. After I started going back to church, I felt happy and well. I had peace in my heart. Persons attending ECB really supported and prayed for me. I feel loved and appreciate belonging to Christ's family.

My baptism today, I believe is God's plan for me. It was the last part of my dream. I thank God for His protection and love.

In conversation, we discovered that she wanted to immigrate to Canada and we agreed to be her sponsor. Finally, in January 2017, our friend was able to immigrate to Canada! We consider her as a daughter and a gift from God.

Flooding in Bangkok

In 2011, we were experiencing major flooding in Thailand, especially in our area. We placed sandbags to block our front door and sandbags at the back door, which made a big step to get into our home. Many people lost their homes on the outskirts of Bangkok because the government was trying to protect the city.

One day, our landlady came, very apologetic, saying that a relative with a newborn baby lost their home: she was obligated to offer accommodation for them and was indirectly asking us to look for another place to live. This actually was a blessing for us. We had returned to Thailand in

2009 for two years, but, at the last APCD meeting, the chairperson had proposed that Aki be approved for another four years as executive director. Aki had not been consulted, but this confirmed that we had to seek other accommodation because his salary did not cover the cost of staying on in the current house. We thought we could manage for two years but this definitely forced us to look elsewhere. This was difficult because many other persons who had lost their homes were also looking for housing at the same time. In fact, many of Aki's colleagues were affected and had evacuated to APCD's training building. Many were still unable to return to their homes so we continued to support them.

In the end, we sold our house in Conestogo, Ontario, and bought a semi-public government condo in Bangkok. We had a choice of three condos in the same building. The one Aki felt was best was a sixty-five square metre unit on the twenty-second floor. I looked out the window and thought there was no way I could live there. Furthermore, the washing machine would be on the mini balcony and I would have to do the laundry there! Aki's reasoning won. It was on the east side, the end of the hall, no building blocking the view, and the emergency steps were around the corner from our door. I can report that I never fainted doing laundry and have to admit the view of Bangkok was fantastic.

In November, Aki was invited to be the keynote speaker at JCSWL's annual conference in Japan where he was able to meet many friends.

Our church in Bangkok was active in social outreach. As chairperson of the Missions Committee, I represented us as part of the ecumenical group that gave a Christmas program at Immigration Detention Centre, in downtown Bangkok. We also distributed a care package to each person because most of them did not have the basic necessities. I vividly remember visiting one room that had 200 women and a few children. A North Korean mother with her two-year-old daughter was in that room. When we sang a song for them, the child was standing at my feet, looking up at my face the entire time we sang. I will always remember her face when she received a child's backpack with goodies. I went home and cried thinking of the future of this dear child. When we visited a men's room, we sang Christmas carols. We had started to sing "Amazing Grace" when one of the men joined in: he knew the words of all the verses and proceeded to sing them alone. It was a moving experience that I wished all our church members could experience to see what their ministry meant to persons in IDC.

Because Thailand did not recognize the status of refugees, law enforcement tried to track down and detain illegal residents. These captured refugees and asylum seekers were sent to detention centres to endure months of inhuman treatment before being deported. The Bangkok Refugee Centre (BRC) became the implementing centre for the United Nations High Commissioner for Refugees, that supported more than 8,000 refugees and asylum seekers living in Bangkok.

In April 2012, Dad's health was rapidly deteriorating, so I returned to Ontario to spend time with him and Anna. The day after I arrived, we helped move Dad to a hospice in Guelph, Ontario. I volunteered to spend the nights with Dad because I had jet lag anyway. Dad kept saying that he wanted to go to the Easter service at church the next day. The administration at the hospice finally relented and said I could take him with the understanding that it would shorten his life! Dad definitely was not well, but there was no way I was going to refuse his last request. So, on Easter morning we left in his van for church and used a wheelchair for mobility.

Dad's eyes were closed during the service, but when the music started his lips moved with the words. Sandy and Sue Shantz, his two daughters-in-law, served him communion, which was so special. My sister Brenda then accompanied Dad to the Shantz home for an Easter dinner and back to the hospice. Needless to say, Dad was exhausted when I arrived for night duty, but we had fulfilled his last request. He passed away thirteen days later. A mentor to many persons, he lived his Christian faith and taught us how to live life to its fullest with a kind generous heart. After the funeral, I returned to Thailand.

The baking project at the Redemptorist Centre continued to expand the menu as well as the market. Besides cookies, the menu included bread, muffins, cakes, and steamed pork buns known as salapao. Pi Moi was an amazing baker and chef. Her salapao became so popular that we usually made 220 at a time. This was a major operation: each one had to be rolled and then gathered in a pinching process to seal it. If it was not sealed properly, the bun would open in the steaming process. In time, we all became professionals at making them. Knowing how much our production was enjoyed, we felt empowered to continue.

Aki continued to thrive on the challenges as APCD Executive Director. The UNESCAP's Asia-Pacific Decade for Persons with Disabilities 2003-2012 had focused on empowerment of persons with disabilities and building networks. For the 2013-2022 decade, UNESCAP had designated APCD as the official international agency to develop capacity-building of persons with disabilities and sub-regional development of emerging groups, particularly related to autism, intellectual disabilities, deaf and blind persons, and psycho-social survivors. Aki was focusing on community-based inclusive development in the Southeast Asian region, involving business sectors to make inclusive barrier-free businesses. APCD would also be serving as the global centre for community-based rehabilitation endorsed by the United Nations World Health Organization (UN WHO.) Aki became Asia-Pacific Community-Based Rehabilitation Network's Secretary General.

Our son, Matt, and daughter-in-law, Katie, became the proud parents of a beautiful healthy daughter, Elle Kioko, on October 4, 2012. Katie was enjoying the privilege of being a stay-at-home mom for a school year. Tim had been called back to work and was happy to be part of the workforce again with his colleagues. Melody was in the third year of her PhD program at the Faculty of Medicine at Memorial University, with research on FASD. Scott was the affordable housing coordinator for the city of St. John's. Maya, in Grade 6, loved lessons in contemporary dance and piano, and was reading Harry Potter! Aidan, in Grade 4, was also a bookworm and was working on drumming skills and karate lessons. Bertha, in Grade 1, was excited to be in school full days in the same school as her siblings and loved singing and playing the violin.

Our work in Thailand continued to blossom. In April 2013, APCD organized the ASEAN Autism Network Conference in Brunei with many participants. It was exciting to see the energy invested in empowering persons with autism. We toured the private centre for persons with autism run by Mr. Malai, a visionary who was committed to providing educational opportunities for autistic children. Because his son was a child with classic autism, he was determined to establish a centre to meet his needs as well as other children: there was no other facility in the country. He resourcefully used local materials to develop a comprehensive program and employed Filipino persons who were educated in the field of special education. Everyone attending the congress left impressed with the centre and was motivated to take action on returning home.

I must share with you about NuNu, employed by APCD as a member of the knowledge management team, especially with the Asian Autism Network, who was emcee for Tim's presentation. Aki and I first met NuNu when she and her mother participated in the second Autism Network Conference organized by APCD in Brunei in 2013. She was so alive and joined the fashion show as a model, wearing the traditional Thai dress. Aki, impressed with her, decided to employ her as staff. In 2018, NuNu was the assistant coordinator for the International Workshop on Autism and Sports in Bangkok, along with Mr. Watcharapol. Activities with AAN began to increase with sports, music, an awareness campaign, and an ASEAN newsletter on autism. NuNu became the AAN secretariat at APCD.

At the opening ceremony for the 60+ Plus Bakery Branch at the United Nations Convention Centre, Aki approached a UN officer in charge of disability about the conference being organized by the UNESCAP and the Chinese government in Beijing for the Mid-Term Evaluation on the Inchon Strategy to Make the Right Real. The Bangladesh government planned to have a side event on autism because the granddaughter of the president of Bangladesh was a person with autism. Aki noted that all the speakers at the event were government representatives, medical doctors, and professionals. Because no person with autism was represented, Aki made an official request to the UNESCAP officer to include NuNu as a speaker for the side event because their motto was "Nothing about Us without Us." The Bangladesh government agreed, but NuNu was told that she only had five minutes to speak and no power point presentation was allowed.

NuNu began her speech by saying Mr. Nino, (Aki) told her that she could take fifteen minutes and have a slideshow, which she did! The daughter of the Bangladesh president, and mother of a child with autism who was the emcee, was scheduled to summarize the side event after NuNu's presentation as last speaker of the day.

NuNu shared her life story with her photos, about her struggles and the discrimination she had experienced. Because her parents had her enrolled in a regular school, she was able to achieve what she had. She said that when APCD employed her in the office, she didn't even know how use the copy machine. Today she can work in an office. She noted that it is important to give children with autism an opportunity to go to regular schools. If companies would employ persons with autism, they could be productive. When NuNu finished her presentation, there was not a dry face in the room. The emcee closed with the words, "NuNu said it all."

NuNu continues to be a valued staff member at APCD today, with her commitment and outgoing personality. She made Tim, our son, feel valued as a person on his visits.

Several months later, APCD organized an autism network meeting in Hanoi, Vietnam for both the North and South. This provided a platform for the leaders to meet each other and begin to work together nationally. Immediately following, The United Intellectual Disabilities Network in the Greater Mekong Subregion met in Bangkok. It was so exciting to see how participants from these countries could work so well together. They were role models for their governments!

APCD's biggest event was to organize and coordinate a side event for the UN General Assembly in New York, in September, focusing on disability and community-based inclusive development sponsored by the Royal Thai and Japanese governments collaborating with the United Nations World Health Organization and Economic Social Commission. Aki invited the Honourable Minister of Social Development and Human Security, Madame Paveena, to be the keynote speaker for this event. She had also been a resource person for the DPI AP Seminar on Women with Disabilities in 2004. Aki had also invited the Thai media, Mr. Krisana, from Nation TV Channel and his crew. This event was later televised in Thailand. Aki was able to meet many global colleagues at this UN event.

In October 2013, I celebrated my seventieth birthday with many friends in Myanmar, attending their first festival focused on art and music by persons with disabilities. It was exciting to meet the artist who drew a bunch of bananas with his feet—the picture hanging on our kitchen wall—that Aki had bought several years earlier. It was one of my favourite pictures. This event gave Aki and me an opportunity to meet many of APCD's ex-trainees in the IL groups, autism, intellectually challenged persons, and many persons in the deaf community. Deaf persons were so thrilled to meet us and share in the joy of their accomplishment to have completed a national sign language dictionary in four years. It was special to see the results of empowered persons with disabilities empowering others: to see resources producing new projects and networking. Nay Lin Soe, my "empowered son," was the key person to organize this arts festival that brought persons with cross-disabilities together to network. It was so inspiring to see the fruit of our labour.

My baking project in Pattaya had slowed down due to changes in location in the project, but I continued to seek to empower persons with disabilities through baking. Commuting by bus every week was tiring. The bakery was not air conditioned: we could not use a fan while baking because the flour would blow away and the flame of the gas oven was also affected, so we sweat it out in mid-thirty-degree temperatures. Guests came to visit but never stayed long due to the heat!

Our church attracted many refugees, of which several were special to us. I invested considerable time and effort in supporting and helping them navigate the system in various ways. God used me in unexpected ways.

Martial Law continued to be enforced after a coup in March 2014, with the military having full power, prohibiting assemblies, and media coverage. Fortunately, visitors were beginning to return because tourism was the major industry in Thailand. With few tourists, the economy was impacted, having a domino effect on tour companies, hotels, restaurants, taxis, and the average person on the street. Because most Thai did not have any savings, it was survival for them. Meanwhile, for us, life went on as usual.

Matt and Katie were blessed with a son, Evan, a brother for Elle: Tim was struggling and in need of additional support. Melody, Scott, Maya, Aidan, and Bertha continued to live in St. John's, with Melody working hard on her dissertation.

In the summer of 2014, we reconnected with Yoshimi Horiuchi, who was special to us. Yoshimi, a Japanese, first came to APCD when she was a student at the International Christian University in Tokyo. She was an exchangee with Thammasat University in Bangkok, where she was teaching

English and Japanese at the Foundation for Employment Promotion of the Blind in Bangkok. Yoshimi had been born with a visual impairment but later became completely blind. In 2009, she knew that she wanted to work in international development so she registered for a one-year program in Kerala, India that cultivated social entrepreneurs. After acquiring skills necessary to establish and operate a NGO/NPO, she returned to Thailand in 2010 and started the forerunner of ARC, Always Reading Caravan Association, which she officially registered in 2014. We supported Yoshimi and went to visit her project about sixty km outside of Chiang Mai. She was amazing, having opened a mobile library and a centre dedicated to the acquisition of basic literacy and numeracy skills for preschool children from hill tribe communities. The ride to the mountain village was a challenge with huge ruts and rocks on the road that also went through a creek. After a performance by the students in the village, we slept on the concrete floor with heavy blankets. Farm animals were part of the landscape. The trip was worth it. Yoshimi's project has since expanded due to her untiring efforts. What an inspiration! Another agent-of-change!

The year 2014 was amazing and exciting: we saw the fruits of our labour with APCD facilitating four significant events in four different countries:

- In March, epoch history was made regarding disability in Mongolia. The prime minister, his cabinet, and 800 persons with disabilities were in attendance to ratify the UN Convention on the Human Rights of Persons with Disabilities (CRPD).
- In June, the prime minister of Cambodia and his cabinet, as well as 3,000 persons with disabilities were present for the adoption of a strategic plan on disability and development.
- In September, the vice-prime minister of Lao PDR made history by adopting a decree on disability with 600 persons with disabilities in attendance.
- And then, in December, the vice-prime minister of Vietnam and his cabinet ratified the CRPD in a launching ceremony in Hanoi.

Seeing the results of our commitment to Asia since 2002 has empowered Aki and myself. We planted the seed, let it germinate, and persons with disabilities were stunned at the power that they were given to change their lives and their families. It took hard work. When the governments saw the commitment of persons with disabilities, they were motivated to make policies regarding persons with disabilities and their human rights.

60⁺ Plus Bakery

Aki, a visionary, had done extensive research for two years regarding a possible community-based inclusive business. He wanted to develop a bakery as a model project and decided in 2014 to pursue his dream. He researched and noted that Thai Yamazaki Bakery had approximately eighty outlets in Bangkok and Thailand alone. He visited the Yamazaki Bakery headquarters in Tokyo, Japan. Aki knew that the president of the Yamazaki Company was a committed Christian, who had founded his business on Christian principles. The Yamazaki International Corporation had bakeries in many countries: in fact, Princess Sirindhorn, APCD patron, and Dr. Tej Bunnag, Chairperson of APCD Executive Board, were impressed with a baguette they had eaten in Paris, France made by Yamazaki Bakery. This was reason enough to approach Thai Yamazaki Company in Bangkok! Aki felt this could be the answer to begin a model project in Bangkok.

In early 2014, Aki met with Japanese Embassy staff requesting their assistance to contact the president of the Thai Yamazaki Company and arrange a meeting. This was the Japanese custom to give credibility to a request. Aki was able to meet with President Saito, who was wondering about the purpose of the appointment. Aki told him that he had come to help him. Mr. Saito called his production and sales managers to join the meeting. Aki proceeded to explain that he was a Christian too, an ordained pastor working with persons with disabilities. They were puzzled, but Aki went on to explain that if Thai Yamazaki would have a joint baking project with APCD to sell bread made by persons with disabilities, it would be good publicity for Yamazaki, showing they valued humanity development. For additional credibility, Aki shared that APCD was a Royal Thai project under the patronage of HRH Princess Sirindhorn. At the end of the meeting, the president of Thai Yamazaki said, "I don't know what step I am taking, but I will collaborate with APCD." Aki's persuasive power had been convincing! That was the first step to develop the model baking project!

After a year of preparation, APCD had renovated a ground floor room with access to a main street into a bakery. Yamazaki provided the interior design, equipment, and two staff. The Japanese Embassy approved a grassroots fund that provided furnishings and a van with a lift to deliver bread to customers.

In March 2015, APCD began recruiting deaf persons who had graduated from the School for the Deaf, intellectually challenged persons, autistic persons, and persons with a psycho-social disability. Fifty persons were selected for a three-week training program after which thirty persons would be in the final selection. APCD invited Mr. Saito and his managers for the opening ceremony for the training workshop for the bakery. About one-third of the trainees came with their families for the starting time at nine a.m.: by ten, two-thirds were present, so the ceremony started. Mr. Saito's comment was, "This is a big challenge." Aki agreed. In Japan, punctuality is important and everything begins on time. By noon, 90 percent of the participants had arrived. At the end of the three-week training, everyone arrived on time, which gave hope!

Because most trainees had spent their time at home prior to their training, basic socialization skills had to be taught, as well as grooming, proper dress, etc. Then the real training began with Thai Yamazaki baking and sales staff teaching basic baking skills. After a month's training at APCD, some trainees were assigned to one of Yamazaki's bakeries for further experience in baking and sales. As a result, after three months the total sales of Yamazaki bakeries rose 3 percent. President Saito was very pleased.

The APCD bakery began with Yamazaki's baking and sales supervisors and two APCD full time staff assigned to the sales section. Of the thirty persons with disabilities who started their training, fifteen were employed by Yamazaki in their different branches within a year.

Bakery staff visited the JICA office, the Thai Ministries of Social Development, Human Security, and Education, as well as other government agencies to sell baked goods for their lunch: a mobile sales unit was kept busy. At the same time, a shop was opened across from the neighbouring hospital. The bakery project caught the attention of the Thai media, with persons with disabilities baking and selling bread in collaboration with Yamazaki Bakery. APCD then employed Chris, a famous TV comedian/actor who had been in an accident several years earlier and was left with minor brain damage and an orthopedic disability. After three years of rehabilitation, he had been looking for employment. The media were familiar with Chris's story and how the queen had covered his medical expenses. He became our mascot!

Chris was very excited to be part of the bakery and attracted many customers. He had been hit by a policeman when he had stopped to help someone with car trouble at the roadside. Chris spoke excellent English because his mother was American—his father was Thai. He would drive to work at six a.m. to avoid the traffic and sleep in his mother's car until eight-thirty when the bakery opened, then return home at four-thirty before the rush hour. He was frequently interviewed by various newspapers and TV reporters. The prime minister, in his weekly program, talked about the bakery

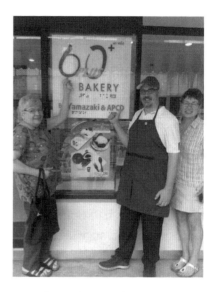

60⁺ Bakery. Left to right: Marcy, Chris and my sister, Brenda.

being a model Disability Inclusive Business (DIB) project. As a result, the bakery has had many orders from Thai parliament, several Ministries, the UN Conference Centre, as well as Thai companies. Chris, ever friendly, blossomed and felt valued for his contribution to the bakery.

In December 2015, HRH Princess Sirindhorn was present for the official opening of the 60⁺ Plus Bakery at APCD, along with the presidents of the Yamazaki Company in Tokyo and Thailand, their representatives, and Thai government officials. The bakery was named in honour of HRH Sirindhorn's sixtieth birthday because she was APCD's patron. Aki wanted to include a Christian symbol in the name because Yamazaki was established by a Christian family, hence the plus sign in the logo after the sixty, signifying a cross. After the official opening, ten persons with disabilities (autistic and deaf persons and one person with a mobility disability) employed by 60⁺ Plus Bakery in production and sales proudly sold their baked goods and had a photo taken with Princess Sirindhorn. Twelve trainees were employed to work daily.

On a visit to Tokyo at a later date, Aki was able to meet the president of Yamazaki Bakery, who promised to continue to collaborate with APCD.

UNESCAP then invited 60⁺ Plus Bakery to open a shop in the United Nations building. It was so well supported that a French Cafe on another floor in the same building was losing a significant amount of their business. We then had to limit the amount we sold there for public relations. Miraculously, a person qualified to be a manager came to APCD seeking employment. He developed this into a model project, attracting customers from everywhere. He was a talented man with managerial skills and was comfortable working with persons with cross disabilities even though he had never done so before. He was truly amazing!

Aki continued to promote accessibility in ASEAN, including rural communities, but DIB became his priority. At the same time, as the bakery was developing, Aki was researching another possible model project—making chocolate. He discovered that there was a factory in Japan where intellectually challenged persons were making chocolate. He kept thinking that this might be a potential project in Thailand because it did not require investing in much equipment. Also, it involved a slow rhythmic mixing process which was ideal for intellectually challenged persons. Aki started buying samples of chocolate on his travels in the hopes of developing a quality project in the future. The manager of 60⁺ Plus Bakery discovered that an agricultural project in Chiang Mai in Northern Thailand had succeeded in developing a cacao farm. This was great news deserving of further research!

In June 2015, Aki and I were invited to Japan by KSSSC to commemorate their fortieth anniversary. Aki delivered the keynote speech, "Prophet Isaiah's Vision and the Future of Kobe Seirei" ("Seirei" meant "Holy Servant"). The Christian organization was established to provide care for persons with disabilities. Aki, noting that few persons with disabilities were present for this event, said he hoped that there would be more representation present for their fiftieth anniversary. I cringed in my seat but felt his comment was right on. I guess being among colleagues we had worked with for almost twenty years, he felt free to honestly speak his thoughts.

After returning to Bangkok, I decided to terminate my volunteer work with the bakery at the Redemptorist Centre in Pattaya. They were very capable of carrying on without me. Because Aki's contract was extended another two years, until September 2017, I decided to visit the Na Kittikoon Foundation in Bangkok: they had expressed an interest in a baking project in 2009, when I had just committed myself to the Redemptorist Foundation.

I am a person who enjoys and needs to be active, so I met with their director, Khun Sontanee to inquire if she still wanted a baking project. Yes, of course she did. Na Kittikoon Foundation was a day care facility for young autistic adults. Their emphasis was on art and music, to enable autistic persons to express how they saw their world, and to give us the opportunity to appreciate their unique art form. They were interested in baking one day per week as a new activity but not to develop a bakery.

I agreed to teach baking one day per week for six young adults with autism and broad-spectrum disorders. They were eager to learn, a delight and challenge to work with. I was back to teaching persons with whom I could not have a conversation, but it was obvious that they enjoyed the challenge of baking. We started with making cookies but expanded our menu to include banana cupcakes, brownies, sesame, and sundried tomato cookies. They were proud of their successful efforts and enjoyed eating their baking for afternoon snacks.

These students were privileged to have such a committed Christian director who valued each person for who they were: she accepted autistic persons who had no other resources available to them. She persevered and her patient, calming support brought results that their parents were stunned to observe. Their artwork has become widely acclaimed as unique and impressive. I have a piece of art that took one of my bakers a year to paint. Only someone with much patience could have stayed focused that long.

People frequently asked me what I did, and I always struggled to give an answer because every week was different, other than the one day per week scheduled for Na Kittikoon Foundation. I continued to be active with the Missions Committee at church and learned much about each project that our church supported.

Georgina Stott was with one such project. She was from Tasmania, Australia and had committed her adult life to Christian ministry in Thailand. She was now the Far Eastern Broadcasting Corporation Director, with much responsibility. When FEBC had first asked her to help them, there were only two shortwave languages and eight stations in Thailand. Much inter-mission work was required to grow the shortwave languages. Her responsibilities included seventeen ethnic languages broadcast over shortwave from the Philippines with listeners in six SE Asian countries. She also had the responsibility for eleven DJ Thai language programs on twenty-nine local AM/FM government stations around Thailand. They also offered several correspondence courses with six lessons each for listeners to the Thai language programs. Her work was part of the world-wide FEBC ministry in 141 languages in fifty countries. Her stories were always fascinating.

Now that Aki's contract was extended to November 2017, he continued to work for the promotion of accessibility in ASEAN, including rural communities with DIB as a priority.

We were excited to have our son Timothy spend a month with us in March/April in Thailand, which included a trip to Hanoi, Vietnam. Tim shared his life story at an epoch-making event, Vietnam's first National Autism Seminar on April 2, 2016, inaugurated by the Vice-Minister of the Ministry of Social Welfare. Tim was reluctant to participate, but, in the end, was glad that he did. He received positive feedback for his excellent presentation. After the formal program in the morning, the afternoon included many different sports activities. In fact, the energy level was so high that a thick rope pulled by opposing sides was torn, sending surprised participants to the floor! It was so much fun watching how the sports activities broke down barriers. I recall one father who approached us with many questions, truly seeking to do his best for his autistic son. He had been moved by Tim's presentation.

In August, Aki and I were able to celebrate our forty-fifth wedding anniversary at Melody and Scott's home in Kitchener where they had moved the year before. It was wonderful to reflect and spend the day with so many family members and friends, including seven persons over the age of ninety who came to share in our joy! It was the first time in many years that all three of our adult children and their families were living in the same area.

Our return trip to Bangkok was via Tokyo, where Aki officiated at the wedding of Maika Tatsuki and Hiroaki Sannomiya on September 4 in Yokohama, Japan, the same date as our wedding in Tokyo forty-five years earlier. We had known Maika since she was a baby because her parents, Shig and Donna Tatsuki, were personal friends. The wedding was beautiful and it was wonderful to meet Shig, Donna, and other friends again from our time in Kobe. We also spent a day visiting friends at Agape Centre where we were first assigned and had lived from 1979-81. They now had a new building with state-of-the-art equipment for their rehabilitation and day care programs for persons with disabilities. What a wonderful reunion with former colleagues!

In October, 2016 Aki was privileged to visit Japan again as the keynote speaker for the JCSWL on the human rights for persons with disabilities. I was well accustomed to filling my days and being independent: with so many friends I was never alone.

When the calendar turned to January 2017, it was the countdown for us, our last year in Thailand with APCD. Knowing this could be the last chance to visit us in Thailand, Matt, Katie, Elle, and Evan, decided to visit us for a few weeks. It was also an excellent place to soak up some sun while saying goodbye to cold Canadian winter weather.

We went directly to our condo in Jomtien, a one-and-a-half-hour drive from the airport. They were enchanted by the lovely long sandy beach, coconuts, fresh seafood, and swimming pools. We visited the Redemptorist Centre and the bakery before returning to Bangkok, where we introduced them to APCD and staff. Using public transportation and shopping in Bangkok was a fun time. A highlight was our trip with the grandchildren to the Bangkok Zoo. Much to our surprise, the reptiles fascinated them the most. A visit to the underground aquarium with all the sea creatures and penguins was also impressive. The time passed by too quickly.

The day after our son Matt's family left Bangkok, Georgina and I went to the airport to say goodbye to our dear friend who was immigrating to Canada. What a shock to see all the refugee Rohingya families also immigrating to the US and Canada. They had probably never seen snow and would have no idea how cold it was going to be at their destination.

Many of these Rohingya families had arrived at the airport from a refugee camp in northern Thailand in bare feet, wearing thin cotton clothing. The International Organization for Migration had staff come with a supply of shoes for the shoeless persons. One young boy, about ten years of age, who was standing near me, was given a pair of lace shoes. Seeing that he did not know what to do with the laces, I taught him how to tie his first pair of shoes. His mother was given a pair of rubber slip-on shoes that were at least three to four sizes too big. I had no idea how she could walk and still keep the shoes on her feet. Another young man, I assume in his late teens, was tagging along with another family sponsored by a church in Canada. He was trying hard to hold back the tears. I have thought of him many times since, wondering how he was doing. He had obviously lost all his family. I wanted to cry with him. After saying our goodbyes to our friend immigrating to Canada, Georgina and I didn't have much of a conversation returning to Bangkok on the airport link.

Aki insisted that I fly to Canada the next day to be sure that our friend was settling into her new country. After three weeks, I returned to Thailand assured that she was doing fine. She was already enrolled in an English language class and was using public transportation.

Believe in the Power of Change

Aki still had projects that he had been working on behind the scenes that he hoped to implement. One was to prepare a musical side event for the Tokyo Olympics and Paralympics scheduled for 2020, with an emphasis on Asian music, using traditional musical instruments such as a variety of drums, bamboo flutes, etc. In preparation for this, APCD visited ten

ASEAN countries to select music groups of persons with disabilities to perform in a drum festival event scheduled for Bangkok in June 2017.

On June 2-3, 2017, APCD and The Nippon Foundation presented the Disability-Inclusive Drum Performance in ASEAN nations—Brunei Darussalam, Cambodia, Indonesia, Lao PDR, Malaysia, Myanmar, the Philippines, Singapore, Thailand, Vietnam, and Japan—with the theme, "Believe in the Power of Change." The event promoted the musical talents of persons with diverse disabilities and increased awareness for a barrier-free, inclusive and rights-based society for all.

The two-day event was held in commemoration of the fiftieth anniversary of ASEAN in 2017 and the 130 anniversary of Thailand-Japan diplomatic relations in 2017. It was generously supported by partners including the Royal Thai Government (through the Ministry of Social Development and Human Security and the Ministry of Foreign Affairs), the Government of Japan, (through the Ministry of Foreign Affairs), the ASEAN Secretariat, Thai Yamazaki) and other supporters.

The festival included thirteen bands from eleven countries, with more than 150 performers with disabilities. Over 1,500 persons with and without disabilities gathered in solidarity to witness an historic, first-of-its-kind musical extravaganza that highlighted an inclusive and accessible community for all.

Because there was no association for deaf persons in the Central Region of Vietnam, APCD used the music event to establish the Central Regional Association of Deaf Persons and provided drums and equipment to form a drummers' group. The drummers admitted that they had a difficult time following the beat and rhythm in the first couple of months, but with the help of their hearing drum teacher and their enthusiasm, they were able to perform impressively. They shared that in their excitement, drumming practices lasted until midnight, until neighbours complained that they could not sleep because of the noise. Of course, the deaf persons had no idea of the volume of noise they were producing! So future practices ended at ten p.m.

The performers captivated the audience with their colourful red and yellow costumes representing the colours of their national flag: they danced with impressive choreography and remarkable drumming skills on big drums. These young artists and musicians saw their participation as a great way to learn new skills and techniques—apart from drumming and dancing together, the members were also into painting, calligraphy, and photography. One of their goals was to be recognized and appreciated for the talent that they offered at the national level. They were already thinking of ways to raise funds for their drum group's performances to achieve their goals.

This event was the first time the young drum performers with autism and intellectual disabilities ages between fourteen and twenty-five travelled out of Cambodia. Their long drums, decorated with a multi-coloured cloth wrapped around, had a string attached to enable the drummer to carry it around the shoulder. They had four or five types, which were used mainly for celebrating happy events. As Cambodians, they thought that the drum was akin to thunder or thunderbolts and signified an important connection to the natural world.

I spent time with their group because the youngest girl needed medical care for a facial injury sustained en route to the airport in Phnom Penh, Cambodia. A dog had run in front of her father's motorbike, throwing her onto the side of the highway. She had major abrasions to her face, but her injuries did not deter her determination: she performed with bandages on her face, which we took off for the official photo.

Groups from Cambodia, Lao PDR, and Singapore represented intellectually challenged persons; persons with autism performed in bands from the Philippines and Thailand; deaf persons performed in bands from Chiang Mai, Thailand, and Vietnam; blind persons represented Indonesia, Malaysia, and Myanmar; members of the band from Brunei Darussalam had cross disabilities. Persons with psycho-social disabilities, representing the Rajanagarindra Psychiatric Hospital Long Drum Group from Nakhon Ratchasima, Thailand, were the last to perform. Under the guidance of the Abbot of the Wang Nam Keaw Temple and with coordination by the head monk, a group of persons with psycho-social disabilities became empowered after learning how to play traditional drums. The aim was to supplement their medications with therapeutic drum practice after seeing the positive changes in the people's disposition and condition. They were exuberant in their performance. The head monk related how the changes were so outstanding that some performers were now back living in their respective communities. One gentleman who sang a song changed from being a recluse to actively participating in the music program.

The drum performance also featured the Fugaku Taiko drummers from Japan. They mesmerized the audience with the thundering reverberating sounds of the taiko drums. The drums were hit so hard that one would have expected the drum to break.

Ms. Petnamnueng Sriwattana, a wheelchair user and TV personality who was emcee for the event, commented, "I am proud to be emcee for this event because I believe that it will change Thai society, and everybody will be able to see the potential of persons with disabilities. This is not just a music event, it is also a place for the self-expression of musical talents of persons with disabilities. Drums are great tools for persons with disabilities to showcase their talent because it has a rhythm that resonates with the beating of their hearts. When we hear drums playing, we are motivated and cheer up."

Although Aki and I continued to be busily engaged, we were becoming aware that our time in Thailand was quickly passing by, and we needed to think about housing upon our retirement to Canada in December. Previously, we had our name put on a waiting list for a condo at the St. Jacobs Meadows in St. Jacobs, Ontario, which was the neighbouring town to the village where I had lived in my growing up years. The Meadows had a unique history. Research undertaken by Reverend Clinton Rohr and Mr. Gordon Hunsberger had shown that there was a need for seniors' housing in the area, so they initiated a community housing corporation, the first in Ontario for community residents to run it themselves as volunteers. It was a committed Christian community that included community health and social programs. Because we thought we would be comfortable joining this community, we had applied for a unit several times but were not successful: I honestly felt that we should consider other options.

At this time, another unit became available. I had given up because we had been unsuccessful five times previously so why try again? My husband pleaded with me to try just one more time. We arranged for our adult children to go to the viewing and take photos. Aki decided to put in a bid, and, much to our shock, we got it! To finalize the purchase, Aki and I made a quick trip to St. Jacobs and were delighted with the condo. My brother Clare kindly agreed to oversee renovations in our absence, so when we arrived in December all the renovations would be completed.

Another big event in September 2017, organized by APCD along with the Thai Autism Association in Bangkok, was the ASEAN Autism Network Sports Festival to commemorate ASEAN's fiftieth anniversary and 130 years of a diplomatic relationship between Thailand and Japan. Approximately 350 persons with autism participated in a variety of games and sports, indoors and outdoors. It was an event in which persons with autism excelled. I vividly recall one female participant from one of the ASEAN countries, who was to compete in a swimming competition. She was an excellent swimmer but refused to swim until NuNu, APCD staff person with autism, jumped into the swimming pool and proceeded to swim with her. One never quite knew what to expect at these events.

Aki was still convinced that chocolate making could be a successful DIB project for intellectually challenged persons. It required patience to mix and no high difficulty techniques. He consulted with the manager of the 60+ Plus Bakery, who agreed to begin a trial project for ten persons with intellectual disabilities, and he stipulated that he wanted quality chocolate made with 60-75 percent cacao and sold at a high price. This would validate intellectually challenged persons, who were capable of producing quality chocolate. It was through connecting with a supplier of cacao based in Chiang Mai—the Mark Rin Company—that APCD was able to develop high quality chocolate products featuring Thailand's own cacao.

There was no such thing as a regular schedule. Neville and Lill Muir, friends from Australia who had been our next-door neighbours before the earthquake in Kobe, shared a day's vacation with us in Bangkok. It was wonderful to meet them again and their son Ian, with Down's Syndrome, who was thriving on his work in a sheltered workshop.

I was becoming concerned with my cataracts in both eyes, and decided it might be easiest to have the surgery done in Bangkok before retiring in Canada in December. I had my right eye done in October and the left eye on November seven. It was amazing how much easier it was to read again! We were excitedly looking forward to having our niece, Heather, and her niece, Briana, come for a two week visit in November before we left for Canada.

I always enjoyed planning an itinerary for our visitors that included APCD, my volunteer work, Thai culture, sightseeing and, of course, some shopping. Briana had done extensive research on the internet before coming. Her priority was to be able to bathe an elephant, as well as visit a coffee shop in Bangkok where the menu and decor was all about unicorns! Unbelievably, on our visit to Koh Chang Island, a four-hour bus ride from Jomtien, a forty-five-minute ferry ride, and another hour by bus to our hotel, we discovered that it was possible for Briana to have one of her wishes fulfilled. She was able to bathe a baby elephant in the sea! On returning to Bangkok, we were finally able to find the unicorn coffee shop too!

Another highlight for Heather and Briana was to be present for Aki's farewell by APCD on November 22, 2017, and welcome to Mr. Piroon, Aki's replacement. The Thai are deserving of accolades in planning such events with good humour. Part of the program included each staff member giving a personal message to Aki. By the end, it almost felt like a funeral! Aki had established APCD and now, fifteen years after working together, it was farewell. Staff with disabilities had been empowered and felt like family. After shedding some tears, we posed for a group photo which holds special memories of working together as close colleagues for many years.

CHAPTER 7

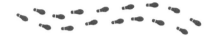

New Life in St. Jacobs

The farewells were leaving Aki and I emotionally drained. It meant saying goodbye to the APCD Foundation, the Ministry of Social Development and Human Security, AAN, the NGOs empowering persons with disabilities, and our many personal friends. The goodbyes were humbling, and it made us realize how much our lives had impacted the persons we came to serve.

We left Thailand on December 14, travelling from Bangkok to Toronto—a twenty-eight-hour day! When we landed in Toronto— the same day we left Bangkok—the temperature was -18—a difference of over fifty degrees!

Two days after our arrival, we hosted a Weber Christmas dinner at the St. Jacobs Meadows Community Centre. It was wonderful to see all of our family again. The biggest challenge was to keep warm. Our bodies were accustomed to a tropical climate.

The year 2018 brought major adjustments: from a busy and productive city life in a concrete jungle in Bangkok to retirement in a quiet rural setting with nature surrounded by many trees: from public transportation of buses and trains to the necessity of owning a car: from a tropical climate to cold winters! For the first time in many years, all of our family members were within easy driving distance of each other. What a blessing to be able to spend quality time with them.

Our condo at The Meadows in St. Jacobs was just two blocks away from St. Jacobs Mennonite Church, the church that I had attended as a child with my parents, grandparents, and now our daughter, as Melody and Scott's family was also attending. We decided to reconnect with this church since they were active with peace and justice issues in the community. It was interesting returning to the Mennonite community that tends to identify through connectivity. To them, I had returned, but Aki was frequently identified as Marcy's husband, Melody's father, or Maya, Aidan, and Bertha's Grandpa. One day during sharing time at church, he stood up and shared the various ways he had been identified and that he had a name. His name was Aki.

Returning to Canada was reverse culture shock. After many years in Asia, I felt like "a fish out of water." My heart was still in Asia, and my interests were different from many friends. The standard of living was also different. Seniors moving into The Meadows were all downsizing, while we were upsizing. Culturally, many Asians were living in the area, enabling us to easily continue eating an Asian diet. All the technicians that did work for our condo were from South Asia. There were many Chinese university students, and Chinese businesses were flourishing.

Of course, we were delighted for the opportunity to return to Asia during the summer of 2018. I accompanied Tim, who was invited as a resource person by APCD in July for an international workshop on autism and sports in Bangkok. Tim was willing to do so because his experience in Vietnam had been so positive. He shared his community inclusive life in Canada with participants from neighbouring ASEAN countries. Because many parents were concerned about their children having to live with autism as adults, his presentation was well received as he helped them understand the life of autistic persons after the age of twenty. This experience empowered Tim to become more active in his community.

Melody, Scott, Aidan, and Bertha travelled to Europe in the summer of 2018 to meet Maya, who was completing her exchange program in France: they decided it was an excellent opportunity to visit us in Thailand because we had adequate accommodation. After the usual tour of APCD and the Grand Palace in Bangkok, we visited the Redemptorist Centre to see the bakery that I had started and meet friends. Some fun time included paragliding and an elephant ride. It turned out that Melody's family visit overlapped with my sister Brenda's trip: she came to accompany Tim back to Canada. Then, poof, everyone was gone, and Aki and I were alone again!

Visit to Myanmar

Aki and I flew to Naypyidaw, Myanmar to visit friends in August 2019. Naoko, a former colleague of Aki's in APCD, had married an ethnic Chin gentleman from Myanmar and was now living there. She requested that I start a cookie-baking project for economically deprived widows in the area to empower families living in poverty. Naoko had done extensive research and discovered that in 2005, the government had begun to shift its administrative centre to Pyinmana City, 320 km north of Yangon, while it bought up farmland in the surrounding area to construct the city of Naypyidaw, which was proclaimed the new capital of Myanmar in 2006. Farmers, with no professional skills, unaccustomed to having cash, drank it away. For many families, the wives became widowed with young children and no means to support themselves. It was this situation that motivated Naoko to begin a baking project.

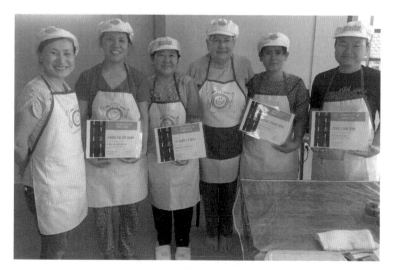

Naoko (far left) and Marcy (centre) with the bakers in Myanmar.

This humble baking project began with five persons who had never done any baking and a small electric oven as a trial. I had taken basic equipment from Bangkok with me. They were eager, quick learners. Again, I was amazed at how easy and fast one could teach persons without an intellectual disability with excellent results. After five days of teaching how to make cookies and banana cake, they needed time to practice on their own. Naoko had done some baking in the past and was able to oversee their production.

Aki and I scheduled a little sightseeing after one week of training. Yvonne Pa, Naoko's brother-in-law, was our designated driver to Shan State, which was his home. While he enjoyed a visit to his home, we stayed in an ecologically oriented hotel beside Inle Lake, a freshwater lake known for over twenty species of snails and nine species of fish found nowhere else in the world.

Our room was on stilts over the water, facing mountains in the distance: behind us was a bird sanctuary with birds filling the trees around four o'clock every afternoon. Most people accessed this hotel by boat but it could be reached by car, which is what we did: the mountain road was very narrow and wound through forest, maintaining an image of living with nature. Aside from the scenic spot, Inle Lake was known for a traditional form of fishing practices by the Intha fishermen (people living on the lake were called Intha). They stood at the stern on one leg and wrapped the other leg around the oar. This unique style evolved out of necessity because the lake is covered by reeds and floating plants, making it difficult to see above them while sitting. Standing provided the rower with a view beyond the reeds and allowed them to have the other hand free to collect the net. The leg rowing style was only practiced by men.

We learned so much on our boat tour on the lake. The Intha people, numbered around 70,000, lived in cities bordering the lake and in numerous small villages along the lakeshore and on the lake itself. Their simple houses were made of wood and woven bamboo on stilts. We learned about their floating gardens. Farmers gathered lake-bottom weeds from the deeper parts of the lake, brought them back in boats, and made them into floating beds in their garden areas, anchored by bamboo poles. These gardens rose and fell with changes in the water level, so they were resistant to flooding. Locals grew vegetables and fruit in large gardens floating on the surface of the lake.

We enjoyed the lake transportation system and went to a "Five Day Market" that rotated amongst five villages. What fun looking at the local goods and wooden souvenirs. Anything in wood fascinated me, so the miniature carved wooden crèches mixed with many wooden carvings caught my eye.

Many ethnic groups lived in the area, the Pa-O (Taungthu in Burmese) being the most obvious with their bright red and yellow turbans wrapped around their heads, signifying a dragon: the women wore black or dark blue dresses. Many Pa-O fled to Northwestern Thailand in 1975 due to the terrible social upheavals and human rights abuses committed by the military junta.

Aki and I flew back to Bangkok from Myanmar on August 23, 2018. We were stunned to read the news that, on August 29, one of the sluice gates of the Swar Chaung Dam in central Myanmar had broken, submerging eight-five villages and affecting over 63,000 people: it had also submerged part of the Yangon-Mandalay Highway that we had driven on several times a week earlier. Thank God for His protection!

Several days after returning to Bangkok, Aki became very ill with a fever of over 104 degrees that would not come down, along with nausea and vomiting. I thought he likely had dengue fever caused by a mosquito infected with the dengue virus. He was hospitalized for two days, until his condition passed the critical stage. We had taken all precautions by using insect repellent and sleeping under a mosquito net while in Myanmar, but I guess a mosquito bypassed our defence. We were so thankful that the doctor on call in emergency specialized in treating persons with dengue fever.

On September ninth, it was time to return to Canada. Happy to return but sad to leave Thailand and Asia, it was back to "home" in St. Jacobs and our family. At this time, Melody was a research scientist with the Centre for Addiction and Mental Health, in London, Ontario. Scott was a PhD student studying environmental sustainability at the Balsillie School of International Affairs, University of Waterloo, in Waterloo, Ontario. Their children, Maya, Grade 12, Aidan, Grade 10, and Bertha, Grade 7, were all enrolled at Rockway Mennonite Collegiate.

Tim was still on a high from being a resource person in Thailand in July, and he was trying to organize an advocacy group in Kitchener-Waterloo.

Matt continued to work as a civil engineer in Kitchener, Ontario. Katie enjoyed sharing and impressing her family and friends with her latest acquired skills in Japanese cooking, which Aki delighted in teaching her. Elle, age six, was passionate about creating things with origami, especially cranes. Evan, age four, couldn't wait to go to school.

The young woman from Nepal whom we helped immigrate to Canada started to work part time at a nearby A & W and hoped to study culinary arts in January 2019.

In October, my sister Brenda invited me to speak to a women's group at the United Church in Holstein. Much to my surprise, over forty women came! In November, a nursing classmate, Bernice Uebele, invited me to speak to the women's group at St. James Rosemount United Church about the baking projects in Thailand.

Soon it was cold weather and the Christmas season. All the festive activities, music concerts, and church activities were amazing. I didn't realize how much I had missed the beautiful Christmas music while in Thailand. I felt so moved hearing the four-part harmony of the Christmas music in the church services! Truly beautiful! Family time over the holidays was a highlight because we were all living within driving distance of each other. Aki enjoyed preparing a Japanese main dish of inari sushi (sushi rice in deep fried tofu sacs), chirashi sushi (sushi rice with veggies, and egg on top) with pickled ginger on the side, and salmon, with the others supplementing the menu. The celebratory meal was followed by fun games with everyone. How blessed we felt to have such a wonderful family!

After Christmas, Aki and I were thinking about Asia. We had already made extensive travel plans using air miles. On New Year's Eve, 2019, we were sitting at Toronto Pearson Airport en route to Bangkok via Taipei, Taiwan, eagerly looking forward to meeting friends again, warmer weather, and returning to Bangkok that was home to us.

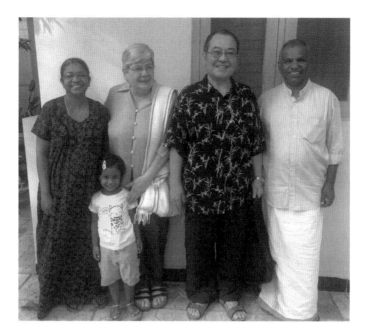

Mr. Abraham's Family in Kerala, India.
Left to right: Sheela, Anahira, Marcy, Aki, and Varghese.

January 17, 2020, Aki and I flew to Trivandrum, Kerala, South India to visit our dear friends, Varghese and Sheela Abraham, who established Seirei Asha Bhavan, a social service residential setting for intellectually challenged persons. The first night we spent at Trivandrum. The next morning, their son, Dilu, kindly picked us up and drove two hours to Punalur, where their centre was located. We had expected to stay in their guest facilities but current government policy made it difficult: it would necessitate registering us with the police, etc., so we stayed at a hotel to eliminate the issue.

What a wonderful reunion to meet Varghese and Sheela who welcomed us to their home in the same compound as their centre. They gave us a tour of the centre, and we visited the various classes and their activities for the different skill levels. One group was sorting colours and shapes: new vocational training programs included making ecological "paper" pens and cloth umbrellas. Some of the higher functioning students were in a computerized "smart" class. Everyone was focused and engaged in their activity. We saw the new hostel building that was inaugurated in March 2018, that was constructed using bricks they had made themselves. It had Spartan furnishings, but it was adequate to meet the residents' needs: each resident had a change of clothing.

Varghese updated us on his community development work. He was a committed visionary who put his Christian faith into action. The government finally acknowledged their efforts in 2018, after many years, and utilized his wisdom by holding a state level seminar and workshop for parents of intellectually challenged persons: his centre found successful job placements for seven persons. They held rural and dental camps and distributed wheelchairs to persons who could not afford to buy one. Mr. Abraham shared how they were able to provide temporary housing and support to flood victims who had lost their homes. Aware of urgent needs in the community, Mr. Abraham's organization was currently renovating a building just outside their property to be a nursery school and kindergarten.

In the afternoon, the centre welcomed us with a formal ceremony, honouring us by draping white shawls over our shoulders while residents and staff entertained us with songs. Mr. Abraham introduced us by narrating projected photos of the history of Seirei Asha Bhavan, which included Aki in many photos because he had been involved with establishing the centre, unknown to the current residents and staff. We were truly humbled. We met Francis, a former resident, who had participated in one of APCD's workshops and was now a staff person, married with a son. He was as excited as we were to meet him again.

The Christmas greetings we had received from Seirei Asha Bhavan prior to coming sums up their sentiments:

"We gratefully remember and thank each and every one who has touched our lives and supported us in various ways. Thank you for your time, thank you for sharing your smile, and thank you for your encouragement and support."

The next day, we declined the opportunity to go to the beach so we could spend more time with Varghese and Sheela. While reminiscing on the history of his project, he suddenly asked Aki if he would be willing to preach at their Mar Thoma Church the next day, which Aki readily agreed to do if the pastor agreed. Varghese said that because his work was in the third decade, most church members did not know the history of Mar Thoma Church's involvement with his project. After the service, the bishop said that he too appreciated learning about the history. In the afternoon, over a cup of tea, Varghese and Aki continued to reflect on the history of their relationship and how their lives had intertwined until the present. . .

It all began when the Archbishop of Mar Thoma Church visited Japan to collaborate with JCSWL because the Mar Thoma Church wanted reformation and chose social action/service as the next major strategy for reformation. They were developing social action for children with disabilities and seniors. JCSWL proposed an exchange of personnel and sent Aki to India.

Varghese Abraham came and spent four months in Japan, observing our social service system for persons with intellectual disabilities: we functioned as his home base. After Varghese returned to Kerala, he continued to work for a large institution for seventy intellectually challenged children. Reverend Koshi, the director, mentioned that he wanted to increase the capacity to accommodate about 200 children. Aki encouraged Varghese to consider community-based inclusive living, beginning with a small group home instead. He also recommended starting in another town to avoid possible conflict with Mr. Koshi's centre.

Varghese took Aki's advice, went back to his hometown, and rented a small home. He married, had a son, and used his dowry to finance his project to live with seven intellectually challenged persons, one of whom had violent outbursts. It was at this time that Aki visited the project and observed Varghese's son slung in a hammock in the centre of the room while one resident was having destructive outbursts. Afraid for the safety of the baby, Aki asked Varghese, "Aren't you afraid for your child?" His response was, "It is not a problem. He will not hurt the baby." Aki was so impressed with his accepting attitude.

All was well until September 2011, when Kuwait was attacked and many Indians from Kerala, who had been employed there, returned home. The owner of the home that Varghese was renting decided to sell it. Varghese informed Aki of the situation. He had just rented another place when Aki arrived for two weeks. Aki felt that for the future it was important to buy a house in the community to avoid being in a similar situation. They found a house with 100 rubber trees on the outskirts of his hometown of Punalur.

The price was $50,000 USD. It was agreed that Varghese would ask his father for his share of his inheritance early, and Aki would return to Japan to fundraise.

When we were reminiscing, we heard Varghese's side of the story. He had trusted Aki to do adequate fundraising due in six months, but the amount kept haunting Varghese. If full payment was not received within the deadline, he would lose his down payment of $10,000 USD. Previously, he had invested in a used three wheeled vehicle and hired a person to provide taxi service in the day time, then parked it at his centre for the night so he would have access to transportation if his residents needed emergency services. He found he suffered from insomnia, thinking of the huge amount of money needed within six months, and he was spending some nights providing taxi service himself. Meanwhile, Aki was fundraising in Japan with Hamamatsu Seirei and Kobe Seirei Associations.

Brazilian residents working in an automobile company in Hamamatsu were very generous. Amazingly, $40,000 USD was raised just before the deadline, much to Varghese's relief. Mr. Tsutomo Hasegawa, Chairperson of Hamamatsu Seirei, Mr. Yoichiro Kanatsuki, Chairperson of Kobe Seirei, and Aki went to Punalur to donate the needed funds to purchase the house and property. They noted the old vehicle used for transportation and decided to return to Japan and also do fundraising for a new Jeep.

While reliving these past experiences, we realized how God had been guiding the work of Seirei Asha Bhavan, whose name had incorporated the name "Seirei" meaning "Holy Servant." Over the years, Varghese had provided learning experiences for some of Aki's university students as field placements. Aki learned later that Varghese and Sheela had given the students their sleeping quarters while they slept on a concrete floor. Such humility. Aki had made numerous trips to Punalur as a mentor throughout the years, but this was the first time for me to visit the Abraham family and their project. My involvement had been limited to correspondence and fundraising. I could feel the commitment and love they felt for their residents, whom they considered family.

Because all of Aki's previous visits were focused on Mr. Abraham's project, this was our opportunity to incorporate some sightseeing on the trip. Aki had done extensive research, as he always does, on the history of this area of India.

We discovered that the Mar Thoma Church sees itself as a continuation of the Saint Thomas Christians, a community traditionally believed to have been founded in the first century by Jesus' apostle St. Thomas. He is believed to have landed in AD 52 in Cranganore near Cochin, which was an important seaport on the Kerala Coast, having trade connections with the Middle East. It was quite natural for St. Thomas to come to India with the Gospel, as the disciples went to different parts of the world in accordance with the commission given to them by Jesus Christ. I was so impressed with the history of the Mar Thoma Church.

The Mar Thoma Church was not known to the Western World until Vasco de Gama visited in 1497. When Vasco de Gama died in 1524, he was originally buried in Saint Francis Church in Cochin, one of the oldest European churches in India. Aki and I felt honoured to visit this historical church and see the tomb of Vasco de Gama in the church.

It was interesting to talk with Dilu, the son of Varghese, who shared that the Mar Thoma Evangelistic Association, the missionary wing of the Mar Thoma Church organized a Maramon Convention annually at the end of January or early February. It is one of the largest annual Christian gatherings in Asia, with up to 100,000 persons attending. Christians go to listen to the gospel as read and expounded by Christian leaders from all over India and abroad. People attending sit on the sandy beach by the sea, with old and invalid persons given chairs.

Mr. Abraham's faith has empowered and impacted our lives over the years, with his unwavering faith in God's guidance as we followed the development of Seirei Asha Bhavan. His family was a pioneer in community-based living for persons with intellectual disabilities in Kerala State. It was such a blessing to finally see firsthand the work of this outstanding project based on Christian principles and commitment. We also learned much about the Christian history started by the Mar Thoma Church in this amazing country.

Kerala State, between the Arabian Sea and Western Ghats' mountain range, is beautiful and steeped in rich history. Dilu kindly drove us to Cochin, five hours away. Although I had lived in different Asian countries, driving in India left me hyperventilating until I devised a system to control my emotions. I noticed that all buses had a religious name written across their front, so, sitting in the back seat of the car, I decided to focus on the names of the buses written across the front of the bus. It worked. We had Gabriel, St. Mary. St. Ann, St. John, etc. I wondered if the symbolic names were intended to protect them from harm because they definitely needed it!

Although the road was divided into lanes, they were simply arbitrary. Traffic would be coming toward you in your lane only to pull into their lane just in time to narrowly miss your vehicle. I learned the necessity of horns in cars. One evening where we stayed, I talked with an Indian mother and her son who were on a visit from Britain. This was the son's first visit to India. I mentioned the driving here in India and that, to my amazement, I had not seen an accident yet in our travels. His response was that in England traffic laws are strictly enforced but he has seen more accidents there than here. Go figure!

We also noticed frequent billboards advertising, "Do you want to go to Canada? Want to study in Canada?" We chuckled when we saw these because when we retired in Canada in December 2017, it was Indians from India who provided technical services. When we asked them where they came from in India, the answer was always, Kerala.

Our travels took us into the Western Ghats to Munnar, one of the prominent hill stations owned by a tea company, with 24,000 hectares of land along the high range of Idukki district in Kerala. The view after climbing the mountainside on some narrow dirt roads with no shoulder or guardrails was spectacular. We safely reached our destination where the tea processing facilities were fascinating.

Aki and I looked forward to our overnight on a traditional house boat in the Cochin backwaters. We floated along a network of waterways for a leisurely ride, observing the rural life along the shore line and stunning nature. Our boat "parked" at a perfect spot to see the sunset and amazing sunrise. What a memorable experience. We also visited the famous Mangalavanam bird sanctuary, a place for many kinds of resident and migratory birds, especially the kingfisher: there are eight species of kingfishers in South India. We enjoyed the quietness, sounds of the wind, nature, and the birds.

Our adventure in Kerala ended at Trivandrum, where we said our goodbyes to Varghese and his son, Dilu, thanking them for their kind hospitality. We felt so blessed to be a cog in the wheel of their pioneer work.

We returned to Bangkok to prepare for our visit to Naypyidaw, Myanmar to follow up on my cookie-baking project for economically deprived widows. We first flew to Yangon on February 8, 2019, where we met with our friend, the director of Eden Centre, a non-profit charity organization established in 2000 to provide education and social services for children with physical and intellectual disabilities in Yangon. We knew the director well because he had been a trainee in one of APCD's training programs. We were impressed with their new facility and vision to meet the needs of children in their care. In the afternoon, we visited the Association for Aid and Relief, a Japanese project in Yangon that runs a vocational training centre for persons with disabilities in tailoring, hairstyling, and computers. They continued to support graduates so they could gain employment, open their own shops, or become teachers at the centre themselves, enabling them to achieve social and economic independence.

They shared that they were having financial difficulty trying to find a market for their tailoring, so they decided to consult with Aki. Aki, always a visionary, immediately suggested thinking outside the box. Because they had several skilled designers in their tailoring program, they might consider designing clothing for seniors and persons with disabilities. They could organize a national fashion show featuring their garments, inviting an internationally, well known Japanese fashion designer, Junko Koshino to participate. This would be an epoch-making project that could generate significant income because there was a market for this type of clothing.

The next day, we were driven five to six hours to Naypyidaw by Yvonne Pa to meet with Naoko, who had started the baking project in August last year. Naoko and her husband, Lian, welcomed us and we prepared for training the next morning. On Sunday morning, I reviewed the baking of scones, etc. with the bakers, who were excited to share their achievements thus far. In the afternoon, we attended their ethnic Chin Church. Even though we could not understand the service, we could feel the power of the spirit moving in their midst. It was a wonderful opportunity to meet their pastor and his wife at Naoko and Lian's home privately after and listen to stories of how Christ had worked in and through their ministry. He was a pastor committed to his ministry, with the community at large as well as his church members.

Yvonne Pa, Lian's brother-in-law, drove us to Mandalay on a public holiday, for a boat cruise down the Irrawaddy River to Bagan, which was on Aki's bucket list. The day began with a beautiful sunrise as we left the dock at six-thirty a.m. for the eleven-hour cruise. It was an excellent way to see the life of people living along the river. Between a delicious breakfast and a lunch of fried rice, veggies, chicken, and fresh fruit, we visited a traditional village where they made beautiful pottery, for a brief glimpse of rural life. A few villagers showed us how to wear the local longyi worn by both men and women.

We enjoyed the leisurely relaxing time on board, having been forewarned that even though the water level was low, they felt it was safe to make the trip. It wasn't until we reached Bagan that staff announced that the cruise ship was unable to anchor at their jetty but they would make it possible to disembark. We were some of the first people to exit the ship, and I looked down at the water and the temporary boardwalk and realized that the only way to leave was to follow the boards, which were at least 190 meters to shore. Aki was behind me, coaching me to be calm and keep on, which I did, until about halfway when the path narrowed to one board with nothing more to hang on to: I froze and could go no further.

Three young ladies who had made it safely to shore were watching and waiting for me to proceed. Everyone else on the ship could only watch and wait. Finally, one crew member, understanding my panic, produced a long bamboo pole and tied it to another at both ends. I was fine then, walking on one narrow board with something to hang on to. On reaching the shoreline, the three ladies clapped and clapped like I had successfully completed a major feat! I must add that after reaching the shoreline, I became aware of a large audience of taxi drivers at the top of the cliff, who had watched the whole scenario while waiting for their passengers. The sunset was beautiful and our driver friend was waiting for us.

The next day, we toured the town of Old Bagan, an ancient city and a UNESCO World Heritage Site. From the ninth to thirteenth centuries, the city was the capital of the Pagan Kingdom, a period in which some fifty Buddhist kings ruled the Pagan Dynasty. It was famous for its thousands of pagodas and stupas stretching into the horizon. We rented a horse-drawn carriage for the day to go around from one pagoda or stupa to another, sometimes following dirt paths winding around shrub-like greenery. We went into pagodas and admired dark crumbling stairwells and thousand-year-old peeling paintings. Grand Buddhas greeted us inside, each a marvellous architectural feat. It was a fascinating city rich in history. People were so polite, helpful, and friendly.

When sightseeing, we got the feeling that life had not changed for the last 2,500 years, as we watched monks burning grasses, women carrying large loads on their heads, oxen plowing the fields at sunrise, monks collecting alms, and gasoline sold on the street in water bottles. Much of the country that was off limits for years could now be freely visited with Myanmar's new leader, Daw Aung San Suu Kyi.

Early in the morning, we watched the procession of monks come to accept alms from the locals. We learned that many children became monks for a free education and could be monks for a short time. Primary children could attend Buddhist monasteries to acquire literacy and numeracy skills as well as knowledge of Lord Buddha's teachings.

We decided to go for a cultural Burmese dinner show that included traditional music, dancing, and puppets. Burmese food was Asian cuisine with Southeast Asian, Chinese, and Indian influences. The country's unofficial national dish, "mohinga," was rice noodles served with fish soup, which I did not learn to appreciate. River prawns were delicious! Rice and tea leaf salad were a major part of the Burmese diet, which I enjoyed. The country was steeped in a rich culture.

Too soon the sightseeing trip was over and then it was back to baking! The bakers had practiced making an apple pie and cheese cake in my absence and were waiting for my comments. They really did very well! The next day, we made brownies and a variety of cupcakes. Banana cupcakes were the all-time favourite. We also made jam. The bakers were eager to learn and were amazing. Naoko and Lian had opened the project at their residence, selling baked goods at local hotels. The "trainees" were now planning to open a small shop in the community. Very impressive!

The next Saturday, Yvonne Pa drove us to Yangon, a five- to six-hour drive, where we were scheduled to meet with Nay Lin Soe, Myanmar Independent Living Initiatives (MILI) Director, who was an ex-trainee of APCD, and my "son." MILI worked to empower and support persons with disabilities for their independent living, as well as advocating and promoting inclusion and the human rights of persons with disabilities. We were impressed with the progress MILI had made, and enjoyed a delicious Burmese meal together. Before our departure the next day, we shared a meal with Lian's parents. We felt honoured and blessed to have so many friends in this beautiful country.

It felt good to be "back home" briefly in Bangkok. Aki reconnected with APCD and I with the Na Kittikoon baking project and Redemptorist Centre in Pattaya, before travelling to Chiang Mai City and Mae Hong Son Province in Northwestern Thailand. We saw this as a last possible opportunity to visit friends there. Asai Shigeo and his wife, Suchitra, were retired agricultural missionaries at McKean Rehabilitation Centre. We attended the church service at McKean Rehab and met some familiar faces. We were surprised when Asai San appeared after the service to sell some fresh vegetables from his garden. In the evening, we celebrated his seventy-seventh birthday with his family. It was the first time to meet all his adult children.

On Monday, we met with our friend Ralf Oberg, another creative visionary I first met when our church in Bangkok helped support his work with ethnic minority children. He now had many projects that worked toward sustainability in Laos, Myanmar, and Thailand. He promoted and installed a simple water system for 2000 families that was invented by a professor in Alberta, Canada. He was planning to install a water purifying system for a village using an old German model that did not require electricity, in addition to an income generating project in Yangon for ten persons that recycled bicycle inner tubes to make belts, purses, backpacks, pouches, etc. There is no waste according to Ralf!

Settling in at The Meadows Residential Community

April 2, 2019, we returned to St. Jacobs for cool spring weather and to celebrate our granddaughter Maya's birthday. In early May, our friends Krisana and Vorayut from Thailand, with a team of six persons, visited our area to learn about Canadian inclusive living and accessibility. Four of the team, as wheelchair users, were impressed with accessibility. They met Mayor Sandy Shantz and community leaders, took a horse drawn wagon tour from St. Jacobs Market to a Mennonite farm, visited the Mennonite Story in St. Jacobs to learn about their roots, and ate pigtails at the Heidelberg Inn. The real highlight was to observe and practice sledge hockey at the Elmira Recreation Centre. Our schedule had not included the unusually cold wet weather that chilled them to the bone! We gave them layers of our winter clothing to wear that we would retrieve on our next trip to Thailand!

In June, Aki was invited as the keynote speaker for Rehabilitation International Asian Conference in Macau, China, and, in September, as moderator and keynote speaker for the ASEAN Accessible Tourism Workshop in Pattaya, Thailand.

We always appreciated family time. Melody was now Assistant Professor at WLU in the Health Sciences Department: Scott continued his PHD studies in environmental sustainability at UW. In June, our eldest granddaughter, Maya, who graduated from RMC, was honoured to be valedictorian, and planned to enroll in the Health Sciences Program at UW. Aidan played his double bass in the KW orchestra, and Bertha was completing Grade 8 at RMC. Matt continued to work as a civil engineer in land development, Katie had returned to the challenge of teaching Grade 6 part time, Elle was in Grade 2, and Evan in kindergarten.

On July 15, Tim and I flew to Bangkok because he was invited by APCD to share his community inclusive life in Canada with persons with autism and psycho-social disabilities in neighbouring ASEAN countries in Bangkok at a ten-day workshop. This time Tim felt more comfortable, and he said he changed his strategy in his presentation. Instead of trying to follow his prepared notes, he decided to focus on narrating his photos, which worked well for him. His presentation was well received, and he felt empowered! He happily took the bus to APCD to join in the daily activities of the workshop. Because Aki had completed his commitments in Macau and Bangkok, he was able to return to Canada with Tim and I on August 8.

What a privilege to travel and have friends in many places. Life continued to be full. St. Jacobs Mennonite Church agreed to sponsor a Syrian family of six, related to the Syrian family already living here, and I agreed to serve on the Refugee Sponsorship Committee. I had always felt strongly about helping refugees feel welcome and adjust to their new home. Having had experience in a war situation, I had empathy for them.

We were back in Canada to enjoy summer weather with family. Spending time with our grandchildren was so precious. Then fall was upon us with the leaves of the maple trees behind our condo turning the brilliant colours of red, yellow, and orange. We were living in a setting where we could enjoy the four seasons. In Thailand, I missed seeing pure white soft fallen snow. Aki and I continue to adjust to living in St. Jacobs with its beautiful seasons.

With our hearts and minds still very much in Asia, we flew to Thailand on January 2, 2020. We had friends in several countries whom we wanted to visit while we still had the health to do so. Asia equated a lot of walking. This time was no exception. After walking 11,000 steps one day, I suddenly developed acute pain in my left knee on January 15, making it very difficult to walk. Before leaving Canada, we had given careful consideration as to whether we should take out a Blue Cross insurance policy because we appeared to be in good health. Thankfully, we did! We opted to go to Bangkok Hospital in Pattaya, which had excellent medical facilities. An X-ray was non-conclusive, so it was medication, rest the knee, and come back in a week. A week later, there was no significant difference: considering we were scheduled to travel to Vietnam in another week for two weeks, I was getting anxious with my dependency on a cane, still with considerable pain. The doctor recommended an injection of cortisone in the knee, which made a significant difference in the next week.

Because we no longer had a one-year visa for Thailand, as Canadians we could stay for up to thirty days without a visa so we spaced our overseas visits within this limitation. We flew to Ho Chi Minh City (HCM) Vietnam, where we stayed at a hotel very near the famous Ben Thanh Market for a few days. We were able to meet with Ms. Tam, President of the Vietnam

Autism Network, and get updated on their activities, followed by a tour in the Mekong Delta. It was fascinating seeing the vibrant green rice paddies between the maze of rivers and canals: boats appeared to be the main means of transportation with motorbikes as a second. It was amazing to see the many "rest stops" at the roadsides for persons travelling by motorbike to take a brief rest. They were easily identified by the hammocks lined in a row, undercover due to the hot sun, with a drink shop attached, often selling a fresh coconut drink. We stopped to use the hammocks, just for the experience. Getting in and out required some help, though! The scene was so unlike the Vietnam I knew. There were many Khmer pagodas. The Cai Be floating market was an interesting, fun experience, with merchants plying the river to sell their produce.

Travel took us to the town of Chau Doc, only thirty km from the Cambodian border. It was a wonderful town, rather unspoiled and very friendly, with a large indoor market. We enjoyed walking around and, in the evening, decided to take a pedicab ride for an hour around the quiet town. The pedicab was unique to the delta but similar to those used in Cambodia. What an experience! Aki and I each hired a pedicab because it was impossible for two Westerners to fold their bodies into one! I needed help to get up and settled with my knees in my face. The driver peddling behind me was rather amused to have a Western female as a passenger and quite enjoyed chatting with me in Vietnamese. We gave our drivers a break by stopping at a small ice cream shop that sold homemade coconut ice cream. Bless our drivers for handing us our ice cream to avoid the embarrassment of getting on and off unnecessarily. That was saved for our disembarking!

It was at this time that COVID-19 in China was in the news. One noon, we were refused service at a restaurant when the owner noticed we were foreigners. We returned to HCM City to our hotel base for a night before taking a train to Nhatrang to meet with former coworkers from the late 1960s. Mr. Bu, owner of La Paloma, a hotel near our hospital, extended a warm welcome as always and helped us contact our friends, who were his friends too. This time was different though. Everyone was aging and many were not in good health, so our gathering at La Paloma was a smaller group, but we still had quality time together. We were able to meet several people at the Vinh Phuoc Tin Lanh Church service on Sunday. Co Thuan and Chi Mai insisted on making a delicious meal for us. Anh Tin, now using a cane, invited us to a new restaurant by the sea, very near the hospital, where we reminisced about our many experiences with the hospital and Yong's family from Pleiku. As usual, Chi Huong invited us to her home for a bowl of pho noodle soup and fun time with her grandson, who recited the Lord's Prayer for us. We were so fortunate to also meet others on what was likely to be our last trip to Vietnam.

On our return train trip from Nhatrang to HCM City, we were met with medical personnel, who were checking everyone's temperature before exiting the station. At our hotel, where we had stayed a few days before, everyone was required to complete a questionnaire related to COVID 19 and a mask and sanitizer were now required. We were amazed how quickly this happened in our four days' absence.

The next day, February 13, we returned to Thailand and decided to spend most of our time in Jomtien near the beach, where there were fewer people around. Due to COVID-19, Chinese and Russian tourists had already returned to their countries or were in the process of doing so. We followed the news several times a day, aware that this was becoming a global concern. Then, on the twenty-fourth, intense knee pain returned, so we went to see the doctor again, who ordered an MRI, which I had the next day. At least I knew what I would have to live with: another injection in the knee joint to gradually reduce the pain: the cane became my temporary companion.

Aki and I had to ask ourselves if we should cancel our upcoming trip to Australia in March. Because we would be staying with friends, we decided to ask them if they were still comfortable with us coming given the present global concern. Their response was, "Yes, definitely come. Welcome!" Truthfully, this was also a trip I had wanted to take for many years. Sachiko Noguchi was in my English language class in Tokyo in 1971, and we continued to stay in contact over the years. Sachiko had married Alan Davidson in Australia and had lived there for about forty years. They had visited us in Kobe, Japan, pre-earthquake, and kept us updated on their lives. We decided that we would continue travelling as planned. It was wonderful to see them in their home in Melbourne.

One day we drove ninety minutes from Melbourne to Phillip Island to see the largest number of little penguins. It was unbelievable to watch these amazing seabirds waddle from the ocean to their burrows at sunset from our viewing platforms and boardwalks. Apparently, over 4,000 of the 32,000 little penguins living in the waters around Phillip Island have their burrows around Summerland Beach, where we were observing them marching in groups. We learned that these little penguins are native to Australia and the smallest of their species are just thirty-three centimetres: they leave their burrows about an hour before sunrise and swim up to 100 kilometres each day before returning at dusk.

This visit was also our opportunity to meet the Neville Muir family with their four boys, who had lived next door to us pre-quake in Kobe. We took the train to their church service and sat in the section for hearing impaired persons with the Muirs, whose ministry had been with deaf persons. The whole service had simultaneous sign language interpretation. After sharing a meal, we drove to their home, where we met all their adult children and their families. We felt so blessed being able to meet everyone and share a prayer with the family knowing it would be the last time to see Neville, who was terminally ill. We always felt connected as families!

Much to our surprise, another long-time friend, Rae, noticed a photo of Melbourne that Aki had posted on Facebook. We had not communicated with her prior to our trip because we thought she was living in Brisbane. She was in Melbourne visiting Frank Hall, with whom Aki had worked in his years with DPI AP. We were able to take the train to Frank's place in downtown Melbourne. Both Frank and Rae were their congenial selves, and we got updated on their activities.

Back to our trip to Australia. We flew to Tasmania and rented a car at the airport in Hobart to be free to go exploring together. The first night at a bed and breakfast, we found ourselves sleeping in what had been a stable for horses. I recognized the wooden trough that was still there! Aki always had a knack for sniffing out points of interest, which included night lodging too.

Hobart, Tasmania, was a beautiful city that began its early life as a penal colony in 1803, making it the second oldest city in Australia. Convicts who had committed serious offences after arriving in Australia were sent to the penal colony from 1804 on and to various stations around the island, most notably Port Arthur. Many of the convicts were young, Irish, and in trouble for believing in a free Ireland. Sending them to far away Tasmania was seen as a solution to their growing demands for independence. The city, abounding in its early convict history, was surrounded by vast wilderness that makes up much of the country.

Our first destination was down south to the Cradle Mountain National Park, home to the mysterious and secretive Tasmanian devil. It was a conservation sanctuary for animals native to Australia. We wandered through the sanctuary with kangaroos who ate from our hands, wombats, and spotted-tail and eastern quolls, about the size of a domestic cat with shorter legs and a pointed face. Unfortunately, wombats and quolls are nocturnal, so we ended up seeing mostly kangaroos.

The town of Richmond was next on our radar, a historic town that had preserved many of the buildings from the 1800s, when convict labour was used extensively. The Richmond Gaol that held many prisoners over time is listed as a World Heritage Site. The town's bridge, built by convict labour in 1823, is Australia's oldest road bridge that is still being used today.

Aki and I drove up the east coast and inland ten kilometres, then crossed the Elephant Pass to the tiny town of St. Marys, nestled beneath the impressive rocky outcrop known as St. Patrick's Head, 2,277 feet high. It was hedged with mountains, rainforests, rivers, waterfalls, and farmland. Our lodging for two nights was a B & B out in the countryside, in the middle of nowhere. Even the GPS had difficulty finding it! The couple, in their sixties, wanted to retire from their farm that had a variety of farm animals, fruit trees, and a vegetable garden. The wife made homemade ice cream, jam, and bread to sell. They were a very friendly couple who thrived on meeting new people. One day we discovered a cheese factory on a local dairy farm way out in the country on a narrow road.

Mount Wellington, a must see, is the summit of the Wellington Range, with the city of Hobart at its foothill. We were able to drive up the narrow winding road to its summit at 4,170 feet above sea level. An enclosed lookout near the summit gave us a spectacular view of Hobart city and, to the east, the Derwent estuary.

There were two people we had dearly hoped to meet on our visit to Australia but sadly did not get to. We had helped to support Thanh and his aunt Minh when they were in a refugee camp in the Philippines, after which they had immigrated to Australia. We had lost contact over the years with all their moves, but, in my mind, they were living in Melbourne. I had asked Anh Tin in Nhatrang, uncle to Thanh, for their address because we were going to Australia; but he didn't have it because they communicated online, so I gave up. Then, shortly after we returned to Canada in March, we had a message on Facebook asking, "Are you the Aki and Marcy that sent me food when I was in the refugee camp in the Philippines?" Thanh's sons had been surfing on their phones and had come across our names, wondering if we were the couple that their dad kept talking about. Yes, we were.

We ended up having an emotional ninety-minute call on Messenger. Thanh was married, had three sons, was living in the outskirts of Melbourne, and drove to his work just five minutes away from our friends' home. We couldn't believe it! Thanh related his life story, how he became an engineer and now had an excellent job. It was through the unfailing support of his aunt Minh that he was able to pursue an education. Besides having a full-time job as a seamstress, she had taken on additional jobs, often working until the wee hours of the morning. He said that his boys had heard our names often enough that they recognized them on Facebook. He told us that his boys would never know the hunger he felt in the Philippines, when he did not always have one meal per day. If they were hungry, they just had to open the refrigerator.

COVID-19 Pandemic

As much as we were enjoying the trip, we were getting concerned with the daily updates on COVID-19. At the international airport in Hobart, on March 13, we were about the only people wearing masks and trying to social distance at the gate area: everyone else seemed to be having a party and looked at us rather strangely. Within days, they were wearing masks too.

We flew back to Melbourne to Sachiko and Alan's home, giving serious consideration about returning to Canada earlier than planned on April second. Then, on March 16, the day we were scheduled to fly back to Bangkok, Melody phoned us saying we should consider returning to Canada because the Canadian doors were already beginning to close, due to the coronavirus: if we didn't return soon, we might find ourselves unable to exit Thailand to return home.

Aki immediately tried to change our flight schedule online, but he was unsuccessful. Because we were flying back to Bangkok that same day, we decided to try again from Bangkok. After trying for about two hours, Aki, exhausted, decided to call it a day and try again in the morning. At two a.m., the phone rang. Both Melody and Matt were concerned that if we didn't soon return to Canada, it might be impossible. I woke up Aki. We agreed that our only chance was to buy new one-way tickets to Toronto. He went online and was just ready to press "confirm," when someone else bought them. Aki started the process all over again and succeeded to get two of the last five economy tickets for Friday, March 20. What a relief! We were fortunate—two days after returning to Canada, the doors closed in both Thailand and Canada.

When we returned home, Aki and I were stunned to learn that the Syrian refugee family in Jordan our church was sponsoring had had their interview with Canadian immigration in Jordan on March 16, which was much earlier than anticipated. Unfortunately, due to COVID-19, the Immigration Department discontinued processing applications two days later, so it was difficult to know when they could immigrate to Canada. But our Sponsorship Committee realized that we needed to start preparing for an earlier than anticipated arrival.

On our return to our condo in St. Jacobs, it was shocking to discover that weekly activities at The Meadows had been discontinued, church services held in the building were no longer allowed, and grocery shopping was limited to one family member. Masks and sanitizer became mandatory, as did physical distancing, and no socializing with more than five persons. We visited our adult children's families, but always outside wearing our masks. We missed spending time with our grandchildren. Zoom became the buzz word, along with virtual online meetings. Aki decided to give Japanese language lessons online to his grandson, Aidan, four evenings a week in July and August. He also started preparing a Japanese meal once a week for a Japanese Canadian resident at Parkwood Assisted Living Residence, in Waterloo, Ontario and our son, Tim, who missed Asian food: Aki continues to make these meals today.

Because various people in the past encouraged me to write a book about my life experiences, I decided that now might be the time to consider doing so, but, truthfully, I was finding it difficult to stay focused. My mind was still in Asia, but the reality was we were living in Canada! Our lives in Asia were busy and active. To suddenly be limited to a quiet life and restricted in movement when we had been accustomed to a busy active city life was stressful for both of us. Nevertheless, the slower paced life in St. Jacobs allowed me time to reflect on my past experiences, how people who walked with me in my life have made me who I am today.

EPILOGUE

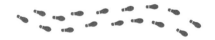

The pandemic has provided me with an opportunity to reflect on and review my life and to seek the ongoing direction of my life journey.

I have observed the four seasons unfold in nature behind our condo. Buds beginning, slowly growing until the bright green leaves appear, and then changing their wardrobe into yellow, red, and orange colours in fall. Now, at the time of this writing, they are barren branches swaying in the breeze, with a blanket of white snow on the ground. God's beautiful and amazing creative power so obvious in spring speaks of resurrection. With a blooming world twelve months a year, I was unaware of how God walks His creation through the four seasons of life in our Canadian climate:

My life journey has taken me from the small village of Conestogo, Ontario, to Vietnam, British Columbia, Japan, Thailand, and full circle to St. Jacobs, next door to the village of Conestogo where I grew up. I have encountered many wonderful people who accompanied me through the seasons of life, and the mountains and valleys I have navigated have made me who I am today. I now realize how much my parents loved me, supported me, helped me, and guided my life journey. I thank God for giving me Aki, such a caring, supportive lifetime companion. God gave us three wonderful children, Melody, Timothy, and Matthew, who have taught me so much! Now they have families and are living within driving distance of the village of St. Jacobs. What a privilege!

I have returned to my Mennonite roots, family, friends, and some nursing classmates, who still keep in contact, although our lives and experiences have been very different. Our paths make us who we are, which makes me feel Asian after spending so many years there.

My journey continues to go forward with God's guidance. I look forward to new opportunities for service that may appear. God's not done with me yet.

ACKNOWLEDGEMENTS

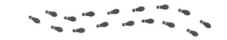

Writing a book is harder than I thought, but it has been rewarding.

The crisis of the pandemic 2020-21 provided an opportunity to write and kept me anchored.

This would not have been possible without the persuasion of Aki my lifetime partner to share my life experiences. My heartfelt appreciation for his unfailing support, wisdom, and advice throughout the whole process that kept me focused to bring the book to fruition. I am grateful to my parents who had the foresight to keep my correspondence from overseas, which helped to refresh my memory. Special appreciation to Charles Kruger who did the first edit of my manuscript and to Patricia Stortz for her professional editorial support. Love and appreciation to Maya Morton-Ninomiya, my granddaughter, who skillfully and beautifully designed the front cover of the book.

Special thanks to family, Melody, our daughter, Timothy and Matthew, our two sons, and Scott and Kate, their spouses, and Maya, Aidan, Bertha, Elle, and Evan, our grandchildren, and to friends and persons whose footprints have accompanied mine on my life journey and enriched my life. Deep gratitude to St. Jacobs Mennonite Church that nurtured my Christian faith and to the Mennonite Central Committee that gave me the opportunity to challenge my faith in service.

Finally, I want to acknowledge the book publishing team at Friesen Press, who made my footprints visible through my book.

BIBLIOGRAPHY

1. *Jimshoes in Vietnam. Orientating a Westerner.* James R. Klassen. Herald Press, 1986.
2. *Harmless As Doves. Witnessing for Peace in Vietnam.* Mary Sue Rosenberger. Brethren Press, 1988.
3. *Seeking Peace.* Titus Peachey and Linda Gehman Peachey. Good Books,1991.
4. *Lucky-Lucky.* Marva Hasselblad with Dorothy Brandon. M. Evans and Company, Inc., 1966.
5. *Vietnam: Who Cares?* Atlee and Winnifred Beechy. Herald Press, 1968.
6. *Vietnam Christian Service: Witness in Anguish.* Church World Service, 1976.
7. *An Enduring Force for Peace.* Ted Allen Studebaker. Gary W. Studebaker, Douglas E. Studebaker. Resource Publications, 2017.
8. *When We Were Hit by the Wind.* Margaret V Fast. FriesenPress, 2021.

ABOUT THE AUTHOR

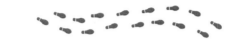

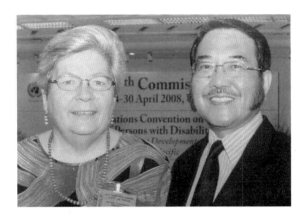

Marcy Ninomiya grew up in Conestogo, a small Mennonite community in Southwestern Ontario, Canada. After completing the three-year Kitchener-Waterloo Hospital nursing program in the early 1960s, she served with Mennonite Central Committee at a medical clinic in Vietnam, during the war. Marcy, and her husband, Akiie, continued to do God's work in British Columbia and throughout Asia for many years.

Returning to her Mennonite roots, she and Akiie now live in The Meadows Retirement Housing Corporation in St. Jacobs Village. She loves spending time with her three grown children, Melody, Tim and Matthew, and five grandchildren.

A piece of Marcy's heart will always be in Asia.

Printed in Canada